Heal Thyself

The Health of Health Care Professionals

Heal Thyself

The Health of Health Care Professionals

Edited by

Cynthia D. Scott, Ph.D., M.P.H.

and

Joann Hawk, Ph.D.

BRUNNER/MAZEL *Publishers* • New York

Library of Congress Cataloging-in-Publication Data

Main entry under title:

Heal thyself.

Includes bibliographies and index.
1. Medical personnel—Job stress. 2. Burnout
(Psychology) 3. Self-care, Health. I. Scott,
Cynthia D. II. Hawk, Joann, 1943-
[DNLM: 1. Health Occupations. 2. Professional Compe-
tence. 3. Stress, Psychological—prevention & control.
W 21 H4316]
R690.H39 1986   610.69   85-22445
ISBN O-87630-406-4

Published by
BRUNNER/MAZEL, INC.
19 Union Square
New York, New York 10003

The Wounded Healer

by Naomi Remen

Illness as altered state:
One emerges as different.
One remembers to let go
A sense of total isolation and helplessness
I am being breathed
Everything that breathes is one.

This illness is a fellow traveller
Where there's judgment there is no healing.

If one has never felt pain
   there is an instinct to avoid it.
The experience of pain
   makes it possible to be there
      and not have to fix it.
There's nothing to do but care.
Not needing to fix pain
   enables pain to change.
The greatest evoking of healing is illness.
Fear is the friction in transitions.

—transcribed by Jay Ogilvy at
Rollo May's house, May 19, 1983

Foreword

There are two reasons to be concerned about the healthfulness of health care professionals' lives. The impaired professional represents an enormous drain on society's assets. When trusted captains put wreck after wreck on the shore without warrant or justification, it is hard to know whom they damage most: their passengers, their crews, or themselves. There is a second reason, equally important for public concern: health professionals' well-being is related to the overall good functioning of the health care enterprise. A close relationship exists between the condition of professionals' lives and how they work, a relationship that is mediated through their life-styles.

While in this volume Scott and Hawk have focused principally on the first set of issues, they are deeply concerned with the second, and this concern shines through their text. From the recruiting and teaching of medical students through the economic arrangements of practice, a set of social arrangements is created that fosters habits of thinking and of personal and professional relationships. Among other things, these are the occupational health habits of the health care profession. It is, after all, a unity to which the authors address themselves: How one lives, how one works, and the state of one's health and well-being are all aspects of the same living whole.

If we consider first the grossly impaired physician, it is evident that we are on this count alone dealing with a problem of considerable proportions. One authority suggests "that the lifetime risk for impairment in M.D.s is about 10%" (see p. 233). Interestingly, this is about what it is computed to be for the rest of us. However one interprets this statistic, it is clear that something is afoot when, as Steindler tells us, "over an 11-year period in Arizona, for example, 3.2% of the physicians in that state had been disciplined because of alcohol problems, 1.7% because of drug problems, and 1.3% because of mental illness" (see p. 222). What does this mean in human terms and what are its costs to society? Most readers of this volume will have their own personal stories. It was a sad event but not a blameworthy one when my mother's aging physician misremembered her diagnosis and medication. One cannot be quite so consoling about his family and professional networks who failed to notice the change in his functioning, or if they did, failed to do something about it.

The most flagrant examples of health profesionals' impairment are instances of alcoholism, drug abuse, sexual exploitation, and major psychiatric breakdown. These are too dangerous to the larger professional community to be tolerated. In recent years there has been more candor about the scope and nature of the problem—about its seriousness and about the need for programs for early detection and rehabilitation. It has not been easy to breach the wall of silence that surrounded these subjects in years gone by, but this has been done with at least moderate success. A key to that has been the rehabilitation efforts through the impaired physician committees of medical societies, whose credibility has improved as their willingness to confront the inevitable denial has grown, and as treatment programs that are demonstrated to be effective have become more available.

These official activities are conducted in the spirit of the title of this book, *Heal Thyself.* The effort of official medicine to put its house in order has been in response to the outrage that attended the puny early efforts of the profession to be self-policing. The rogue doctor was presumably held in check by the threat of a malpractice suit, a deterrent that in addition to being ineffectual created its own vicious spiral of increasing costs and stressful mechanization of the practice of medicine.

The contributors to this volume have a number of important perspectives on this subject that may be summarized under two headings:

> The impaired health care professional is the symptom carrier for a malfunctioning work system;
> An ounce of prevention is worth a pound of cure.

Burnout is a particularly important instance of breakdown, with behavioral expression both in the work and personal realms. It is now well known that some work situations are so stressful and unsupportive that depression and apathy become epidemic. An escalating cycle of low morale, poor work performance, health problems, and absenteeism develops that can immobilize potentially competent staff groups. It is particularly by contrasting such demoralized settings with those doing similar work without similar difficulties that one can learn what factors devitalize these work situations.

As always, the existence of the symptomatic few points to the unmet needs of the many. For each frank clinical case of malnutrition there are many undernourished; for every poisoned worker there are a dozen with subclinical toxicity; gross stress breakdown in a few leads to excessive burdens on the multitude. This takes us squarely to the institutional question: What is there about the organization of the practice of health care that puts its practitioners at risk? Does this tell us something about the ordinary ills, indeed the ordinary health, of the health care establishment? Does it perhaps bring us a step closer to identifying issues that impede progress towards a health care system that is more workable for both consumers and practitioners?

I think it does and for that reason feel this volume has implications that extend beyond the troubling and still largely unresolved questions raised by the existence of frankly impaired physicians. In order to see those implications we can sketch quickly some of the current problems of the health care scene as they might relate to the subject in hand. My intention here is not to suggest a cause and effect relationship, but rather to draw attention to a systemic interlock as in a jigsaw puzzle, where each piece holds the others in place and is in turn held in place by them.

Of all the stress factors identified in this volume the one that recurs most frequently is shortage of time. For example, from early days as a medical student through internship, residency, and on into practice, the doctor is acculturated to living in a world where there is never enough time. For the reasonably ambitious young doctor everything falls before the inexorable demands upon his time made by professional duties. Women physicians are even more vulnerable to the accusation that they cannot get their time priorities straight—simply another way of expressing the role conflict for both genders torn between a profession and attention to other more personal needs. Thus, time being the ultimate commodity becomes a currency in which all these transactions are finally settled. This volume is replete with statistical and anecdotal expressions of this theme. Over and over we hear from respondents that time pressures stress them most and easing of time constraints would be a great gift.

Let me pick up a second strand and try to weave it with the first: perfectionism, and its associated demon, fear of failure. Health professionals are held, and for the most part hold themselves, to extremely high standards of performance. It is believed that they should always be at the peak of technical proficiency, emotionally available, straightforward, clear, and compassionate. The rewards for this are high status, admiration, respect. Lapses are in two directions: cynicism and money grubbing, or despair, feelings of failure, and disgrace. This latter triad is often associated with the more frank and overt symptomatic breakdown into addiction and substance abuse.

Of course, time is money, particularly in a fee-for-service environment.

The lords of medicine in the high-priced surgical specialties have largely retained control of their own time allocations through various licensing, hospital access, and other territorial operators. The primary care physician, on the other hand, as well as many lesser specialists, needs to make each minute count. The quid pro quos do not always work out to the doctor's benefit. The price of high status and high income may be unprotected availability (the telephone at mealtime), self-criticism ("I botched that procedure") and social criticism (rising malpractice insurance rates).

We are presently witnessing a vast reupholstering of the medical furniture. The marketplace and the computer are both being invoked in service of the new goddess, the reduction of health care costs. A major transformation of medicine, much of it apparently heartless, is under way. It is against this background that the most beneficial consequences of the preventative and remedial strategies advocated in this volume should be evaluated. By paying attention to the health and well-being of health care personnel, we may be developing a strategy that will be of considerable benefit to consumers as well. Health care students can be taught from the beginning of their careers that they have as much responsibility for their own sanity and physical well-being as they do for those qualities in the lives of their patients. They can pay as much attention to their connections with their own families as they ought to pay to those life-giving structures for others. The fulfillment of their gender roles in positive terms and their connection with their own sexuality can invigorate their work. The luxury of an ecologically sound, contextual view of their own lives as citizens, husbands, wives, parents, and lovers cannot help but correct the boredom that goes with ecology chopping and fragmentation. It is a good bargain to trade deification for humanizing, and unforgiving schedules for a balanced use of time by this route. The injunction "Physician, heal thyself" may thus reveal the full depth of its wisdom to us.

Donald A. Bloch, M.D.
Director
Ackerman Institute for Family Therapy

Contents

Foreword by Donald A. Bloch, M.D.   vii

Contributors   xiii

Introduction   xvii

I. UNDERSTANDING IMPAIRMENT: A GENERAL FRAMEWORK

1. Cultural Antecedents Promoting Professional Impairment   3
   John-Henry Pfifferling, Ph.D.
2. Who Is to Blame for Helpers' Burnout? Environmental Impact   19
   Ayala M. Pines, Ph.D.
3. The Impaired-Physician Syndrome: A Developmental
   Perspective   44
   Robert H. Coombs, Ph.D., and Fawzy I. Fawzy, M.D.
4. Risk Factors: Predictable Hazards of a Health Care Career   56
   Nancy C.A. Roeske, M.D.
5. A Case of Family Medicine: Sources of Stress in Residents and
   Physicians in Practice   71
   Joann Hawk, Ph.D., and Cynthia D. Scott. Ph.D., M.P.H.
6. Role Conflict for Women Physicians   86
   Dalia G. Ducker, Ph.D.
7. Physicians, Stress, and Family Life: A Systemic View   110
   Shae Graham Kosch, Ph.D.
8. Physicians in Transition: Crisis and Change in Life and Work   134
   *Dennis T. Jaffe, Ph.D., Michael S. Goldstein, Ph.D., and
   Josie Wilson, M.A.*

II. INTERVENTIONS FOR PREVENTION

9. Faculty Interventions: How Far Should You Go?   147
     Gerald Bennett, Ph.D., R.N.
10. Clinical Behavioral Scientists: Consultants and Teachers in
     Family Practice Residencies   161
     Sylvia Shellenberger, Ph.D., and Gary Wellborn, M.D.
11. Coping with Stress During Internship   174
     John L. Ziegler, M.D., and Nick Kanas, M.D.
12. The Health Professional in Treatment: Symptoms, Dynamics,
     and Treatment Issues   185
     Herbert J. Freudenberger, Ph.D.
13. The Inner Strains of Healing Work: Therapy and Self-Renewal
     for Health Professionals   194
     Dennis T. Jaffe, Ph.D.

III. EMERGENT STRATEGIES: DESIGNS FOR THE FUTURE

14. Health Promotion—A Challenging Approach to Health Care   209
     Cynthia D. Scott, Ph.D., M.P.H.
15. The Role of Professional Organizations in Developing Support   221
     Emanuel M. Steindler, M.S.
16. State Medical Societies: Their Perceptions and Handling of
     Impairment   228
     Robert C. Larsen, M.D., M.P.H.
17. Implementing a Self-Care Curriculum   235
     *Janet Mentink, R.N., M.H.S., and Cynthia D.
     Scott, Ph.D., M.P.H.*
18. Caring for the Health and Wellness of the Healer Within the
     Health Care Institution   257
     Esther M. Orioli, M.S.
19. A Health Awareness Workshop: Enhancing Coping Skills in
     Medical Students   269
     Leah J. Dickstein, M.D., and Joel Elkes, M.D.
20. Developing a School of Dentistry Wellness Program at the
     University of California, San Francisco   282
     *Lewis E. Graham II, Ph.D., Cary E. Howard, Ph.D.,
     Jared I. Fine, D.D.S., M.P.H., Larry Scherwitz, Ph.D.,
     and Samuel J. Wycoff, D.M.D., M.P.H.*

Index   297

Contributors

Gerald Bennett, Ph.D., R.N.,
Chairman and Associate Professor,
Department of Mental Health-
Psychiatric Nursing,
Medical College of Georgia,
Augusta, Georgia

Robert H. Coombs, Ph.D.,
Professor and Director,
Office of Education,
UCLA School of Medicine,
Los Angeles, California

Leah J. Dickstein, M.D.,
Associate Professor,
Department of Psychiatry
and Behavioral Sciences and
Department of Community
Health; Associate Dean
for Student Affairs,
University of Louisville
School of Medicine,
Louisville, Kentucky

Dalia G. Ducker, Ph.D.,
Associatee Proffesor,
California School of
Professional Psychology,
Berkeley, California

Joel Elkes, M.D.,
Distinguished Service Professor
Emeritus, The Johns Hopkins
University, Baltimore, Maryland;
Professor Emeritus, Department of
Psychiatry and Behavioral Sciences
and Department of Community
Health; Director, Division of
Behavioral Medicine, University of
Louisville School of Medicine,
Louisville, Kentucky

Fawzy I. Fawzy, M.D.,
Associate Professor of Psychiatry
and Chief of Consultation-Liaison
Psychiatry Service,
UCLA School of Medicine,
Los Angeles, California

Jared I. Fine, D.D.S., M.P.H.,
Visiting Lecturer in Behavioral
Sciences and Wellness,
University of California,
San Francisco, California

Herbert J. Freudenberger, Ph.D.,
Private practice,
New York, New York

Michael S. Goldstein, Ph.D.,
Associate Professor of Public
Health and Sociology,
UCLA School of Public Health,
Los Angeles, California

Lewis E. Graham II, Ph.D.,
Visiting Lecturer and Researcher in
Behavioral Sciences and Wellness,
University of California,
School of Dentistry,
San Francisco, California;
Partner and Director of Consulting
TSA Management Consultants,
Palo Alto, California,

Joann Hawk, Ph.D.,
Faculty Member,
Family Practice Residency
Training Program,
Community Hospital;
Private Practice,
Santa Rosa, California

Cary E. Howard, Ph.D.,
Coordinator,
University of California Wellness
Program, School of Dentistry,
San Francisco, California

Dennis T. Jaffe, Ph.D.,
Co-Director,
Health Studies Program,
Saybrook Institute,
San Francisco, California

Nick Kanas, M.D.,
Assistant Chief, Psychiatric Service,
Veterans Administration
Medical Center;
Associate Professor,
Department of Psychiatry,
University of California,
San Francisco, California

Shae Graham Kosch, Ph.D.,
Associate Professor,
Department of Community Health
and Family Medicine,
University of Florida,
Gainsville, Florida

Robert C. Larsen, M.D., M.P.H.,
Assistant Clinical Professor,
University of California
School of Medicine,
San Francisco, California

Janet Mentink, R.N., M.H.S.,
Director of Behavioral Science,
Family Nurse Practitioner/
Physician Assistant Program,
Family Practice Department,
University of California
School of Medicine,
Davis, California

Esther M. Orioli, M.S.,
President, ESSI SYSTEMS,
San Francisco, California

John-Henry Pfifferling, Ph.D.,
Clinical Associate Professor,
University of North Carolina;
Director, Center for Professional
Well-Being,
Durham, North Carolina

Ayala M. Pines, Ph.D.,
Social Psychologist,
Department of Psychology,
University of California,
Berkeley, California

Nancy C.A. Roeske, M.D.,
Professor,
Department of Psychiatry;
Director of Undergraduate
Curriculum,
Indiana University
School of Medicine,
Indianapolis, Indiana

Larry Scherwitz, Ph.D.,
Assistant Professor,
Department of Dental Public
Health and Hygiene,
School of Dentistry,
University of California,
San Francisco, California

Cynthia D. Scott, Ph.D., M.P.H.,
Research Associate, Department of
Family and Community Medicine,
University of California
School of Medicine;
Director of Pro-Health Programs,
ESSI SYSTEMS,
San Francisco, California

Sylvia Shellenberger, Ph.D.,
Director,
Behavioral Science Program,
Department of Family Medicine,
Medical Center of Central Georgia,
Macon, Georgia

Emanuel M. Steindler, M.S.
Director, Department of
Human Behavior,
American Medical Association,
Chicago, Illinois

Gary Wellborn, M.D.,
Associate Director of Family
Practice and Assistant Professor,
Mercer University
School of Medicine,
Macon, Georgia

Josie Wilson, M.A.,
Graduate Student,
University of South Georgia,
Atlanta, Georgia

Samuel J. Wycoff, D.M.D.,
    M.P.H.,
Chairman, Department of Public
Health and Hygiene,
School of Dentistry,
University of California,
San Francisco, California

John L. Ziegler, M.D.,
Associate Chief of Staff/Education,
Veterans Administration Medical
Center,
San Francisco, California

Introduction

It is ironic that the professionals who are supposed to teach about health and assist us when we ourselves become sick often have a difficult time doing just that for themselves. There is increasing recognition of the problems of burnout, alcohol and substance abuse, and suicide among health professionals. In response to the recognition of these problems there has been an increasing emphasis on teaching self-care skills in health professional training, to ensure that the individuals who are trained will continue to be available to serve those who need them. This problem of diminished capacity affects patient care. Truax and Mitchell (1971) showed that when physicians are able to be friendly and caring, their patients exhibit a greater probability of recovering from illness. It is becoming increasingly clear that the most important "instrument" in the health care system is the health professionals themselves.

The emphasis on prevention at both the individual and organizational levels represents a shift in the development of approaches to impairment. Graduate and professional training institutions are becoming more involved in bridging the gap between current and future practice. A research symposium of the American Medical Association (Doub et al., 1980) listed a broad range of studies undertaken on the impaired physician. What was strikingly missing was information on prevalence and incidence of impairment and the primary and secondary preventive approaches. Professional organizations are also starting intervention programs for impaired colleagues, and mental health professionals are struggling to adapt treatment models to produce effective interventions. Not only are there shifts inside the health

The editors wish to give special acknowledgment and thanks to Dr. Herbert Freudenberger for his support in the design of this introduction.

xvii

professions, but outside regulatory agencies, boards of medical quality assurance, and even insurance companies are beginning to see the possible relationships between impairment and malpractice suits.

This volume has been designed to be a collection of original papers that address all aspects of the health and well-being of health professionals. Professionals in the fields of medical anthropology, medical sociology, health psychology, behavioral medicine, and psychiatry have long been interested in the individual patient as the population of interest. This book will focus on the impact on the individual clinician, on training organizations, and on professional relationships with other disciplines. Both organizational and clinical approaches to these issues are explored.

This book marks a transition in the exploration of stress and burnout. When Freudenberger (1975) first began his inquiry into burnout, the concern was primarily with the health professional in drug and alcohol abuse programs, initially the observations sought to understand the paradigm of the individual. The approach was clinical and predominantly psychoanalytic, using the application of case studies and clinical observations of staff members in treatment programs. Subsequently, Maslach (1978) and Pines and Kafry (1978) broadened the approach to burnout by adopting a research-oriented perspective using both questionnaires and interviews. Over a period of time, the concern with seeking to understand the dynamics of the burned-out person expanded to include how an individual perceives stress. Questions were raised about how cognitive appraisal mediates stress and burnout and what objective factors need to be present in the environment of the individual in order for burnout to occur.

Next the exploration focused on causes and related factors within the work environment. The work of Maslach (1978) on how people cope with burnout became important. At the same time studies with the numerous helping professionals were completed. Clark (1980) wrote of nursing administrators; Daniel and Rogers (1981), of the pastorate; Cunningham (1983), of teachers; Farber and Heifez (1982), of psychotherapists; Battle (1981), of women physicians; Radde (1982), of pharmacists; Suran (1982), of judges; and Freudenberger and Robbins (1979), of the psychoanalyst. Many others wrote of librarians, child care workers, attorneys, physical rehabilitation workers, dentists, and social workers.

Concomitant to this concern with the helper and his/her work environment, the emphasis began to shift to the social, economic, political, and historical factors that might have an impact on the helping professional. Cherniss (1982) commented that "part of the answer to the economic, political and social roots of stress might lie in the nature of our political system and the policy making process." This approach was further articulated by Sarason (1982), who said, "Burnout is never a characteristic of or within an individual but rather, it is a complex of psychological characteristics that reflect features of the larger society."

It is the intent of this book to provide background on the contextual factors that contribute to the continuation of organizational structures and philosophical viewpoints that foster the burnout and impairment of health professionals. Specific interventions that individuals and organizations can take will be highlighted. The major portion of this volume describes programs that are currently under way to make changes in professional organizations, work settings, training processes, and individual career development.

It is our desire to take the temperature and blood pressure of the health of health professionals and provide some prescriptions for self-care. We intended this book to be of interest to educators in academic training and continuing education in nursing, medicine, dentistry, and technical specialties; to clinicians seeking to understand the needs of health professionals in treatment (psychologists, psychiatrists, social workers, and family counselors); to administrators responsible for the design of work settings and the management of treatment programs; to employee assistance professionals who are involved in the design and implementation of intervention programs and policies; to researchers and consultants who work in the health system (anthropologists, sociologists, management and organizational development specialists, and human resource managers); and to all levels of health professionals who are seeking to understand and shape their careers and personal lives.

The three sections of this book combine theory and practice. The first section focuses on understanding impairment from a cross-disciplinary perspective. Pfifferling, one of the pioneers in developing wellness interventions for impaired professionals, presents a broad overview of the philosophical underpinning of the development of the health care system and the process of training health care professionals. Pines follows with a suggestion that "the dispositional weakness of the individual helper may not lie within the individual but rather with the situational stresses in the service-providing environment." Using a case study, she suggests that we need to take into account the bureaucratic features, institutional policies, role conflicts, and ambiguity as significant contributors to individual burnout. Coombs and Fawzy explore the impact of the educational matrix on physician impairment. They examine student expectations versus medical school realities. Too often medical students are severely shocked when they find that their status deprivation, the quality level of teaching, and their role-relevant levels of learning are not only at odds, but may not have really prepared them for their professional future.

Roeske speaks sensitively to four areas that may assist the professional in assessing risk factors in his/her life that increase vulnerability for impairment. The four areas are the social transformation of health care, the function and meaning of the health care provider/consumer relationship, the health care professional's personality, as well as current social support system and professional satisfaction.

Hawk and Scott use family medicine as a field to further understand the extent and prevalence of stress and burnout. They examine the coping styles of residents and physicians and target some specific areas of personal and professional stress. They draw out differences between male and female physicians in levels of stress and its impact over time.

Ducker presents the thesis that "there are two major differences between the situations of male and female physicians . . . the societal norms about the proper relationship between women's professional and family lives . . . and the attitudes of their professional colleagues about the suitability of their professional involvement." She presents interesting statistics that suggest that "women trade career advancement for time to raise their families."

Kosch discusses the impact of society's contribution to the role model development of the physician, e.g., the physician as "a special person," as the person from whom perfection is expected. There is little doubt that these expectations are further reinforced by a family's often verbalized value on "my daughter or son the doctor." The need for "super Doc" provides fertile ground for future impairment. Kosch illustrates the importance of preventing physician family dysfunctioning.

The final chapter in this section, by Jaffe, Goldstein, and Wilson, examines physicians who are in a life transition. They focus on helping these physicians to develop a holistic orientation to their work as an alternative to previous work styles. They utilize imagery as a technique for self-exploration on this voyage of self-discovery.

The second section pulls together different levels of intervention strategies that have direct impact on the individual health professional. The issue that may have faced as faculty in training settings is to what degree do we as faculty have a right and duty to intervene in the identification of and assistance to impaired students. Gerald Bennett explores the ethical and legal considerations for faculty intervention. Questions are raised and answered of how to mobilize the institutional structure to work for the best interest of the student and diminish the impact of burnout during training.

Shellenberger and Wellborn discuss the advantages of having behavioral scientists as permanent members of the health care team. They talk about specific skills contributed by the behavioral scientist to the practice setting as clinicians and consultants and of the importance of their support for the practitioner. Ziegler and Kanas summarize the impact of a residents' support group on stress and burnout. They discuss the planning and implementation steps of developing this program in a large institutional setting.

Freudenberger's chapter deals with practical, useful therapeutic intervention techniques that may be utilized with impaired professionals in an independent practice setting. He talks of the personality dynamics of the impaired, their presenting symptoms, as well as the difficulties of treating this population. He presents specific checkpoints for therapists to watch for in the treatment of impaired professionals. Jaffe's contribution suggests that "working as a health professional . . . creates a unique set of inner pressures and demands." Health professionals need to cope with their proximity to suffering and death and the great emotional and physical needs of their patients. The negative effects of this exposure are numbing, denial, deadening, and turning away from feelings in an effort to cope with burnout. Jaffe recognizes that this continued pressure will ultimately have its impact on the health professional's self-awareness, family, and ability to communicate.

The third and largest section provides information on recent developments in policy, training programs, courses and curriculum design, and value shifts. Scott's chapter sets the tone for looking toward the future of health care. She emphasizes the need to explore basic assumptions about the provision and structure of health care, as well as the need to prepare to respond to environmental pressures in the financing and structure of health care practice. She makes a case for an increased emphasis on health promotive education for health professionals, both for their own health and to respond to the shift in consumer interest.

Steindler provides a retrospective review of the development of the committee on well-being and its current and future role within the American Medical Association. He points the direction to further developments that will guide and shape the future of organized medicine. Larsen summarizes an extensive study of the characteristics of state committees on impairment and their policy influence on national issues. The pattern of response he notes is a key to designing intervention structures in the future. Mentink and Scott provide a comprehensive outline of the design and implementation steps for the introduction of a self-care curriculum within a health sciences campus. This effort encompassed a large-scale organizational development effort undertaken to clarify the values and objectives of a health science faculty. This curriculum had a long-lasting effect on the practice of the students and faculty.

Orioli provides a call to action for health care institutions to establish Employee Assistance Programs (EAPs) for their own staff members as they develop these services for the community. She reviews the development of EAP models and offers specific suggestions for implementing them in health care settings. Dickstein and Elkes share their design and implementation strategy for a self-care workshop. They have gone far beyond a "survivalist" mentality to offer an opportunity to learn through continued self-exploration. They discuss a number of research projects that could provide data for preventive interventions all through the training period.

The faculty of the Dentistry School at the University of California, San Francisco, provide a carefully constructed design for an institutionally based wellness education program. They discuss strategies for implementation as well as assessment research. Their program consists of several different interventions; student curriculum, educational forums, research, and intensive stress groups. To be effective, they say, health promotion programs must "get into the university drinking water . . . just like fluoride."

This book is based on our combined 11 years of teaching and designing behavioral science curriculums for health science students and practicing professionals, conducting research on the sources and levels of stress among health care professionals, providing policy analysis and consultation on the provision of patient services, and giving clinical consultation to health care professionals and their families in educational and private practice settings.

We have each spent extensive time directly observing practitioners working in a wide variety of settings and have used our clinical skills in formulating interventions in educational organizations and private clinical practice. It is our belief that the well-being of health professionals does affect their ability to deliver quality patient care and that health professionals are not given adequate preparation and support for self-care skills to enable them to practice well-being in their personal and professional lives. We hope this book will give direction and courage to rethink, design, and implement programs that assist health professionals in being careful of themselves and their patients.

Cynthia D. Scott
Joann Hawk

REFERENCES

Battle, C. V. (1981). The itrogenic disease called burnout. *Journal of the American Medical Womens Association, 36*(12), 357–359.

Cherniss, C. (1982). Cultural friends—Political, economic and historical roots of the problems. In S.P. Whiton (Ed.), *Job stress and burnout: Research, theory and intervention perspectives.* Beverly Hills, Calif.: Sage.

Cherniss, C., & Kane, J. S. (1977). Public sector professionals: Satisfied but alienated from work. Unpublished paper. Ann Arbor: University of Michigan.

Clark, C. C. (1980). Burnout: Assessment and intervention. *Journal of Nursing Administration, 10*(9), 39–44.

Cunningham, W. G. (1983). Teacher burnout—Solutions for the 1980's. A review of the literature. *Urban Review, 15,* 37–51.

Daniel, S., & Rogers, M. (1981). Burnout and the pastorate: A critical review with implication for pastore. *Journal of Psychology and Theology, 9*(3), 232–249.

Doub, N. H., Warschawski, P., & Kessler, I. I. (June 1980). Summary of the epidemiologic research on the impaired physician. *First International Research Symposium on the Impaired Physician.* Baltimore.

Farber, B. A., & Heifez, L. J. (1982). The process and dimensions of burnout in psychotherapists. *Professional Psychology, 13,*(2), 293–301.

Freudenberger, H. J. (1975). The staff burnout syndrome in alternative institutions. *Psychotherapy: Theory, Research and Practice, 12,* 73–82.

Freudenberger, H. J., & Robbins, A. (1979). The hazards of being a psychoanalyst. *Psychoanalytic Review, 66*(2), 275–296.

Maslach, C. (1978). Job burnout: How people cope. *Public Welfare, 36,* 56–58.

Pines, A., & Kafry, D. (1978). Occupational tedium in the social services. *Social Work, 16,* 499–506.

Radde, P. O. (1982). Recognizing, reversing and preventing pharmacist burnout. *American Journal of Hospital Pharmacy, 39,* 1161–1166.

Sarason, S. B. (1982). Foreword. In B. A. Farber (Ed.), *Stress and burnout in the human service professions.* New York: Pergamon.

Suran, B. G. (1982). Psychological disabilities among judges and other professionals. *Judicature, 66*(5), 184–193.

Truax, C. B., & Mitchell, K. M. (1971). Research on certain therapist interpersonal skills in relation to process and outcome. In A. E. Bergin & S. L. Hartfield (Eds.), *Handbook of psychotherapy and behavior change.* New York: Wiley.

I
Understanding Impairment: A General Framework

Chapter 1

Cultural Antecedents Promoting Professional Impairment

John-Henry Pfifferling, Ph.D.

The medical profession has become intensely concerned with the problem of impaired health professionals. As with diseases or conditions that do not have a single cause, there are multiple suggestions as to the origin, contributing factors, and types of susceptible hosts. It is therefore urgent that the overall problem, its component parts, and the numbers of affected professionals be defined. These epidemiological factors must be established if we are to develop successful primary and secondary prevention programs. The following analysis will indicate both the nature of the dilemma and why potential remedies and preventive measures may be so difficult to apply.

DEFINITION OF IMPAIRMENT

The American Medical Association (AMA) defines the impaired physician as "one who is unable to practice medicine with reasonable skill and safety to patients because of physical or mental illness, including deterioration through the aging process or loss of motor skill, or excessive use or abuse of drugs including alcohol" (Shortt, 1979). The Resident Physician's Section (RPS) of the AMA expands the definition, considering a physician impaired when a personal problem interferes with the quality of his/her medical care. The RPS Workgroup on Physician Well-Being also extends this definition to include the interference of this personal problem with his/her education

3

or family life. The American Pharmaceutical, the American Dental, and the American Nurses Association all use a definition similar to the AMA's and have recently (1984, 1985) published handbooks on the impaired professional.

Based on their definition, the AMA conservatively estimates that one of every 10 physicians is at risk to impairing conditions. The impaired physician characteristically denies that he is disabled in any way. It is generally agreed that impaired physicians persist in their professional activities or do not perceive their impairment, and if they do, they usually do not seek help. The culture of medicine aggravates these tendencies.

American physicians are trained and practice in a society that allows the physicians, their families, and patients to idealize them. In addition, the newly developing physician accepts an unrealistic, perfectionistic self-image which often interferes with coping abilities (Tokarz et al., 1979).

Physicians, like all other people, experience the stresses, problems, and losses of life that may lead to poor coping, but too often their cultural and personal values deny them the opportunity for personal and professional support (Donnelly, 1979; Pfifferling, 1980). Furthermore, American culture imposes such tremendous expectations on physicians that they are less able to reconcile the needs of their own personal lives because of the strenuous service expected of them. House staff, for example, work in a fatigue-prone environment pervaded by role conflicts and ambiguity as to the appropriate coping response (Donnelly, 1979).

The studies on house-staff training suggest that efforts to reduce these conflicts, such as (1) teaching effective coping strategies, (2) reducing call schedules, and (3) providing administratively sanctioned support and insight sessions, are discouraged in house-staff programs (Berg & Garrard, 1980; Donnelly, 1979; Elwood & Barr, 1973; Kahn, 1964). If the availability of support, insight into effective areas, and opportunity for rest and reflection during residency is negatively sanctioned, the probability of developing inappropriate coping mechanisms and future impairment is greatly increased.

Physician impairment is a study in extremes. The American work ethic is epitomized by the total immersion of the medical trainee in professional preparation. This apprenticeship exacts a personal and societal cost. Traditionally, physicians are considered more dedicated and harder working than their peers in other occupations, but physicians also run a higher risk of developing disabilities, including chemical dependency and depression, which interfere with the quality of care they render and the quality of their personal life (Tokarz et al., 1979).

The philosophy of most medical training programs model overwork. Since the demands of the profession are so great, students should overwork themselves as a preliminary test of their mental and physical endurance potential. Most students and residents already have unrealistic expectations for their performance which predispose them to burnout. Medical students and house staff are unaware of the potential effects of the accumulating stresses of clinical training.

The medical student and house-staff training environment generally neglects the personal growth and development of the physician and fails to provide effective and nonstigmatized assistance during times of stress. This combination of factors, namely, an unaware population subjected to conditions of overwork, neglect of personal growth, and inadequate personal support with unrealistic performance expectations, often leads to inappropriate coping responses and subsequent burnout and impairment.

THE SCOPE OF IMPAIRMENT

Physician impairment is a generic concept in which personal problems interfere with the reasonable performance of medical activities including a continued ability to keep up with medical advances and a personal capacity to contribute to health promotion through interpersonal skills. Physicians are highly susceptible to the development of overt symptoms such as chemical or alcohol dependency. This usually develops in a progressive manner. Talbott et al. (1980) found that 12 to 14% of physicians have had, currently have, or, in their opinion, will have problems with alcohol or drugs. The incidence and prevalence of other impairing conditions—such as psychiatric or emotional problems—is thought to be high, but the epidemiological data are inadequate to define the extent of the problem (Pfifferling, 1980).

Clues to physician impairment are found in both preclinical and clinical settings (symptoms may be marked and severe or may be subclinical). Medical students may be using mind-altering substances on a regular basis to gain added energy, to relax, or for relief of stress. Residents may indulge in consistent use of mind-altering substances, repeatedly make errors in cases requiring routine clinical judgments, avoid experiences that are relevant to their stated practice specialty, and make apparently illogical changes of training paths. Both young and more mature physicians may self-prescribe and use drugs; alienate themselves from family, community, and colleagues; display marked changes in office, hospital practice, or duties; and demonstrate deteriorating physical or personal care (Talbott et al., 1980).

It appears that the probable history of generic impairment includes a vulnerable individual selected by (1) an admission process oriented to technical and academic achievement; (2) a societal role strain that demands unrealistic behavior; and (3) a professional culture that disallows open discussion of physician role stresses —particularly the needs of the physician as a person (Vaillant et al., 1972). As the American way of life reduces social support from continuity of community, family, and work, greater stresses are added.

Physicians pay more attention to their patients' medical needs than they do to their own (Bradshaw, 1978). Seventy percent of physicians in one study did not receive regular checkups (Sharpe & Smith, 1962). In another study, it was reported that 60% of family physicians do not have regular personal physicians (Tokarz et al., 1979). When they are patients, male physicians are often overdiagnosed, and their surgical-use rate is three times that of the general male population of the United States (Bunker & Brown, 1974).

Ironically, physician compliance with medical treatment modalities is extremely poor. As patients they refuse, ignore, or deprecate their own treatment. This is well documented for alcoholic physician patients. For example, once they have begun treatment for alcoholism, they are often treated for illnesses other than the alcoholism, which is their primary problem (Bissell & Jones, 1976; Goby et al., 1979). Physician patients, especially those diagnosed as alcoholics and/or chemically dependent, routinely leave treatment centers against medical advice and before the completion of their treatment (Jones, 1975). Fortunately, increased publicity and training workshops for physicians engaged in treating physician patients are beginning to change the overall prognosis to a more positive view. Treatment centers that routinely incorporate the physician's family in treatment through an ecological approach are also guardedly optimistic. (Talbott [1980] claims 90% of his physician patients return to their practices.)

As patients, physicians are poor role models. Many physicians are too harried and too busy to lead balanced and satisfying lives. According to Vaillant et al. (1972), physicians are overburdened by perfectionistic, mythologized self-images. In the areas of cancer and mental illness, they are slow to seek treatment for themselves (Vaillant et al., 1972).

Mental Illness

Recent reviews suggest that the incidence of mental illness is higher among practicing physicians than among members of similarly educated groups (Bissell & Jones, 1976; Scheiber, 1977; Shortt, 1979). Vaillant et al. (1972) in their longitudinal study found that twice as many physicians as matched controls sought psychiatric treatment. Both Waring (1974) and Vaillant et al. (1972) suggest that male physicians may be less fit in terms of mental health than either the general male population or members of other professional groups. Their familiarity with psychiatric treatment modalities may also explain why physicians seek treatment more than members of comparison groups.

Chemical Dependency

There is much confusion about the extent of chemical dependency, including alcoholism, among physicians. Often, chemical dependency is not separated from alcoholism. Numerical estimates range from the AMA's (Steindler, 1975) figure of 17,000 disabled by alcoholism and chemical dependency, to Green et al.'s report (1978) of approximately 25,000 disabled by alcoholism.

Estimates of the extent of chemical dependency among physicians are widely divergent. Commonly cited estimates vary, but are 30 to 100 times greater than for the general population. Scheiber (1977) states that 1.5% (50 times the United States norm) of physicians are "addicts." Reviews of general physician populations indicate that a majority of physicians use an excess of drugs (Vaillant et al., 1970). Compared with socioeconomically matched peers (lawyers and engineers), practicing physicians are twice as likely to misuse mood-altering drugs (Shortt, 1979). Treatment center estimates differ markedly according to the physician's specialty, though.

Compared with the lay drug-abuse culture, physician addicts may be even more isolated. Their dependency level is high, they use purer drugs, and peers ostracize and stigmatize them. Nationally, through the AMA's efforts, this ostracism is beginning to be replaced with increased understanding and support as they try to deal with their dependency.

Suicide

Physicians take their own lives with greater frequency and generally at an earlier age than do members of the general population. Suicides account for between 33 and 38% of all premature deaths among physicians (Steppacher Maussner, 1974; Thomas, 1976). Suicide rates for female physicians are the highest reported for any occupational group of women. They are nearly four times higher than for women in the general population who are 25 or more years old (Ross, 1971; Steppacher & Mausner, 1974).

In reviewing the literature on the correlates of physician suicide, the most commonly described are (1) a sense of hopelessness associated with their medical practice, (2) depression, (3) drug dependency, (4) chronic disease, (5) failure to cope with the loss of the practicing physician role through retirement, and (6) professional success with personal failure. Why female physicians, particularly residents, should be so suicide prone is unexplained.

Postmortem psychological autopsies of physician suicides reveal some probable suicidal indicators. Included in this composite lonely pattern are (1) a hurried existence, (2) indecision about ordinary medical procedures,

(3) marked indecisiveness when confronted with difficult diagnostic problems, and (4) gradual neglect of their medical practice.

These physicians often leave regular colleague contacts, retreating from a hospital association to a solitary office practice. Colleagues of the doctor who has committed suicide often recall having observed indecisiveness, disorganization, and depression. Since colleagues rarely discuss their concerns with the potentially suicidal doctor, they often suffer consequent feelings of guilt. These doctors need support and the opportunity to talk to others to relieve the considerable burden of unresolved guilt.

MEDICAL EDUCATION

Premedical Education

Premedical students quickly learn that they must be achievement oriented and acquire an outstanding scholastic record. Competition for grades becomes a way of life among premedical students who allocate time for studying first and for other life-maturing experiences last. Their social experiences are generally limited, and they often feel restricted by guilt feelings that someone else is studying and will get the coveted place in medical school. Socializing experiences as a "premed" prime the student's ego for overachievement, ego recognition through grades, and a workaholic life-style.

Medical and Residency Education*

Traits that help earn entry into medical school, such as self-sacrifice, perseverance, competitiveness, and denial of personal feelings, are magnified by the typical medical school experience. The preeminent cultural value allegorizes devotion to work and the internalization of the work role as the student's self-image. For example, in their first clinical rotations, medical students joust with each other as to who had the least sleep or the most "workups." The denial of weakness is a first lesson that homogenizes most medical education. It has a pervasive existence which shapes the affective conditions that later cause colleagues to conspire in silence when a physician is troubled or vulnerable. Dealing with serious issues, such as helplessness and hopelessness, exposes students to constant emotional challenges. They respond by feeling fear, anxiety, insecurity, and frustration. Often these emotions are combined into a single encompassing term—dread.

---

*Currently Dr. Pfifferling is finishing a book devoted to nonchemical coping skills for residents. It will be published by the American Medical Association. Its working title is *Residency: A Personal Guide.*

Medical students leave the premedical environment feeling ecstatic at their success with medical school admission. They achieved a difficult goal, maintained a hard pace, and can congratulate themselves on their discipline and single-minded purpose. When they enter medical school, they are suddenly confronted by a subordinate status. Their desire for adult independence conflicts immediately with their dependence on faculty for positive strokes, on patients for ego gratification ("you cured me"), on peers for social support, and on nurses for learning routine procedures.

Only gradually do they begin to feel more comfortable as doctors; then they enter internship where they are often unable to cope with the different and greater responsibilities that are encountered. Both medical students and house staff are debilitated by sleep deprivation and social isolation, test or board anxiety, fantasies of making a mistake, and their seemingly eternal student status. Thus dread, dependency, and debilitation describe part of the process of becoming a physician in most American medical schools.

In many medical school environments a system of reinforcement fosters the development and exaggeration of traits and behavioral patterns that may later become debilitating, e.g., a tendency to develop an excessive work load, self-denial, repression of feelings, inattention to personal needs, and intellectualization of emotions. Medical school is hard, which we may not want to change, but do we want the driving hardness to damage our doctors for life?

The detached hardness of medical training facilitates an attitude toward the use of mental health services and mental health professionals that compounds the difficulty of treating physicians when they do request it. Their treatment is often inadequate because physician-patients need to maintain a façade of adequacy and control. Their therapists, likewise, often have difficulty in managing physician-patients because they identify with the therapists and use defensive denial to conclude that they are more well than ill.

Medical training also fosters an attitude that idealizes technical and scientific management, perhaps to the detriment of the clinical, human encounter between doctor and patient. Academic medical centers uniformly favor the scientific experience over the clinical; the specialist over the generalist; the bench researcher over the clinical teacher; the completeness of the "workup" over the benefit of the patient's emotional well-being. It may be that these values predispose trainees to become technologically astute but clinically rigid.

Attitudes of technical mastery and omnipotence over the ambiguous subject area of the human condition predispose the physician to *predictable* feelings of dread that he/she cannot master. Physicians are constantly involved in transference feelings, one minute being the resident-learner and the next being the resident-physician. Physicians must simultaneously learn to protect themselves from their patients who tantalize them with ego rewards and dependency needs in a circadian rhythm that would fatigue even the super-human physician of popular myth. The support of the public and medical media manipulate this greater-than-life image. The faculty, the trainee, and the public lose sight of everyday limits on the physician. All are convinced that he/she deals in everyday miracles.

The paradoxical aspects of medical training extend from training programs to a physician's personal habits. For example, medical trainees cope with patient illness in tertiary-care hospitals and are taught by tertiary-care faculty, but only 5% of these young physicians will ever go into academic medicine. Both the diseases they encounter and the technology and medical resources at hand in training differ widely from the everyday problems they must attempt to resolve without resources when they are in practice. The conflict between their expectations and the reality of practice mirrors the initial discomfort they felt when they euphorically entered medical school only to learn that humanistic clinical practice is an ideal unattainable to most. The separate perfectionistic demands of the technological training world, along with an ever-increasing amount of "necessary" information, produce an accommodation that allows no opportunity for synthesis.

Socialization for physicianhood discloses two especially salient themes for young physicians. First is a recurring confusion between personal identity and career identity. Second, an exaggerated competition between time for work and time for self and independence that is often expressed as a fear of acknowledging any need for care (Lander, 1978). Coombs (1978) notes, "The subjective features of medical education, if discussed at all, are usually covered on an intellectual level. So unless students have informal channels to unload, personal feelings are routinely suppressed. Because of this . . . some clinicians are needlessly hampered in their ability to provide healing aid. . . . How can a doctor allay the fears and anxieties of others if his or her own feelings have never been resolved?" (p. 252).

Partly because so many expectations are placed on the medical educator, the medical trainee, and the academic medical setting, a clearly shared vision of the end product of medical education does not exist. Though most medical schools state their goal as teaching physicians to care for the whole person, they fail to recognize that medical students and house staff are no less whole people than are the patients, and most often deal with them only in terms of their professional roles. The personal development of providers, including the acquisition of personally destructive habits during and subsequent to training, is viewed by most medical educators as irrelevant to their professional functioning.

Educational Values That Reinforce Impairment

Many educators view stress and overburden as part of the curriculum and argue that responsibility is learned by stressful testing. Others believe that a content core of information must be imparted to students based on the belief that success is measured by the student's factual knowledge. Each discipline and each faculty member, therefore, believes that this core is essential for a (future) practice. Because of this belief system, students are expected to become walking computers and to synthesize from an over-abundance of disparate facts the information that is essential to the field.

Students and educators believe that their specialized knowledge will somehow be integrated into a comprehensive whole for a lifetime of behavioral practice. Testing of this integrating process, however, should be on a piecemeal basis, not on the overall concept or body of knowledge. This conflict results in examinations that translate into union cards which reinforce the current educational structure even if it has no impact on the individual's capacities to integrate or maintain lifelong learning attitudes.

Faculty rarely share the logic behind their conclusions nor the mistakes they made as they learned new problem-solving skills. They are in such a rush to impart information that they forget that lifelong learning requires independent manipulation of constantly changing variables. Students learn that factual mastery equates with competency and emulate this behavior when they, in turn, become teachers. The tyranny of memory fuels unrealistic expectations in high achievers and fosters dependency on subspecialization to the exclusion of generalists. Pecking-order hierarchies leave room for personal devaluation.

Many educators emphasize teaching of factual learning and understanding in the absence of real work and real responsibility (Weed, 1975). Thus, much of clinical learning takes place without the excitement of solving real patient problems. The answers, instead, are given without the student seeing how one searches for answers. Under these circumstances, students learn without feeling responsible because the answers are already known. As the professor presents problems with worked-out solutions, the students either emulate the professor or risk being cut down when they offer unacceptable solutions.

Professional education focuses on ingestion of massive amounts of facts and theory without equivalent regard for its relevance to real work and real problem solving. Reality in clinical care means that every situation has some attribute of novelty and every patient is a new "textbook." When students finally begin to deal with these real problem-solving situations, they have often become so dependent on theoretical answers to old problems that they fail to adapt to the new situation. One significant outcome of this confrontation with reality is professional burnout and/or reality shock.

The belief that the number of academic courses and the rapidity of completion, disregarding the end result of the content, is what counts is held by many educators. Some students learn some of the material well and others learn less of it. Each may pass the course on some gradient. Passing each course reinforces mediocrity since passing is rewarded rather than mastery. This educational system is based on the constants of time (everybody takes histology or anatomy) and the number of courses required. The message to students is clear: perserverance is more important than achieving mastery of the content at the appropriate pace for each student.

Finally, many educators believe that passing one large examination is sufficient insurance for a lifetime of practicing in that specialty. Students therefore are not prepared for a lifetime of audit and maintenance of lifelong learning skills.

These beliefs reinforce individual valuation based on (1) static tests, (2) single-time examinations, (3) facts as more important than problem solving, and (4) an attitude that engenders obedient student behavior. The obedient student works hard and waits for a recognition of merit, while feeling tremendous resentment because that reward rarely arrives. If success professionally is based on lifetime flexibility, independent networking, generalist risk taking (connecting in areas outside of your subspecialty), learning from real work with real responsibility, and using connections and mentors (Scheele, 1979), then our educational values predispose our students to impairment.

SOCIETAL FACTORS

Physicians are socialized in an occupation that promises technological solutions to problems on a level that cannot be solved *solely* by technological interventions. Both consumers of medical services and providers expect the latest available technology and that the providers are competent in its use. The bulk of the problems that are present in ambulatory contexts require nontechnical interventions. Physicians worry about the potential errors associated with more and more complex technologically derived data. Time spent coordinating, managing, and interpreting biomedical data ruthlessly becomes symbolic of working as a physician. In addition, patients expect physicians to be freer to spend time with them, instead of as reported in a study where physicians physically spend an average of less than a minute with each of their patients (Duff and Hollingshead, 1968). Working hard in an ever-expanding biotechnical world means more interprofessional communication for the physician and less time reaping the rewards of the healing bond.

Society demands a medicalized world view (an orientation that emphasizes health and orthodox definitions of health) of physicians. Trainees in medicine adopt this unitary stance—the primacy of the medical model—but lose their humanism in the process. Society loses the nurturant, altruistic healer because the training process commodifies and distances the student physician. The biomedical focus (what we call a medicalized world view) discounts qualitative human variables, because they are patently difficult to measure, and resorts to substituting science as the arbiter of human meaning in illness. The "noise" in the system often loses the patient, and his or her essential aloneness and experience of illness are rarely understood by his or her physician. Unaware physicians usually become technocrats, sick people become disease entities, and the healing bond becomes a commodity transaction.

PREVENTION

In order to prevent physician impairment, several efforts must be made. A model for the physician role must be developed that allows many options for the medical graduate. This could include practitioners who practice augmentative medicine focused on a health orientation and not disease centered. The risks of emotional disability associated with medical training must be publicized. Concern for the well-being of medical trainees must be continuously modeled in medical training. Rituals of education must be purged so that training is efficient and emotionally rewarding. Students must be rewarded for displaying behavioral patterns that characterize efficient problem solvers not memorizers. Clinical skills including interpersonal affect must be monitored, emphasized, and rewarded. Prestige must accrue from many avenues, especially from positive medical outcomes. Physicians who share responsibility with colleagues and patients should be granted both professional and societal status. A new-age physician can and must be trained so that needless human wastage is reduced.

Our approach to the problem must then necessarily be twofold. First, we must move beyond the acknowledgment to confrontation of the problem. Second, we need to focus on methods of prevention, early correction, and modification of the population at risk.

If personality and family background factors are partially etiological in impairment problems among physicians, we can screen out or modify the population-at-risk. Screening out assumes that individuals with given risk factors will necessarily develop the problem, and that tests measuring these risks are valid and specific. Both assumptions can be faulted.

Modifying the population-at-risk entails teaching and rewarding nonchemical models of training, such as values clarification, support groups, and stress management techniques. Many of these models have been validated, and several of them are now being added to programs that stress interpersonal skill training. Some programs combine several models and apply them to both medical trainees and faculty. The goal of such attempts is to set feedback loops into motion.

In the wider context of medical education, the most difficult factors to change relate to the common training model that relies on memorization, overwork, and audit by default. Yet there are educational values that would reduce the risk to students. The following suggestions for changing educational values are all based on innovations made in some medical school already.

Students need to be exposed to the whole of the field of medicine before immersion into the individual intricate parts of the curriculum. This can be done by careful orientation to research questions, service demands, and the needs of individual patients. As the student shadows physicians involved in solving problems in sectors of the whole profession, the student gains insight into the variety of definitions associated with professional roles. Many medical schools ask students to be patient advocates or primary health educators to a healthy family before they begin solving pathological problems.

Students' examinations should be oriented toward problem solving for problems without accepted solutions. In this way, the faculty member can assist students in the development of problem-solving approaches applicable to a lifetime of novel situations. The faculty and student would then be able to jointly share in the discovery process of learning. In addition, it is essential that examinations be based on mastery of content with time as the variable rather than as a constant. For example, what is important in medical care is not that the student passed an examination with mediocre technical skills, but that when he applied the skills, the problem had a high probability of being solved. If it takes one student two hours and another 10 hours to master a task, it is important to focus on the mastery and, thus, a positive outcome for the patient.

Students can be exposed to the mistakes made by their faculty so that errors in problem solving can be used to improve learner behavior. Faculty self-disclosing behavior and modeling of personal/professional humility to a student, reinforce the necessity to be on guard against medical arrogance that can cost a patient his life. By self-disclosing mistakes to their students, the faculty prevent the student from becoming too arrogant or too distanced from the troubles of their patients, and provider/patient bonding is strengthened and improved. Failure to address this fundamental provider/patient relationship issue results in distancing that can lead to intensification of adversarial position taking and elimination of a major source of positive feedback.

Students must be rewarded for cooperation and collaboration since quality medical care is based on teamwork, not isolated interventions. Examinations that are based on establishing strategies for dealing with unsolved clinical problems will teach the students collaborative work habits and prevent some of the destructive territoriality that allows nurses and physicians to needlessly dump on each other. All too often, physicians and nurses are ignorant of each other's strengths and skills.

From the beginning of the educational process, students can be exposed to faculty members solving real problems with real patients. Students can then internalize similar values of humility and responsibility that will assist them in dealing with a lifetime of uncertainty.

Of equal importance is early student exposure to professionals who have suffered from the stress syndromes that plague professionals, including burnout, impairment, and job dissatisfaction. Contact with professionals who can honestly discuss how stress was managed in dysfunctional ways can reduce student reality shock and disillusionment. As students are exposed to recovered professionals, they will learn both positive and negative coping strategies. Exposure to recovered professionals will also allow them to feel the human cost of professionalism and to ask themselves questions about their personal risks. The University of Tennessee Medical School in its AIM programs has already implemented this model (1985).

From the beginning of school, students can be given access to memory-relieving tools, such as coupling databases on computers, so that overburden and the resulting lower self-esteem associated with memory failure is reduced. Facts are changing so rapidly that examinations based on memorization are inefficient and wasteful of the student's ability to think and solve problems.

Most important, the faculty must incorporate community practitioners to help establish curricular objectives. In addition, students should be rewarded for learning behavioral patterns that establish lifetime learning skills.

If greater participation by patients in medical decision making will lead them to accept some of the responsibility now borne by the physician, the physician can continue to have authority but in a more limited sphere. Patient responsibility will place control where it legitimately belongs. Patients live with the variables all the time. If they are aware of these variables as risk-enhancing factors, they can initiate coordinated care plans better than anyone else. Physicians see only a fragment of the total picture, as they are exposed to only a fragment of the patient's life. Why demand responsibility from the physician for comprehensive care when he can never know or control most of the variables?

If patients and society take and share responsibility, then dependency states that lead to inefficient utilization of the medical care system are not reinforced. Only then the interactions between the patient and the physician can facilitate the celebration of each other's dignity, autonomy, and self-worth.

CONCLUSIONS

The prevention of physician impairment with the simultaneous enhancement of well-being is not only necessary, but crucial, if we are to reduce professionally and personally crippling distress, burnout, and impairment among health professionals.*† Impaired professionals use defensive denial to discount their disability and commonly fail to reach for help when they are troubled. Efforts to reduce the problem of impairment must, therefore, be well supported and well funded.‡ Professional and nonprofessional organizations and individuals must cooperate in raising the consciousness level about the prevalence of impairment and publicize the resources available for support.

The costs of physician impairment are socially, economically, and professionally staggering. Rehabilitation is costly, lengthy, and extremely difficult, although major gains have been made in the last few years with aggressive intervention programs. These few successful programs are well funded, led by committed physicians, and supported by a combined effort including state medical societies, auxiliaries, state medical boards, and other professional groups.

Medical students and residents will have access to many of the changes suggested in this chapter, but they must be helped in instituting awareness and supportive programs. Practicing physicians must initiate these programs themselves. Meetings can be planned with colleagues where the primary objective is to share the stresses and conflicts of physicianship in a supportive and open environment. A time-management plan can be structured so that "instant vacations" (five minutes of quiet time) are allotted for every three patients seen in an office visit, or they can redesign their practice so that the most difficult (to the physician's emotional health) patient visits are followed by positive health visits (where well patients learn to augment their wellness).

---

*We have suggested similar profession-specific well-being interventions for dentistry: "The Well-Being of Dentists," by J.H. Pfifferling, 1985, *North Carolina Dental Journal*, 2(2):3-6.

†The same issues for pharmacy are addressed in our six articles on pharmacy burnout, well-being, and prevention. See J.H. Pfifferling, et al. "The Well-Being of Pharmacists, Parts One and Two," *Michigan Pharmacist*, April and May, 1985.

‡As of July 1985, following the lead of the New Jersey Medical Society, several other medical societies in conjunction with other health professional societies are now hiring full or part-time medical directors to oversee help for the impaired professional in their state. Write Dr. David Canavan in New Jersey for more information.

Continuing education meetings can be planned so that colleagues and families can participate in problem-solving sessions on the stresses of their role.

The prevention of physician impairment should be a high priority in allocating resources in the health care sector. Currently, efforts are at a rudimentary level. Continued support is needed to bolster the work of the Department of Health and Human Behavior of the AMA, its associated state medical society committees, the Committee on Mental Health of the American Academy of Family Physicians, and the Center for the Well-Being of Health Professionals in Durham, North Carolina.

The next step is for the profession to confront the fear of acknowledgment that surrounds troubled physicians and their families. The stigma of betrayal to self and to the profession must be confronted when one wishes to aid the impaired physician. Professionals openly admit the fear of contagion in order to truly listen, hear, and respond with empathy and compassion to a troubled physician. The key thing to remember is that physicians are individuals first and health care workers second.

REFERENCES

Berg, J. K., & Garrard, J. (1980). Psychosocial support in residency. *Journal of Medical Education, 55*, 851–857.

Bissell, L., & Jones, R. W. (1976). The alcoholic physician: A survey. *American Journal of Psychiatry, 133*, 1142–1146.

Bradshaw, J. S. (1978). *Doctors on trial.* New York: Paddington press.

Bunker, J. P., & Brown, J. P., Jr. (1974). The physician patient as an informed consumer of surgical services. *New England Journal of Medicine, 290*, 1051–1055.

Coombs, R. H. (1978). *Mastering medicine.* New York: Free Press.

Donnelly, J. C. (1979). The internship experience: Coping and ego development in young physicians. Unpublished doctoral dissertation, Harvard University.

Duff, R. F., & Hollingshead, A. B. (1968). *Sickness and society.* New York: Harper & Row.

Elwood, J., & Barr, R. (1973). A new work schedule for interns. *Lancet, 18*, 371–372.

Goby, M. J., Bradley, N. J., & Bespalec, D. A. (1979). Physicians treated for alcholism: A follow-up study. *Alcoholism: Clinical and Experimental Research, 3*, 121–124.

Green, R. C., Jr., Carroll, G. J., & Buxton, W. D. (1978). *The care and management of the sick and incompetent physician.* Springfield, Ill.: Charles C Thomas.

Jones, R. E. (1975). Do psychiatrists cover-up addiction of physicians? *Psychiatric Opinion, 12*, 31–36.

Kahn, R. (1964). *Organizational stress.* New York: Wiley.

Lander, L. (1978). *Detective medicine: Risk, anger, and malpractice crisis.* New York: Farrar, Straus and Giroux.

Pfifferling, J. H. (1980). The problem of physician impairment. *Connecticut Medicine, 44*, 587–591.

Ross, M. (1971). Suicide among physicians. *Psychiatry in Medicine, 2*, 189–198.

Scheele, A. (1979). *Skills for success.* New York: Ballantine.

Scheiber, S. C. (1977). Emotional problems of physicians: Nature and extent of the problems. *Arizona Medicine, 34*, 323–324.

Sharpe, J. C., & Smith, W. W. (1962). Physician heal thyself. *Journal of the American Medical Association, 182*, 234–237.

Shortt, S. E. D. (1979). Psychiatric illness in physicians. *Canadian Medical Association Journal, 121,* 283–288.

Steindler, E. M. (1975). *The impaired physician.* Chicago: American Medical Association.

Steppacher, R. C., & Mausner, J. (1974). Suicide in male and female physicians. *Journal of the American Medical Association, 228,* 323–328.

Talbott, G., Benson, D., & Benson, E. (1980). Impaired physicians—The dilemma of identification. *Postgraduate Medicine, 68,* 56–64.

Thomas, C. B. (1976). What becomes of medical students: The dark side. *John Hopkins Medical Journal, 138,* 185–195.

Tokarz, J. P., Bremer, W., Peters, K., Pfifferling, J. H., & Viner, J. (1979). *Beyond survival.* Chicago: American Medical Association.

Vaillant, G. E., Brighton, J. R., & McArthur, C. (1970). Physicians' use of mood-altering drugs: A 20-year follow-up report. *New England Journal of Medicine, 282,* 365–370.

Vaillant, G. E., Sobowale, N. C., & McArthur, C. (1972). Psychological vulnerabilities of physicians. *New England Journal of Medicine, 287,* 370–375.

Waring, E. M. (1974). Psychiatric illness in physicians: A review. *Comprehensive Psychiatry, 15,* 519–530.

Weed, L. L. (1975). *Your health care and how to manage it.* Burlington, VT: Promis Lab.

Chapter 2

Who Is to Blame for Helpers' Burnout? Environmental Impact

Ayala M. Pines, Ph.D.

In recent years there has been a growing awareness of the stresses involved in the helping professions and the resultant phenomenon—burnout. Burnout is a state of physical, emotional, and mental exhaustion. It is marked by physical depletion and chronic fatigue, by feelings of hopelessness and helplessness, and by the development of a negative self-concept and negative attitudes toward work, life, and people. The negative self-concept is expressed in feelings of guilt, inadequacy, incompetence, and failure.

Burnout results from long-term involvement with people in situations that are emotionally demanding. These kinds of situations are particularly prevalent in the helping professions, where hour after hour, day after day, professional helpers are exposed to physical, psychological, and social problems and are expected to be both skilled and personally concerned. Almost every job in which a person helps others involves a certain degree of stress. The specific degree and kind of stress depend on the particular demands of the job and the resources available to the individual.

Although each occupation has its unique pressures, anxieties, and conflicts inherent in the work itself and in the context in which the work is done, there are certain generalizations that can be made across occupations. The generalizations apply mostly to the process of burnout. At the end of this process professionals who started out idealistic and caring end up resenting their work and their co-workers and losing concern for the people in need of their help. Helpers who reach this state may come to treat their service recipients in a detached and even dehumanized way. Thus, although burnout is a very painful experience for the individual experiencing it, it also represents a great loss to the society as a whole.

If intense involvement with people in situations that are emotionally demanding causes burnout, and if such involvement is characteristic of most human service professions, it should come as no surprise that burnout is very prevalent among such helpers.

This conclusion is based on a decade of research involving well over 5,000 participants representing a wide range of human service professionals, including physicians, nurses, medical and dental personnel, psychologists, psychiatrists, social workers, counselors, teachers on all levels from kindergarten to college, probation officers, police officers, managers and supervisors, journalists, lawyers, politicians, and others.

Participants in the research came from different cultural backgrounds and included, in addition to Americans, Israelis, Australians, Canadians, and Japanese. The research utilized a variety of research strategies: human service professionals were observed at work, they responded to extensive questionnaires about themselves and their work environments, they were interviewed in depth, and they participated in both short-term and long-term experiential workshops. The research resulted in the publication of two books, 15 book chapters, and numerous articles (e.g., Pines & Aronson, 1981).

Burnout, in all these studies, was measured by a 21-item questionnaire representing its three components: physical exhaustion (e.g., feeling weak, tired, rundown); emotional exhaustion (e.g., feeling depressed, trapped, hopeless); and mental exhaustion (e.g., feelings of worthlessness, disillusionment, and resentment). (For further information about the measure, including validity and reliability data, see Pines, 1985.) All the data to be presented in the rest of this chapter were collected using this questionnaire.

The conceptual framework for all this work on burnout was a social-psychological model (see Figure 1). The model assumes that most human service professionals start their careers with a high level of motivation. When they work within the context of a supportive environment, they can achieve peak performance. This in turn strengthens their initial motivation. The result is a positive motivational loop that can be sustained indefinitely.

On the other hand, when the same highly motivated individuals confront a stressful environment in which failure is built in, the result is burnout. The experience of burnout in turn weakens their initial motivation. The

The Job Burnout Model

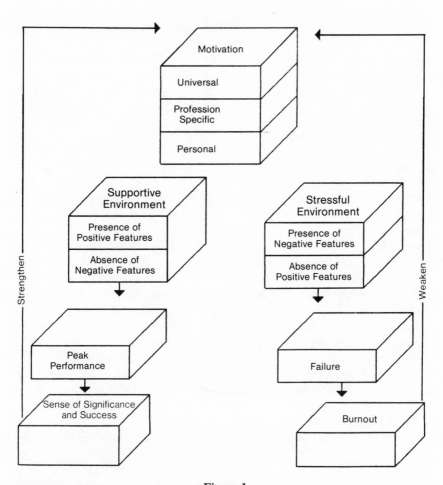

Figure 1

result is a negative motivational loop that turns some people into "dead wood"; makes some people quit their jobs; and causes others to leave their career altogether and look for work in a field that does not involve stressful work with people.

In this model, the crucial determining factor in deciding whether a certain individual will burn out or reach peak performance is the specific characteristics of the work environment.

It is important to note that the model does not apply to those professionals who start out alienated or cynical. An initial high motivation is a prerequisite. The initial motivation can be divided into three major components: universally shared work motivations (such as money, significance, autonomy, growth, and social networks); profession-specific motivations (in the case of human service professionals these include such things as humanitarian people-oriented orientation and a dedication to service); and personal motivations (inspired by an influential person, home background, or some special element in the personal history). (Further discussion on this subject can be found in Pines, 1982c.)

As for the features distinguishing between a supportive and a stressful environment, a supportive environment is characterized by the presence of positive work features (such as autonomy, variety, significance, actualization, growth, challenge, support, and participation) and the absence of negative work features (such as overload, noise, service recipients with severe problems, "red tape," paperwork, and communication problems). A stressful work environment, on the other hand, is characterized by the absence of positive features and the presence of negative ones. (Further discussion of this topic appears in Pines, 1982b.)

The emphasis on the work environment in determining the likelihood and intensity of the experience of burnout is not shared by most of those who studied the subject matter. Even David Harrison, who recently proposed a similar motivational model of burnout, emphasized instead, the role of social competence (Harrison, 1983).

In the Harrison's model, the assumption has been that burnout is the psychological price helpers pay for their involvement and care. It is their high need for achievement, their need to express social competence, their overinvolvement, and their unrealistic expectations of themselves and of their service recipients that cause their burnout.

In many of the discussions that followed the publication of the books and articles about burnout since 1974, the blaming finger has been pointed at the helpers—"The reason why they burn out," the typical argument went, "is because there is something wrong with them"; and the ready proof—"Why are there people in the same occupation who even after many years love their work and show no signs of burnout?"

What both critics and sympathizers have in common is a focus on the dispositional attributes of the helpers, whether described positively as a special personal ambition or negatively as a special weakness. The focus of the social-psychological model presented in this chapter, on the other hand, is on the situational attributes of the work environment. How is it possible to test what has more effect—a helper's personality or the work environment?

One possible answer is to put the same helper one time in a positive environment and a second time in a negative environment and observe what happens. If burnout is primarily a function of individual dispositions, the different environment should make very little difference. On the other hand, if burnout is primarily a function of situational determinants, the individual can be expected to burn out in one environment and flourish in the other. This kind of experiment could never be carried out for obvious ethical reasons.

But life is less concerned with ethical issues than most research psychologists, and as we all know, there are cases in which the same individual ends up, because of a particular set of circumstances, working in two environments differing radically in terms of the relative presence of positive and negative work features. These kinds of cases are important because they demonstrate the effect of the work environment independently of the individual. The following case study demonstrates this point very well.

The case involves two special-education classes for severely handicapped children, both taught by the same teacher. Both classes were serving suburban neighborhoods under the auspices of the same county government and within the limits of the same budget. Yet the work environment—psychological, physical, social, and organizational—and, as a result, the staff burnout in them were vastly different.

It is important to emphasize that although the particular case study involves a teacher-counselor, the conclusions drawn apply to all human service professionals. The work environment of a hospital, for example, may be very different from that of a special-education class, and yet it can be similarly analyzed in terms of such positive features as autonomy, significance, challenge, and support or, conversely, such negative features as overload, red tape, and paperwork. In other words, the question of who is to blame for a helper's burnout applies to all helpers independently of their particular work.

TWO SPECIAL-EDUCATION CLASSES: A CASE STUDY

Carol, a special-education teacher, always liked children and for as long as she can remember thought about becoming a teacher. For five and one-half years she worked in a small school for retarded children, leaving only because of personal reasons.

Physical Environment

The physical layout of the school was designed by teachers. The teachers knew what they and the retarded children needed and helped the architects

plan the school according to those needs. It was a new building. Each classroom was very spacious and had a lot of light. One wall in every classroom
was all windows. On the other side of the windows were play areas so children
could be outside and inside at the same time. The play areas were fenced so
it was safe for the children to wander around. Another wall in each classroom
was all mirrors so the children could get to know themselves and develop
their self-image. There were big movable cabinets so the room could be
divided as needed. It was also possible to move the walls dividing the classroom and open up the whole school. The colors of the rooms were bright
and cheerful; the particular colors for each class were chosen by the teachers.
The furniture was all new and color coordinated. Different size chairs were
in different bright colors. There was a lot of equipment because the budget
was adequate and there was enough space.

There was a big area for physical activities in the middle of the school. It
allowed for socializing activities such as parties, plays, and joint lunches.
The support staff—such as speech therapists and physical therapists—had
their own rooms so they could work individually with children without
disturbing the rest of the class. There was a staff room so the teachers had
a place to go to during their breaks. The staff room was very close to all the
classrooms, so when a crisis occurred the teachers were right there. Since
the school was small and built as one unit, the staff could supervise each
other's children during breaks. There was always someone close by in case
of an accident to watch the other children.

Effects of Physical Environment on Children and Staff

The children loved the physical environment of the school and felt safe
in it. They were free to move around and to go to other classrooms. They
were close to other children and to other staff members. The school felt
almost like a home. There was a lot of community feeling. The physical
environment enabled teachers to be responsive to the children's needs.

Since the school was in one building, it felt like a community. The teachers
could watch out for other children. When a child left his classroom, he was
still in the school building, so other teachers could keep an eye on him. After
two and a half years and after many staff meetings, the teachers got together
and decided to work as a team. All the children in school were divided into
groups according to their age and ability ranges. Each teacher then chose an
area to teach. There was a lot more variety and challenge in the team teaching
because of the different age and ability groups and because the staff could
go in depth into areas they liked. Since the teachers worked as a team, they
had total control on assigning children to the program. When a child who

was sent to the school was clearly misplaced, the teachers had the power to affect the placement decision. Staff members felt they had a lot of autonomy and a lot of support and felt that their work enabled them to grow as professionals and have real impact on the children they were teaching.

Carol was heartbroken when she had to leave the school and soon discovered that work environments can be very different.

Physical Environment in the Second School

Carol's new class was housed in a little theater building on a regular elementary-school campus. There were two special-education classes in the same room that was all together of the same size as the classroom she herself had in the other school. The difference was that now she had to share the same space with another teacher so that actually she had half the space. The other teacher was someone she did not know, and someone who was very resentful about Carol's being there, against her strong objections, and having half of her space. The building was old and always seemed dirty and dark, even after being cleaned up. The floors were scratched. The furniture was mismatched, left over from other classes. The tone of the environment was depressive. Even though Carol had the same budget she had had in the previous class, there was no point in purchasing equipment because there was no place to put it. There were not enough storage cabinets and no space to put things away. The playground was a walk away from the classroom. It was not fenced and was next to a parking lot with many cars going in and out. The staff had to watch the children constantly. It was frightening because it took a child only a second to run to the street. Even though there was a teacher's room on the school grounds, it was too far away from the classroom and Carol was afraid to go there in case something happened.

The support staff did not have their own space and worked with children in the classroom; as a result there were always many people in the classroom: an occupational therapist, a speech therapist, a physical therapist, and the two physical education teachers. The therapists complained about having to work with the children when there was so much noise and so many distractions. The noise was horrible. Carol felt she was under observation all the time, with other people constantly telling her how to teach her class. Their presence added a lot of stress to a situation that was already quite unbearable.

Effects of Physical Environment on Children and Staff

The staff recognized the need for some modifications in the classroom and wrote a four-page letter requesting change; they even found other classrooms

better suited for the children's needs, but there was never a response. The
staff had no say about which children would be placed in each class or how
many. One day the school bus driver pulled over and said to Carol, "You
are getting another child tomorrow." She had no say! That totally pushed
her off, at a time when she felt she could hardly keep up with things anyway.
There was no understanding of the fact that this was a particularly difficult
situation, no sympathy, no compassion.

After six months on the job Carol started coming home from school totally
exhausted, physically, emotionally, and mentally. "I would walk in and
collapse, sleeping 10 to 12 hours every night. I had a lot of back problems
caused by tension. I felt depressed, trapped, and very inadequate. I felt
scared. Teaching was something I loved, and I was afraid that I would never
love it again, that that was the end of my career."

The doctor Carol saw for her back problem suggested that she take some
time off from work. She started by taking a month off, but after a month
still was not ready to get back, so now she is taking two more months off.
During this time she is looking for other jobs and talking to other teachers
who left the same school. Most of the other teachers who left the school took
a drop in salary and benefits, but felt that the work environment they now
have was more than worth their money losses. The specific lessons from
Carol's case study will be extensively discussed later in this paper.

FEATURES IN THE WORK ENVIRONMENT THAT MAY
AFFECT BURNOUT

While discussing work environments, it is possible to start at a very general
level of analysis and thus include variables never even mentioned in the
previous case study, for example, the particular country or culture in which
the work environment is placed; the particular social, political, and economic
climate; the particular location; and the particular organization. Membership
in religious communities, the military, the public sector, the private sector,
or the nonprofit sector can also have a major impact on the work environment
and consequently on the perceived stress of the individual.

In addition to work environment, every discussion of burnout has to include a consideration of both the human service professionals in danger of
burning out and the recipients of their services; just as certain personality
or problem-related features of service recipients can make helping them more
stressful emotionally and thus more likely to produce burnout, there are
certain personality characteristics that can make some people burn out faster
than others.

And yet, as the example of the special-education classes presented earlier shows, even the same person, working with children exhibiting similar problems, in two schools similar in function, location, budget, and sociopolitical environment, will burn out in one and not in the other. The example of the two classes, supported by extensive research, suggests a number of variables in the work environment that play an important role in promoting or preventing burnout. The variables represent four different dimensions of the work environment: psychological, physical, social, and organizational (see Table 1). The *psychological* dimension of the work environment includes features that can be emotional or cognitive in nature. Examples of variables that affect the emotional sphere are the sense of significance and personal growth provided by the work environment. Examples of variables that affect the cognitive sphere are the variety provided by the work environment and the frequency of cognitive overload.

The *physical* dimension of an environment includes on the one hand such fixed features as space, architectural structure, and noise and on the other hand the flexibility to change fixed features and make them suited for one's own taste and needs. The *social* dimension of the work environment includes all the people coming in direct contact with the individual including service recipients (their number and the severity of the problems they present); coworkers (work relations, work sharing, and availability of time out); and supervisors and administrators (feedback, support, and challenge they provide). The *organizational* dimension of the work environment includes such bureaucratic hassles as red tape and paperwork and such administrative features as rules and regulations and the role of the individual within the organization.

The Psychological Dimension of the Work Environment

The emotional and cognitive spheres of work have a major impact on psychological well-being. Emotional and cognitive features can be inherent in the work itself, but the focus of this chapter is the environmentally induced sense of significance in burnout. The psychological dimension of the work environment includes the cognitive and the emotional spheres. The cognitive sphere will be discussed first. It includes such variables as autonomy, variety, and overload.

Autonomy

The extent to which a certain work environment provides discretion and enables people to decide on their own how to do their work determines to a large extent their sense of power and control over that environment. The sense of control mediates against stress and prevents burnout.

Table 1

Work Environment Features That Are Burnout Correlates

Psychological	Physical	Social	Organizational
Cognitive	Fixed	Service recipients	Bureaucratic
Autonomy	Structure	Numbers	Red tape
Variety	Space	Problems	Paperwork
Overload	Noise	Relations	Communication problems
Emotional	Flexibility to change	Co-workers	Administrative
Significance	fixed features	Work relations	Rules and regulations
Actualization		Sharing	Policy influence
Growth		Time out	Participation
		Support	
		Challenge	
			Role in the organization
		Supervisors and	Role conflict
		administrators	Role ambiguity
		Feedback	Status disorder
		Rewards	
		Support	
		Challenge	

Source: A. Pines, "Changing Organizations: Is a Work Environment Without Burnout a Possible Goal?" In W.S. Paine (Ed.), (1982b), *Job Stress and Burnout* (p. 192). Beverly Hills, CA: Sage.

In the first special-education class presented earlier, teachers had a lot of autonomy—they designed the school, they could affect placement decisions, and they eventually decided on their own teaching style in the school. In the second class, one of the most stressful aspects was the fact that teachers had almost no autonomy at all; the administration ignored the teachers' repeated complaints about the classroom and they had no say in the placement of children.

Perceived control over one's work environment is a powerful mediator of stress, associated with feeling able to cope effectively, predict events, and determine what will happen.

Not surprisingly, autonomy was found in several of our studies to be positively correlated with job satisfaction and negatively correlated with burnout. That is to say, the more autonomy, the less burnout. For example, in a sample of 198 mental retardation workers, the correlation was $r = -0.32$; in a sample of 52 Social Security Administration workers, the correlation was $r = -0.35$ (both $p < 0.05$).

Variety

All higher organisms actively seek variety in their environment and avoid monotonous environments. A rat in a maze will use different routes to food, if they are available, rather than the same one all the time. It will tend to avoid areas in which it spent considerable time and to explore less familiar areas.

Variety in the work environment enhances interest and challenge. It has been identified by industrial psychologists as a key factor in employee satisfaction, performance, and attendance. In the example of the special-education class, Carol noted variety as one of the positive aspects of team teaching because of the different age and ability groups.

Variety was found in several of our studies to be negatively correlated with burnout: the more variety there was in the individual's work environment, the less likely was that individual to report experiencing burnout. For example, in a sample of 294 psychology students, the correlation between variety and burnout was $r = -0.35$; in a sample of 277 professional women, the correlation was $r = -0.32$ (both $p < 0.05$).

Overload

A work environment can impose two different kinds of overload on the individual: a quantitative overload and a qualitative overload. A quantitative overload is the result of having too many tasks to accomplish per unit of time, whereas a qualitative overload is the result of having tasks that are too difficult for the individual.

In Carol's case the work environment imposed both qualitative and quantitative overload. She not only had too many children but also children with very serious problems she was never trained or felt qualified to treat. Carol's feelings of inadequacy about treating the special problems presented by the children were amplified by the fact that there were so many of them, and so many different problems.

Overload was repeatedly found in our studies to be a positive correlate of burnout: the more overload in the work environment (both quantitative and qualitative), the more likely were individuals to burn out. For example, in a sample of 52 Social Security Administration workers, the correlation was $r = 0.30$; in a sample of 725 human service professionals, the correlation was $r = 0.35$ (both $p < 0.05$).

The second sphere in the psychological dimension is the emotional sphere, which includes such variables as significance, actualization, and growth.

Significance

One of the most common reasons for job dissatisfaction and subsequent departure from a job is the belief that the work has no significance, that it is meaningless and futile. And indeed lack of significance was found in several of our studies to be a major cause of hopelessness, depression, and burnout. For example, in a sample of 267 police officers and in a sample of 101 Israeli managers, the correlation between significance and burnout was $r = -0.27$ ($p < 0.05$). The more sense of significance individuals have in their work, we found, the less likely they are to burn out.

As noted earlier, some jobs are inherently more significant than others, yet within a given job, different work environments can enhance or diminish the individual's perceived sense of significance. Noting the case study, in the first school Carol felt she was having a major impact on the children's lives, that she was more than a teacher, that her work was extremely significant; whereas in the second school she felt inadequate, hopeless, and scared. She could hardly deal with the children's physical needs and felt she failed to fulfill her teaching objectives. Her feeling that no matter how hard she tried she could not affect her work situation and have more of an impact on the children under her care was one of the major causes for her subsequent burnout.

Actualization and growth

The human need for self-actualization and growth is a major theme in the writing of humanistic psychologists and several personality theorists. According to Maslow, people's drive toward actualization of the human potential is a central personality tendency, and the highest need is the human hierarchy of needs. Thus a work environment that enables individuals to actualize themselves and grow professionally is a work environment that should reduce rather than produce burnout. This contention was supported by several of our studies (Pines, 1982b). In all these studies self-actualization on the job was negatively correlated with burnout (i.e., the more self-actualization, the less burnout). For example, in a sample of 52 Social Security Administration employees, the correlation between self-actualization and burnout was $r = -0.40$; in a sample of 205 professionals, the correlation was -0.28 (both at $p < 0.05$). And in the case study presented earlier, Carol noted that one of the things she enjoyed most about the team teaching on her first job was the fact that it was challenging "because of the different age and ability groups." Her second job provided no opportunities for actualization and growth.

The Physical Dimension of the Work Environment

There is growing evidence that the physical quality of the work environment can have a major impact on mental and physical health. The whole field of environmental psychology was developed to deal with the interplay between environmental problems and human behavior. A work environment can be a source of numerous stressors; the ones mentioned most often and thus chosen for discussion here include architectural dysfunction, crowding, and noise. For example, in one study involving 205 professionals the correlation with a comfortable environment was $r = -0.29$ ($p < 0.05$), while environmental pressures at work such as noise and uncomfortable setting were positively correlated with burnout (i.e., the more noise, the more burnout [$r = 0.27, p < 0.05$]).

Architectural structure

Zimring (1981) views stress as resulting from a misfit between the individual's needs and environmental attributes. The severity of the stress and its long-term consequences for the individual are affected by such issues as the importance to the individual of the misfit, the chronic or acute nature of the misfit, and the strategies available to the individual for solving it. The environment can stress us both directly and indirectly.

The design of the physical environment affects individuals directly by supporting or thwarting their work-related goals. For example, since the retarded children in Carol's class needed a lot of one-to-one work, the windows by the outside enclosed play area were very important because they enabled her to keep an eye on the other children while she was working with one child.

The design of an environment can also indirectly influence the person-environment fit by making desired social interaction easier or more difficult to achieve. For example, given the openness of the school building, children felt free to move around and go to other classrooms; as a result they developed close relationships with children in other classrooms and with other staff members.

Some scholars argue that vandalism is a symptom of stress caused by designs that destroy social networks. When individuals do not have a sense of belonging and mutual support, they will not care for their space. And indeed, the example of the two schools indicates that whereas the first school felt "almost like a home," and the children liked it and felt safe in it, the second school was a very stressful environment and had a very negative effect on the children. "They would run around, climb on tables, run to the other side of the room and disturb the other class, and throw toys when they got angry."

Space

In any given work space individuals must manage the physical environment in order to achieve their goals. When other people are a part of that given space, there must be a coordination of everyone's needs for resources, activities, interaction, and space. As the number of people populating a certain space increases, the task of managing and coordinating that environment becomes more difficult and more likely to drain energy that otherwise would be available for attainment of work goals.

In the special-education school described by Carol, lack of space had a major negative impact on both the teachers and the children. Sharing classroom space with another teacher, and with all of the support staff, resulted in the teachers and therapists feeling resentful. The children, who needed a lot of space, felt trapped in the small space of the classroom. "No matter what they did they were in somebody's space. Everybody was always tripping over toys." The crowded, inadequate space of this classroom increased the tension and the stress experienced by students and staff.

Noise

Noise is a psychological concept and is defined as sound that is unwanted by the listener because it is unpleasant or bothersome, interferes with important activities, or is believed to be psychologically harmful (Kryter, 1970).

Two field studies have artifically increased classroom noise levels and assessed the effects on student behavior and performance. In one study highway traffic noise was broadcast outside a large university classroom building. As a result, less student participation and attention were observed when compared to a no-noise control group (Ward & Suedfeld, 1973).

In the second study the noise level of several fifth- and sixth-grade classrooms was increased by adding a white noise background (Ward & Suedfeld, 1973). Results of the study indicated that children tested in the classrooms with the additional noise showed impaired auditory discrimination, visual motor skills, and visual discrimination as compared with children tested in classrooms without the additional noise.

In the second class cited earlier, the noise was horrible. For both pupils and teacher the noise constituted a chronic stressor that added to the noxious classroom environment. Numerous studies, cited by Ward and Suedfeld (1973), indicated that there are negative effects of noise that occur after the noise exposure is terminated, and indeed, Carol reported that often the screams of the children and the other noises would continue ringing in her ears for hours after she left school.

Flexibility to change fixed features

In addition to the absolute quality of the fixed features, another crucial element in the physical dimension of the work environment is the flexibility to change those fixed features. Some people are more sensitive to noise than others; some like large, open areas whereas others feel comfortable in small, enclosed areas. The best physical environment is one that is flexible enough to accommodate the individual, rather than forcing the individual to accommodate. In the first example, the flexibility was maximized: The physical layout of the school was designed by teachers; it was possible to move the walls dividing the classrooms and open up the whole school.

In our research physical environments that were pleasant and designed to meet workers' tastes, needs, and preferences were found to be negatively correlated with burnout. Physical environments that were pleasant and designed to meet workers' tastes, needs, and preferences were found to be negatively correlated with burnout. For example, in the study of 205 professionals mentioned several times earlier, the correlation was $r = -0.29$ ($p < 0.05$). To protect against burnout, working and living spaces should accommodate as much as possible the individual's needs and preferences and be as personalized as possible.

The Social Dimension of the Work Environment

Most human service professionals, by definition of their occupational choice, are oriented more toward people than toward things and tend to view themselves as caring, sensitive, and understanding. Because of this orientation, human service professionals are extremely sensitive to the social dimension of their work environment. When the social environment is noxious, burnout will occur even if other things are acceptable, and vice versa—if the social environment is very supportive, burnout will not occur even if the work itself is extremely stressful.

The social dimension of the work environment includes all the people coming in direct contact with the individual as part of his/her work. For most human service professionals, the social environment includes service recipients, co-workers, supervisors, and administrators. Each of these people can impose certain demands on the individual and provide certain rewards. The ratio of demands to rewards is an important determinant of burnout.

Service recipients

There are many different ways in which service recipients can influence the physical, emotional, and mental well-being of a service-providing individual. The most straightforward impact results from their number, the seriousness of their condition and the relationship between them and the service provider.

Number. The quality of interactions in many human services is affected by the number of people for whom the professional is providing care. As this number increases, so does the cognitive, sensory, and emotional overload of the professional.

Problems. The severity or complexity of the problems presented by the service recipients can have a negative effect on the human service professional especially when the service involves prolonged and direct contact. One of the most stressful work environments for nurses, for example, is the burned-children's unit.

Relations. The relationship between the professional staff and the service recipients affects the work atmosphere and thus can produce or reduce the staff's work-related stress.

Co-workers

Several components contribute to the atmosphere of the work environment: work relations, sharing, time out, support, and challenge.

Work relations. The nature of the relationship between co-workers either can be a major source of stress at work, or else it can be a central factor in individual and organizational health. Difficult relationships at work were reported by Yates (1979) as causing symptoms associated with extensive stress such as diarrhea, pain in the neck or lower back, anxiety, and insomnia. As Yates (1979) noted: "Certain associates can *literally* be a 'pain in the neck.' "

Work relations were consistently found in our studies to be negative burn-out correlates—i.e., the better the relations, the less burnout. In a study of mental health settings (Pines & Maslach, 1978), it was found that the better the work relations, the more professionals liked their work ($r = 0.38$, $p = 0.001$), the more they felt free to express themselves ($r = 0.41$, $p = 0.001$), the more they were likely to be staying in mental health for self-fulfillment ($r = 0.41$, $p = 0.040$), the more successful they felt on the job ($r = 0.31$, $p = 0.008$), the more "good days" they had at work ($r = 0.27$, $p = 0.025$), the more likely they were to confer with others ($r = 0.27$, $p = 0.025$), the higher they rated their particular institution ($r = 0.49$, $p = 0.001$), and the more consistently positive they were in their descriptions of patients.

In Carol's case the fact that both she and the other teacher sharing the little theater building with her did not know each other, had nothing in common, and very much resented being thrown together in the confining classroom area, undoubtedly contributed to both their work stress and dis-satisfaction. A trusting and caring relationship with one's co-workers and colleagues can make a world of difference, especially when the work is otherwise stressful.

Sharing. Sharing and teamwork can help diffuse many work stresses. In addition to serving the function of diffusion of responsibility, work sharing can increase challenge, variety, and power. Work sharing was found in every study in which it was measured to be a significant negative correlate of burnout: the more work sharing, the less burnout. For example, in a sample of 87 American managers, the correlation between work sharing and burnout was $r = -0.37$; in a sample of 129 social service workers and in a sample of 205 professionals, it was $r = -0.28$ (both at $p < 0.05$).

Also, in Carol's case team teaching meant that each teacher could choose an area he/she particularly loved. And because the teachers worked as a team, they had complete control over assigning children to the program which they would not have had otherwise.

Time out. One of the things that makes the work so stressful for many professionals is the lack of a break. Carol reported that after working straight through for five hours, she "felt like she couldn't breathe."

In contrast, one of the things that made the work in the first setting so enjoyable was the fact that the school structure enabled teachers to supervise each other's children. The staff room was very close to all the classrooms, so the teachers had a place to go to during their breaks, but when a crisis occurred, they could be right there.

Support. One of the most important functions co-workers can provide for each other is support. Everyone needs support during times of crisis and appreciation during times of success. These kinds of support and appreciation are most valuable when they come from someone who understands all the intricacies of the work one does. Whether or not co-workers provide each other with support and appreciation determines whether the work atmosphere will be hostile, stressful, and burnout producing or else friendly, supportive, and burnout preventing.

Challenge. Although it can be comforting to be in a work environment where one is the sole expert and no one challenges or can potentially challenge that expertise, unfortunately too much comfort of this sort is stifling. Colleagues can challenge each other and enhance each other's creativity, excitement, and continuous growth. The crucial element that will determine whether a certain challenge will be a positive feature in the work environment and a negative correlate of burnout, or a negative feature and a positive correlate of burnout, is the absence or simultaneous presence of support. Thus the best challengers are co-workers who also provide each other with support and appreciation. Challenge enhances significance, learning, and growth, which are important aspects of the psychological dimension of the work environment and powerful buffers against burnout.

Supervisors and administrators

The relationships between individuals and their supervisors and administrators are an important part of the social dimension in a work environment. The study of House et al. (1971) focused on the impact of leadership on workers' work stress and satisfaction, exploring the relationship between individual's perceptions of their immediate supervisor's behavior and their satisfaction from their work and organization. House et al. found that supervisors demonstrating consideration for their subordinates was highly correlated with the various indices of job satisfaction. The degree to which supervisors set clear objectives and procedures on the job *with* their subordinates was also positively related to satisfaction. Democratic leadership style was another variable found to be correlated with job satisfaction.

By providing feedback, recognition, challenge, and support supervisors and administrators can influence the psychological well-being of workers and the general atmosphere of a work environment.

Feedback. In psychology, feedback is any kind of direct information from an outside source about the effects and/or results of one's behavior. The best feedback is immediate, appropriate, and provided by someone who is in a position to understand the full scale of one's performance, i.e., a supervisor or an administrator. Feedback about work, especially when coming from a supervisor, provides individuals with information about their levels of performance and success and as such is crucial for their sense of meaningfulness and achievement at work.

Lack of feedback from supervisors and administrators is a particularly damaging organizational stressor. Yates (1979) notes that when the upper echelon of management are simply unresponsive to the requests and reports of lower-level employees, they create stress in them. "Nothing seems to bother people more than just being ignored. We appear to prefer any response—even a negative one—to no response at all. Not only are people distressed when they are met with unresponsiveness; they are also discouraged from taking any initiative in the future." The more feedback received from supervisors and administrators, the less burnout.

Rewards. In addition to providing straight feedback about performance, supervisors can affect organizational morale by adequate distribution of rewards. A reward is defined as an object, situation, or verbal statement which is presented upon completion of a successful performance of a task and which tends to increase the probability of the behavior involved. Rewards include pay, benefits, security, and promotional opportunities, as well as appreciation and recognition. Lack of rewards was found in several of our studies (Pines & Aronson, 1981) to be highly correlated with burnout; the less rewards, the more burnout.

Support. Another crucial function for supervisors and administrators is providing their staff and organization with professional and administrative support. This support is independent of the support provided by colleagues and is equally important.

In Carol's case, the fact that she got no administrative support greatly increased her stress. Both Carol and the other teacher sharing the classroom space wrote several letters requesting classroom change; they even found other classrooms better suited for the children's needs, but there was never a response. Because the work environment was so negative they needed more administrative support than they otherwise would, but they got almost no support at all.

Challenge. When supervisors or administrators are consistently supportive of their staff, they can enhance significance, learning, and growth by constructively challenging their subordinates. Like challenge by co-workers, a challenge by a supervisor needs to be for the benefit of the person being challenged rather than the person doing the challenging. Supervisors who challenge themselves before they do it to their staff can provide a positive role model.

By utilizing feedback, rewards, support, and challenge appropriately, supervisors can have a major impact on the social dimension of any work environment and thus have a major impact on the likelihood that their staff will either burn out or cope with burnout successfully.

The Organizational Dimension of the Work Environment

The organizational dimension of the work environment and its effect on workers' performance and job satisfaction have been the focus of most writings in the field of industrial and organizational psychology. Variables that are burnout correlates and that are built into the organizational dimension of the work environment include bureaucratic hassles, administrative features, as well as the role of the individual in the organization.

Bureaucratic features

Bureaucracy is defined as "a government by department officials following an inflexible routine" (Webster's Dictionary). The word bureaucracy acquired a negative connotation as a dehumanizing work environment marked by a rigid hierarchical structure and many unnecessary rules and regulations, a cumbersome and inefficient paper-eating monster.

Most human service professionals, without proper warning and training, end up working some kind of a bureaucratic organization. By definition of their size and complexity, most of these bureaucratic organizations are slow and unresponsive. They tend to be more self-serving than public serving and thus are blamed for causing burnout in idealistic and caring human service professionals. The problems mentioned most often as causing burnout among the bureaucratic features of the work environment include red tape, paperwork, and communication problems. All three have been found to be significant correlates of burnout.

Paperwork. Bureaucratic organizations often generate so much paperwork that employees complain they are shuffling papers instead of treating or serving people. The official concern for forms and routines creates special problems for the more caring and idealistic professionals, who feel they are becoming clerks instead of social scientists. Paperwork becomes a needless waste of time and emotional energy and is viewed as a senseless obstacle to goal achievement.

Communication problems. Bureaucratic organizations are often built as rigid hierarchical structures that create communication problems between staff members. Many times there are many levels of administrators and many levels of front-line workers in the organization. Because of inadequate communication, individuals feel isolated and undervalued. It often happens that two people who are doing similar work and can potentially provide each other with professional support and challenge do not know about each other's existence. The problems can be on vertical communication lines or on horizontal communication lines between co-workers. Both kinds are well-known bureaucratic hassles, both are stressful, and both can, and often do, enhance the process of burnout. In a sample of 724 human service professionals, the correlation between bureaucratic interference and burnout was $r = 0.24$; in the sample of 101 Israeli managers, it was $r = 0.31$ (both $p < 0.05$).

Administrative influence

The administrative influence in a certain work environment is often transmitted via rules and policies. When these regulations are excessive, senseless, and arbitrary, the likelihood of burnout is greater.

Rules and regulations. Typically when one examines bureaucratic rules and regulations one often discovers that although some are too vague, others are too detailed. Both excesses frustrate the goal achievement of the individual, and thus enhance burnout.

"Every organization of any size has a myriad of rules, policies, and procedures that make sense only to the person who created them. . . . There may have been problems that arose because of a lack of a specific procedure, so several procedures and rules were created to cover a situation that probably would occur only with the greatest infrequency" (Yates, 1979). Ridiculous rules, policies, and procedures constitute one form of bureaucratic pettiness that is a well-known antecedent of burnout.

Policy influence. In any large bureaucracy it is often difficult to identify the source of certain regulations or policy influences. This unclear responsibility keeps workers from effectively stating and correcting their grievances.

Participation

Another common antecedent to burnout revolves around not having the opportunity to participate in decisions that affect one's work. The effect of participation on job satisfaction is related to a perceived sense of control. Studies demonstrated that the greater the belief in the ability to influence the environment, the lower the reported job strain and the higher the reported work satisfaction (Maslach & Pines, 1977).

Role in the organization

In the organizational features discussed previously the focus was on the organization. The next section will focus on the individual. A work environment characterized by role conflict or role ambiguity and inadequate career development also influences the individual's level of performance.

Role conflict. Role conflict exists whenever an individual in a particular role is torn by conflicting demands. There are different kinds of role conflicts, and they can be imposed by the same source. For example, in Carol's case the demand from the administration was that she teach the children while attending to their physical and psychological needs. Yet given the number of the children and the seriousness of their problems, there was no way Carol could comply with both demands. Feeling torn between those conflicting demands was experienced as extremely stressful by Carol and clearly contributed to her burnout.

Conflicting demands can be imposed by different people such as a supervisor and an administrator both demanding, at the same time, different tasks to be accomplished.

Role conflict has serious consequences for the individual's subjective experience of stress. In several of our studies it was found that the more conflicting demands imposed by a certain work environment, the more individuals in that environment were likely to burn out. For example, in two studies, one involving 724 human service professionals and the other involving 87 American managers, the correlation between conflicting demands and burnout was $r = 0.31$ ($p < 0.05$).

Role ambiguity. Role ambiguity exists when individuals have inadequate information about their work roles, when there is lack of clarity about the work objectives associated with the role, about colleagues' expectations of the work role, and about the scope and responsibilities of the job. Robert Kahn and his colleagues at the University of Michigan found that people who suffered from role ambiguity experienced lower job satisfaction, higher job-related tension, greater futility, and lower self-confidence (Kahn, 1978).

Status disorders. A different set of environmental stressors built into the role of the individual in the work environment is related to status disorders in career development. Career development refers to the impact of overpromotion, underpromotion, status incongruence, and lack of job security. Status disorders can have a negative effect on both the psychological and social dimensions of the individual's work environment and thus increase the likelihood to burnout.

BURNOUT FROM A SOCIAL-PSYCHOLOGICAL PERSPECTIVE

The preceding discussion of work environment and burnout represents a social-psychological perspective. Rather than explain burnout in dispositional terms (such as the particular vulnerabilities or weaknesses of a certain individual helper) it focused attention on situational factors (those environmental features that cause almost all helpers to burn out).

It was suggested that in addition to such general variables as culture-specific influences and economic and political considerations, every work environment has four dimensions: psychological, physical, social, and organizational. Throughout the chapter a case study was presented in an attempt to demonstrate the specific effects of a variety of environmental factors within those four dimensions. However, it is important to note that the discussion did not take into account the individual helpers in the particular work environment, their personal histories, physical and emotional makeups, their strengths, their vulnerabilities, and their strategies for coping with burnout. And yet, as the case study suggests, in spite of all individual differences, the work environment has a crucial effect on helpers' burnout. Although individual differences may determine how soon one helper will burn out, how extreme the experience will be, and what its consequences will be, the work environment determines the likelihood that burnout will occur across the board.

The case study also provides a demonstration of the social-psychological model of burnout. It shows how a highly motivated individual, when working in a supportive environment, achieved peak performance and consequently felt a sense of significance and success. These, in turn, strengthened the initial motivation and created a positive motivational loop that could have been sustained almost indefinitely. The same highly motivated individual, when working in a highly stressful environment, inevitably failed. Her failure and the emotional turmoil surrounding the failure caused her burnout and the negative motivational loop that eventually made her quit her job. The case study is important because, as noted at the beginning of this chapter, it demonstrates the effect of the work environment independently of the individual since the same individual flourished in one environment and burned out in the other.

REFERENCES

Harrison, W. D. (1983). A social competence model of burnout. In B. Farber (Ed.), *Stress and burnout*. New York: Pergamon Press.

House, R. J., Filley, A. C., & Gujarati, D. N. (1971). Leadership style, hierarchical influence and dissatisfaction of subordinate role expectations. *Journal of Applied Psychology, 55*, 422–432.

Kafry, D., & Pines, A. (1980). The experience of tedium in life and work. *Human Relations, 33*(7), 477–503.

Kahn, R. L. (1978). Job burnout prevention and remedies. *Public Welfare, 16*, 61–63.

Kanner, A., Kafry, D., & Pines, A. (1978). Conspicuous in its absence: The lack of positive conditions as source of stress. *Journal of Human Stress, 4*(4), 33–39.

Kryter, K. D. (1970). *The effects of noise on men*. New York: Academic Press.

Maslach, C., & Pines, A. (1977). The burnout syndrome in day care settings. *Child Care Quarterly, 6*(2), 100–113.

Paine, W. S. (1982). *Job stress and burnout*. Beverly Hills, CA: Sage.

Pines, A. (1981). Burnout: A current problem in pediatrics. *Current Problems in Pediatrics, 11*(7), 1–32.

Pines, A. (1982a). The buffering effects of social support. In B. Farber (Ed.), *Stress and burnout*. New York: Pergamon Press.

Pines, A. (1982b). Changing organizations: Is a work environment without burnout a possible goal? In W.S. Paine (Ed.), *Job stress and burnout*. Beverly Hills, CA: Sage.

Pines, A. (1982c). Helper's motivation and the burnout syndrome. In T.A. Wills (Ed.), *Basic processes in helping relationships*. New York: Academic Press.

Pines, A. (1985). The burnout measure. In J. Jones (Ed.), *Police burnout: Theory, research, application*. Park Ridge, IL: London House Press.

Pines, A., & Aronson, E. (1980). *Burnout*. Schiller Park, IL: MTI Teleprograms.

Pines, A., & Aronson, E. (1981). *Burnout from tedium to personal growth*. New York: Free Press.

Pines, A., & Aronson, E. (1983). Combating burnout. *Children and Youth Services Review, 5*, 263–275.

Pines, A., & Kafry, D. (1978). Occupational tedium in social service professionals. *Social Work, 23*(6), 499–507.

Pines, A., & Kafry D. (1981a). Coping with burnout. In J. Jones (Ed.), *Selected readings in staff burnout*. Park Ridge, IL: London House Press.

Pines, A., & Kafry, D. (1981b). The experience of life tedium in three generations of professional women. *Sex Roles, 7*(2), 117–134.

Pines, A., and Kafry, D. (1981c). Tedium in the life and work of professional women as compared with men. *Sex Roles, 7*(10), 963–977.

Pines, A., Kafry, D., & Etzion, D. (1980). Job stress from a crosscultural perspective. In K. Reid (Ed.), *Burnout in the helping professions*. Kalamazoo, MI: Western Michigan University.

Pines, A., & Kanner, A.D. (1982). Nurses' burnout: Lack of positive conditions and presence of negative conditions as two independent sources of stress. *Journal of Psychosocial Nursing, 4*(20), 30–35.

Pines, A., & Maslach, C. (1980). Combating staff burnout in a child care center. A case study. *Child Care Quarterly, 9*(1), 5–16.

Pines, A., & Silbert, M. (1984). Burnout of police officers. In J. Jones (Ed.), *Police burnout: Theory, research, application.* Park Ridge, IL: London House Press.

Stress. (1980, January). *New York Teacher,* 1B–8B.

Ward, L. M., & Suedfeld, P. (1973). Human responses to highway noise. *Environmental Research, 6,* 306–326.

Yates, J. (1979). *Managing stress.* New York: AMACOM.

Zimring, C. M. (1981). The stress in the designed environment. *Journal of Social Issues, 37,* 145–171.

Chapter 3

The Impaired-Physician Syndrome: A Developmental Perspective

Robert H. Coombs, Ph.D.,
and Fawzy I. Fawzy, M.D.

The problem of physician impairment has recently attracted widespread interest and concern. Local and national conferences have highlighted a variety of personal problems that can afflict physicians. During recent years the number of published articles on this topic has grown at a rapid rate. To date, however, most of the literature is descriptive in nature with few systematic explanations.

A developmental perspective of physician impairment is the intent of this chapter. Our data derive from two longitudinal studies and are supplemented with a number of shorter-term analyses. The first prospective study was based on serial interviews during each year of training with an entire class of medical trainees over a seven-year period—from the time they first received letters of admission to medical school until they were in their residency training programs. The second study consisted of in-depth interviews with the spouses of 150 medical trainees together with a follow-up interview a decade later.

IMPAIRED VERSUS "COMPLEAT" PHYSICIANS: A TYPOLOGY

The personal lives of impaired physicians are typically dominated by career involvements. So much time has been devoted to their careers that outside activities are minimal. Living an imbalanced life-style, they gradually become drained, physically and emotionally exhausted, depressed, addicted, or even suicidal.

In short, a single-minded devotion to career is impoverishing. By gradually severing ties with family members and neglecting restorative activities that offer rest and diversion, physicians diminish their emotional resilience. When this occurs, the technical quality of work suffers, as do interpersonal relationships with patients, family members, and others. These unrewarding social encounters contribute to further stress, thus bringing about a vicious cycle.

If impairment is to be correctly understood, the opposite must also be understood (Coombs et al., in press). "Compleat physicians" is the label we give to those physicians who, in contrast to impaired doctors, provide complete medical care (for emphasis, we use the Old English spelling). Realizing that warm sensitivity is important to patient care as well as technical competence, compleat physicians make an effort to understand and implement these subjective qualities in their own lives.

Dealing sensitively with others' feelings, the affective components of illness, cannot, of course, be achieved if, in the pursuit of career excellence, one's own emotional well-being has been neglected. Compleat physicians offer complete medical care, interpersonal sensitivity, as well as technical competence, because they have paid the price in time and effort to nurture affective qualities and have successfully avoided the degenerative processes that detract from them. They have not been swept along by social forces that promote career attainment at the expense of personal and family well-being.

"The longer I live," observed Oliver Wendell Holmes, "the more I am satisfied of two things: first, that the truest lives are those that are cut rose-diamond fashion, with many faces answering to the many-planed aspects of the world about them; secondly, that society is always trying in some way or other to grind us down to a single flat surface. It is hard work to resist this grinding down action."

"Impaired doctors" and "compleat physicians" are, of course, ideal mental constructs. Only a relatively few doctors actually fit either of these extreme descriptions—they vary on a continuum. That is, most physicians vary in degrees between these opposites. Yet all are gradually moving toward one type or the other, toward impairment or completeness; professional careers are dynamic, not static. Impairment is a developmental process, not a cataclysmic event.

Our thesis is that (1) the system of medical training as it is now constituted includes built-in reinforcers for emotional impairment, and (2) those who successfully avoid these debilitating processes must generally do so on their own without much encouragement. If one is to maintain personal well-being during the rigorous years of medical training, thoughtful effort is required. Continuous reflection and planning must be followed by assertive efforts to enhance personal growth and well-being. Time and energy must be devoted to activities that promote physical and emotional fitness, spiritual and cultural sensitivity, and social and familial vitality.

EMOTIONAL VULNERABILITY DURING MEDICAL TRAINING

Stress has typically been held accountable for physician impairment. Although not discounting the well-established link between stress and emotional and/or physical disorders, this seems to be a simplistic explanation. Clearly, some stressors, those that are role relevant, can be precursors to professional development, not the opposite. When handled properly, role-relevant stress can promote feelings of progress and fulfillment, even exhilaration.

Some stressors, however, contribute little, if anything, to either career or personal development. The only functional value of some stressors (sleep and status deprivation, for example) is to test, sometimes excessively, the trainee's physical and emotional stamina. Impairment statistics document that some do not survive these rigors, whereas others develop unhealthy work styles and psychological inhibitions. Role-irrelevant distress, when added to an unbalanced life-style and emotional unexpressiveness, promotes emotional vulnerability.

In our view, three socializing conditions in the medical training milieu contribute substantially to the gradual erosion of emotional well-being: status deprivation, imbalanced life-styles, and emotional isolation.

Status Deprivation

Gaining a place in medical school is one of the most coveted achievements attainable by young men and women. It all but guarantees a professionally stimulating life, one characterized by status, power, and affluence. Those who aspire to this goal, often as early as childhood or early youth, usually do so single-mindedly, possessing no alternative career ambition. For them, the years of arduous academic performance are unmistakably worth the effort.

Because of the fierce competition involved in securing one of the relatively few available openings in medical school, high anxiety typically grips applicants who await notice of admissions committees. Small wonder that success in this regard is marked by personal exultation and celebration with friends and loved ones, while those who are rejected simply try and try again.

Yet, amazingly, many students, four out of 10 in our own study, consider dropping out of medical school during their first year (Coombs, 1978). Although the number has recently decreased to negligible proportions, 5 to 10% have traditionally withdrawn, and those who remain are often discontented, frustrated, disillusioned, and angry. Why?

A major reason for this surprising dilemma is, in our view, the disillusioning realities of an authoritarian environment that typically strips trainees of their status and fails to meet their expectations.

Acceptance in medical school symbolizes entrance into America's most prestigious profession, so students naturally anticipate that this achievement will enhance their status, not diminish it. After all, doesn't a proven record of high motivation and academic attainment indicate that they, the "cream of the crop," have risen to the top?

Upon entering medical school, many feel that they have fallen, not risen, in status, and this status deprivation recurs regularly throughout the long and arduous years of training. Expecting to be regarded as an elect group, these new recruits are surprised, in fact, stunned, to find themselves treated as "undergraduates or less." When asked, "How high or low are you on the status ladder of the teaching hospital?" 9 out of 10 freshmen indicated a very low status, some saying, "on the bottom," "the lowest of the low," "zero," "even lower than the orderlies," "you just can't get any lower" (Coombs & Boyle, 1971).

After being accustomed to considerable personal freedom, a symbol of status and self-worth, premed students anticipate that medical school will offer more, not less, independence, initiative, and responsibility than they had as undergraduates. Not surprisingly then, as freshmen medical students, they are taken aback when authoritarian mentors project a view of them as immature, irresponsible, lacking in motivation, and even stupid. Repeatedly, students complain about being made to feel like "dodos," "high school kids," "children," or "infants" (Coombs & St. John, 1981).

Since medical school has higher status than college and is so much more difficult to get into, premed students also expect a proportionately higher quality of instruction. Medical-school professors are envisioned as being top-notch persons primarily oriented toward helping students learn. As compared with college instructors, they are viewed as being smarter, more interested in their particular fields, better able to inspire students and to convey an interest in the subject matter. In addition, they are imagined as being more professional, more comprehensive, and better organized.

It does not take long in medical school, however, to realize that many instructors are primarily interested in research rather than teaching. Disillusionment is high when students find out that such instructors regard teaching as a chore, a job to be done, a necessary evil. "I get the feeling that every second spent away from their research is considered a waste of time."

In this regard, a sharp contrast can be noted between student expectations and actual experience as measured first before entering medical school and again at various times during training.

- "Teaching in medical school is generally superior to college teaching." (Only 11% of the premed students who had just received acceptance letters disagreed with this statement. Yet, after one year's exposure, 43% disagreed, and the proportion rose even higher to 57% and 61%, respectively, in the sophomore and junior years.)

- "The medical-school faculty places much more importance on helping students than on performing their own research or other activities." (Sixty-six percent agreed before entering medical school, but after a year's experience, only 16% did so, and this latter figure remained constant in subsequent years.)

- "There is little waste of time in the medical curriculum." (Before coming to medical school, 70% of the students agreed; after one year the number dropped to 20%, and then to 4% during the following years.)

As physicians-to-be, students naturally expect to concentrate on clinically relevant topics, those that have clear applicability for patients and their problems, but, as longitudinal results indicate, these expectations are not realized.

- "Everything that happens to a student in medical school will be important in learning to be a doctor." (Whereas only 15% disagreed with this statement before coming to medical school, 44% did so after a year's exposure; in the sophomore year, 57% disagreed, as did 63% in the final year.)

- "Much of the subject matter is irrelevant to the practice of medicine." (Only 20% of the uninitiated agreed, whereas 44% did so a year later; the number increased to 63% in the sophomore year, and this proportion remained constant.)

It is disillusioning, as a student points out, to find oneself "sitting behind a desk memorizing minutiae; the good stuff doesn't come until the third year." "It is like going to college all over again," another complained, "taught by professors who have never practiced medicine and who approach the material like we are graduate students rather than prospective doctors."

A variety of unflattering terms are used to express disenchantment with the academic detail that must be memorized, described in such terms as "insignificant, ridiculous minutiae," "junk," "Mickey Mouse," "baloney," to mention just a few.

Because so much of the assigned material seems of questionable relevance to their future careers, students complain of "not getting anywhere, just not accomplishing anything." "I feel like I am just staggering along, not really taking a definite step in a positive direction," one said. "I didn't expect to waste time on rinky-dink stuff in medical school."

The drive to be successful, to feel good about oneself, is of course not unique to those who choose medical careers. John Dewey observed that "the deepest urge of human nature is the desire to be important." Few other careers, though, seem to create as much status anxiety. The seesaw course of medical training recurrently strips young men and women of most of their hard-earned status and starts them again at the bottom. Trainees barely achieve one height, one peak in their career, and then they must begin again as fledglings to prove themselves. In few occupations does a person intermittently occupy the position of neophyte over such a lengthy period. Even after residency training is completed, usually in the third decade of life, there are board examinations to pass, a practice to build, and a reputation to be established.

To outsiders, it seems that medical students "arrive" when they receive their M.D. degrees. Within medical circles, however, this is just the beginning. The young doctor, of course, gains satisfaction from family, friends, and others in the nonmedical community who acknowledge their hard-earned medical degrees, but they look to other physicians for their feeling of worth as a physician. The latter have become a "reference group," one that critically evaluates the fledgling doctor by standards of excellence. There is little opportunity to rest on one's laurels, because there are always new emergencies to cope with, new knowledge to acquire, and new techniques to master. Small wonder that conscientious physicians are described as "perpetual students." Neither is it surprising that many physicians are willing to sacrifice personal pleasures to work excessive hours and to neglect family affairs in the interest of career success, for this dedication wins them the approval of their colleagues and thereby gives them self-esteem.

Imbalanced Life-styles

The recruitment process favors those who are willing to sacrifice personal pleasures in order to earn the credentials necessary for admission to medical school (high scholastic grades and scores on the Medical College Admission Test). Such individuals seem extraordinarily motivated for career attainment. Rather than floundering in search of a meaningful career, like so many of their youthful peers, most medical students decide to be physicians at an early age. Even before entering college, three out of five in our study population had a clear vision of a medical career; 21% could not ever recall a time that they had not wanted to be a physician. Moreover, when asked what career they would have selected had medical school been inaccessible, three fourths (76%) could not think of an alternative career (Coombs, 1978).

As mentioned, entering medical students are often surprised and disillusioned by what they find at medical school, such as status deprivation, relatively poor-quality teaching, and the apparent clinical irrelevance of materials they are required to learn. There is no error in their expectations that hard work will be required to master the assigned materials (Coombs & Boyle, 1971). They fully expect and have been "programmed" by their premed training to put in long hours of study.

Excessively long work days result not only from external demands, but from trainees' inner quest for approval and high attainment; their own competitiveness, thoroughness, and idealism contribute to an excessive work style. Idealistic trainees worry that if the materials are not mastered, someone might die. Consequently, recreational and social life, so essential for mental health, are typically delayed and then take the form of binges.

At all stages of training, during medical school, internship, and residency, trainees report that they not only work hard but also play hard. Work schedules exceeding 80 hours per week are typical. As many as 120 hours per week are worked by some residents, leaving less than seven hours a day for all other activities, including sleep (Schaff, 1981). Since sleep deprivation has been demonstrated to affect psychological well-being (Valko & Clayton, 1975), it is not surprising that nonmedical observers have asked whether such training is preparation or hazing (Cousins, 1981).

"Whatever men attempt, they seem driven to overdo," Bernard Baruch noted. Attainment in any endeavor requires balance and moderation. For this reason, moderation has been described as "the silken thread through the pearl chain of all virtues."

In the pursuit of excellence, in constantly attempting to impress critical colleagues, and thereby feel good about oneself, a physician's life-style can become skewed and imbalanced. When one is overworked and preoccupied with career, physicial and emotional exhaustion are likely. This condition is exacerbated when, in order to project a proper image, personal feelings of doubt, uncertainty, fear, and personal inadequacy are chronically suppressed.

Emotional Isolation

The medical school recruitment process favors those who are emotionally inexpressive. Recruits have traditionally been male rather than female, self-sacrificing and bookish rather than balanced, and devotees to scientism (only things measurable are considered real or important), rather than psychologically minded. Lief's (1971) psychiatric study of an entire class of medical students reinforces that medical students tend not to be subjectively oriented. All but a third of the trainees were found to be emotionally constricted or uncomfortable with their own feelings. Lief explains that the medical school environment reinforces tendencies toward social isolation and emotional constriction: "Medical school is in many ways a closed society; it limits the student's chance to travel, to meet new friends, to have experiences outside the classroom, laboratory or hospital. The medical student becomes so immersed in his work that he hardly has time to keep up with the major news events of the day."

Although the competitive nature of the grade-oriented training experience creates anxieties for most medical trainees about personal deficiencies, these anxieties and self-doubts are rarely expressed openly. Trainees typically judge their own academic performance by a self-imposed norm which we label "relaxed brilliance." Consequently, each trainee thinks that he or she is the only one who feels inadequate and under emotional duress. This has been made abundantly clear to us when interviewing medical trainees. Although almost all trainees experience profound feelings of self-doubt and inadequacy, most are unaware that these feelings are not unique. They have emotionally isolated themselves by projecting a calm exterior.

Despite this ubiquitous problem, relatively little is done to meet the emotional needs of trainees. Instead, neophyte clinicians are expected to remain analytical and emotionally aloof. In this male-dominated milieu, such composure or *machismo* is highly valued. To openly express personal feelings among scientifically oriented associates is to risk the appearance of being "soft" or "weak," in short, "nonprofessional" (May, 1978). This is readily apparent in anatomy and autopsy rooms where human bodies are dissected with apparent tranquility. As a coping technique, trainees learn to chronically suppress or intellectualize their feelings. The challenge for the neophyte clinician is to privately maintain personal sensitivity while publicly carving a dead human body. Many find relief by losing themselves in the work. The pressure to learn a myriad of body parts in a limited time reinforces the tendency among students to occupy themselves with the details of the dissection process and memorizing scientific nomenclature. In so doing, dissection can become a mechanistic exercise rather than an emotional experience. This absorption in work, as Lief and Fox (1963) have noted, acts as a "psychic counter-irritant."

It is significant that, although a vast block of curriculum time is devoted to the anatomy laboratory, most medical schools devote little or no time to discussing the impact of these experiences on personal feelings. This omission, coming early in medical training, sets the stage for students to objectify and intellectualize living bodies while suppressing personal feelings.

When the scene shifts from the lecture room and laboratory to the hospital, students, lacking opportunities to verbalize their feelings, utilize their newly acquired coping strategies. In order to protect themselves from the human tragedies that frequently confront them, students develop a "protective shield" by, as one said, "busting up the human organism into pieces and dealing only with the pieces—then you don't have to see the whole picture." It is this orientation, so offensive to patients, that expresses itself in such comments as "the gallbladder in Room 114." Referring impersonally to patients as "cases," rather than people, is often a manifestation of intellectualization and emotional suppression.

Although clinicians are rarely given praise for a job well done, they are fiercely criticized for haphazard clinical performance. Clinical pathology conferences provide a forum for such expression. Such critiques reinforce the idea, one physician remarked, that "if we were just smarter and had not made this or that mistake, the patient would still be alive." The impression is that death is preventable and is not supposed to happen to good doctors; as least, this is the idea typically left with medical trainees. No wonder doctors often exert heroic efforts to keep a body going, despite contrary wishes of the family, and feel personal defeat when a patient dies.

Our interviews with practicing physicians about death reveal rather dramatically how much suppressed emotionality exists among practitioners (Coombs & Powers, 1975). When probed, most of them disclosed unresolved psychic problems such as having a sense of helplessness in dealing with hopeless disease or guilt regarding the disquieting experience of inadvertently "killing" a patient through error or bad advice, for example. A significant number of physicians we interviewed wept during our conversations, apparently for the first time. Our interviews apparently provided the first opportunity for them to openly unload their pent-up feelings. "We were never asked to express our feelings or discuss how we felt about death," one observed. Nor could any physician recall a single experience where a mentor openly revealed his own feelings about emotionally poignant situations, such as, frustration, anger, or the feelings of hopelessness that occur, for example, when a patient dies.

Physicians who feel anxiety and self-doubt have learned to conceal these emotions from others. "I've had a lot of training in putting up a good front so that others can't see what I am feeling inside," one reflected. "I've learned to keep this cool façade of being in control, but inside I'm feeling a lot of stress." Another added, "I can speak for myself and possibly for a lot of other physicians. In my younger years, my professional self-image wouldn't permit me to be slowed down or have my efficiency reduced by my feelings, so I evolved into a condition of what I now call 'disembodied intelligence.' " The result of this emotionally sterile state of affairs is not only to rob patients and their families of the warm sensitivity they seek, but also to deny a doctor a rich personal life.

BALANCING HANDS, HEAD, AND HEART:
AN EDUCATIONAL MODEL

Lengthy personal interviews with medical students reveal the ubiquitousness and depth of pent-up frustrations, anxieties, and resentments. Knowing how busy medical trainees are, we anticipated that our requests for in-depth interviews would be met with resistance. To our surprise and delight, however, our fears were in vain; all willingly participated. After giving lengthy responses to our questions regarding their feelings and circumstances (lasting from one and a half to three hours), they typically remained another 15 to 20 minutes informally discussing their views and circumstances. Then, upon leaving, they thanked us for *our* time!

Apparently, we had inadvertently met their need to ventilate about their experiences, a need that is not met elsewhere. Most remarkable was the fact that almost all trainees reported similar feelings of anxiety and inadequacy, yet each assumed that he or she was the only one so afflicted. None of the interviewees seemed aware that his feelings were typical. In an effort to appear "cool," "intelligent," and "professional," they had become emotionally isolated from one another.

These in-depth interviews, which began in the first year of medical school and spanned a number of subsequent years, convinced us that trainee affect is a neglected aspect of medical training. This lack has adverse consequences for physicians and those whom they serve.

Although the medical-school curriculum is organized to teach clinical skills and the basic sciences, little emphasis is given to the affective dimension of patient care. Mental health programs for medical trainees and practicing physicians generally consist of crisis intervention approaches (the medical model) or diversion approaches (a combination of the criminal justice and mental health models). Unexplored and generally inaccessible areas of study are preventive approaches based on a developmental or social learning model.

In our view, what is needed is a balanced emphasis in all aspects of medical training—the intellect (head), clinical skills (hands), and patient/physician affect (heart). Figure 1 illustrates this model (Coombs, et al., in press).

If trainees are to become compleat physicians, every discussion pertaining to a clinical problem, whether in classroom or clinic, should include consideration of the affective component. This is important because it affects not only the patient, but the clinician as well. Trainee clinicians should be rewarded, not looked down upon, for insightful observations and open expressions about the subjective milieu and those factors that affect the patient's health and the practitioner's effectiveness.

Because medical training typically emphasizes only two of these domains, the head and the hands, emotional constriction among trainees is inadvertently reinforced. In our view, emotional exploration should be encouraged in ongoing "bite-sized" doses, not saved for massive ventilation when trainees require psychotherapy. There needs to be adequate opportunities for physicians-in-training to ventilate and explore personal feelings, their own and those of their patients, and to discuss with their mentors the socioemotional

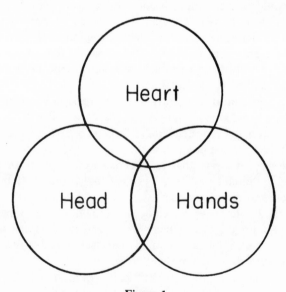

Figure 1

dilemmas that regularly and urgently confront them. To fail to do this impairs, by degrees, their personal lives as well as inhibiting their capacity to deal sensitively with patients.

A personal life devoid of emotional sensitivity is not likely to be one that contains the range and depth of experience necessary for a humanistic clinical practice or for a personal life characterized by growth and fulfillment. The emotionally uneducated, those who have developed only the "head" and "hands" but neglected the "heart," will, as Donald Arnstein has said, "live most of their emotional lives as children, taking seriously what deserves a smile, laughing at what deserves respect, and floating on the surface of experience, the depth of which is hidden to them" (quoted by Mason, 1979).

In our view, medical education will come of age when the affective aspects of medical training and patient care receive a proper emphasis. At that time, we predict, the concern will shift from the rehabilitation of obviously impaired doctors to the most effective techniques for educating compleat physicians.

REFERENCES

Coombs, R.H. (1978). *Mastering medicine: Professional socialization in medical school*. New York: The Free Press.

Coombs, R.H., & Boyle, B.P. (1971). The transition to medical school: Expectations versus realities. In R.H. Coombs & C.E. Vincent (Eds.), *Psychosocial aspects of medical training*. Springfield, IL: Charles C Thomas, pp. 91–109.

Coombs, R.H., & Powers, P.S. (1975). Socialization for death: The physician's role. *Urban Life: Journal of Ethnographic Research, 4*(3), 250–271.

Coombs, R.H., & St. John, J. (1981). *Making it in medical school*. Los Angeles: Medicine and Society Press.

Coombs, R.H., May, D.S., & Small, G.W. (Eds.). (in press). *Inside doctoring: Stages and outcomes in the professional development of physicians*. New York: Praeger.

Cousins, N. (1981). Internship: Preparation or hazing? *Journal of the American Medical Association, 245*(4), 377.

Lief, H.I. (1971). Personality characteristics of medical students. In R.H. Coombs & C.E. Vincent (Eds.), *Psychosocial aspects of medical training*. Springfield, IL: Charles C Thomas, pp. 44–87.

Lief, H.I., & Fox, R.C. (1963). The medical student's training for "detached concern." In H.I. Lief, V. Lief, & N.R. Lief (Eds.), *The psychological basis of medical practice*. New York: Harper & Row, pp. 12–35.

May, D.S. (1978). On my medical education: Seeking a balance in medicine. *Medical Self Care*, Summer, 37–41.

Mason, J. (1979). Brigham Young University Forum lecture.

Schaff, E. (1981). Paper presented at annual meeting of the American Medical Student Association, Houston, Texas.

Valko, F.J., & Clayton, P.J. (1975). Depression in the internship. *Diseases of the Nervous System, 36*(1), 26–29.

Chapter 4

Risk Factors: Predictable Hazards of a Health Care Career

Nancy C.A. Roeske, M.D.

Being at risk for illness or disability is an inevitable hazard of being a health care provider. The hazards are ubiquitous. They originate in factors as varied as the personality structure of the health care provider and the accelerated social transformation of the American health care system during the past 20 years. The purpose of this chapter is to help the health care provider assess the risk factors in his/her life that increase vulnerability for personal and professional impairment. Such an analysis includes four major areas: (1) the social transformation of health care; (2) the function and meaning of the health care provider/consumer relationship; (3) the health care professional's personality and family of origin life experiences; and (4) current social support system and professional satisfaction. This list of factors that can place a person at risk for physical or psychological impairment emphasizes the diversity and unavoidability of stressors.

The essential issue in predicting whether or not a factor is a hazard is role strain. This sociological term describes the conflict that can develop within the health care professional as he/she strives to meet both the demands of the professional role and the need for personal gratification (Etzioni, 1969). Role strain occurs when the health care professional believes that he/she must function at a maximum level of competence at all times, even when the social institutions needed to support the performance are missing or inadequate. The professional is unable to derive satisfaction either from realization of a job well done or acknowledgment of internal feelings of pleasure.

SOCIAL TRANSFORMATION OF THE HEALTH CARE SYSTEM

The discussion in this chapter will begin with a brief overview of major social factors that promote a milieu of uncertainty for current and future health care careers. Beginning in the late 1970s cost containment became the buzz word of American health care. Health care spending had increased sixfold between 1965 and 1981 to 9.8% of the gross national product, or $362 per capita. Cost containment legislation, methods for service delivery, and reimbursement have heightened competition among health care providers and strengthened business administrators' roles in the world of the hospital, outpatient clinics, prison systems, and private practice. The expansion of the "for-profit motive" of business executives has prompted concern in many that this value system may be displacing the traditional value system of providing care (Roeske, 1984). Analysis of products and markets is a concept borrowed from more traditional industry and utilized in contemporary health care administration. Market analysis looks at the number of potential users of a service, the demand, the utilization rate, the share of the market one must be able to obtain, and the competition. The education of the public for whom the product is directed and the promotion of a need to purchase services are also essential elements in marketing. Thus, the health care provider must analyze the needs and demands of the marketplace and provide a product that will be bought. In his brilliant book, Paul Starr (1982) points out that "even the response to rising costs cannot be entirely understood apart from a diminishing faith in the efficacy of medicine and an increasing concern about its relationship to other moral values"(p. 380).

Public opinion polls and marketing surveys report that health care consumers have inadequate information about the professional capabilities and the wide variety of types of health care providers. One of the major reasons for this lack of understanding has been the burgeoning of the health care field to the point where there are now more than five million persons in the health professions (U.S. Department of Health, Education, and Welfare, 1976–77).

Prior to the 1970s social workers, nurses, and psychologists were traditionally defined as paraprofessionals. The word was defined as "para" meaning "beside" or "parallel." Para may also mean "associated with" in a subsidiary capacity (Glasscote et al., 1980; Roeske, 1979a). In the early 1970s new health care workers, for example, indigenous workers, health care specialists, and health care assistants or associates, e.g., physician assistants and nurse practitioners, were regarded by the medical profession as new paraprofessionals. Within this definition the term paraprofessional suggests an intermediary role between the established professional and the consumer. A decade later we are confronted with the tension that has evolved from the rapid evolution of multiple health care roles and unclear, unstable definitions of these careers. Competition for the increasingly controlled health care dollar and the personal psychodynamic meaning of selling oneself may be additional sources of anxiety for the health care professional. These factors may be particularly stressful for women.

Every society shapes and is shaped by the demands made upon it. In the United States the political system and the judiciary's distinctive roles in interpreting the constitution encourage the dissatisfied to organize in social movements and to present their demands as claims covered by the Bill of Rights. These tendencies were never more evident than during the 1970s. Health care was seen as a major right over which the individual had ultimate control. Three forms of the social reformation have significantly changed health care. The first encompasses patients' rights: informed consent, the right to refuse treatment, the right to see one's own medical record, the right to participate in therapeutic decisions, and the right to due process in any proceeding for involuntary commitment. Folk medicine is another part of this social movement that presented itself as a humane alternative to an overly technical, impersonal, disease-oriented medical system. Finally, the women's movement expressed a generalized distrust of professional male domination of women as patients and as professional persons. A direct consequence has been the sharp increase in the number of women entering medical school. In 1970–1971, 9.8% of medical students were women. In 1983–1984, 33.6% were women. A similar increase has been seen in the law profession, which has served as a supportive and increasingly more active, directive role in the health care delivery system.

The social forces that reinforced growing acceptance of the right of equal access to health care meant that the cost control had to be built into the system. The concerns of government and business and the demands of the public have set the stage for the current reform proposals and actions regarding third-party coverage for health care. In turn, this change in coverage has intensified professional and personal tensions between health care providers.

Starr points out that the history of health reform is characterized by a little-known law of nature which seems to require that every movement toward regulation be followed by an opposite movement toward litigation.

Doubt about whether medical care causes more problems than it cures is reflected in a spectrum of patients' behavior from requests for drug information to malpractice suits. These attitudes are part of a broad current of skepticism about the value of social services. Furthermore, education has been as much the target as medical care. Schooling, rehabilitation, and medical care are seen as interrelated forms of social control. Thus, health care providers and others, for example, school psychologists and social workers, may find themselves in the suspect group.

All of these changes reflect the fact that we live in a democratic capitalistic society and are confronted with the hazards inherent in its social structure (Roeske, 1979b). This social structure fosters the development of individualism, which resonates with the goal of the health care provider. Yet, sociological theory points out that any society functions most smoothly when the individual is assigned a potential adult role at birth and when the life experiences are designed to educate the individual to eventually fulfill the adult role. Every society is confronted with the dilemma of maintaining the status quo through role induction and at the same time fostering the unique capabilities of its members. Sex and race have always been power attributes around which the concept of role and eventual status in a society have evolved. A person's status and role are essentially equivalent to one another in most social groups.

The stability of the society is always threatened if it wishes to use the talents of its members and examine without bias the traditional stereotypic roles in order for individuals to have opportunities to achieve status and role through competition as well as through assignment. Yet all societies fear the social chaos and anarchy that could occur with unrestrained role fluidity. This fear is currently being expressed in numerous ways varying from concern about financial loss to a sense of personal threat.

In conclusion, an individual may fear that if he/she discards a role, there will be such a modification of role that a psychological identification with the person in power is required, for example, the health care professional's fear of becoming too business oriented. Therefore, inherent in these sociological concepts are two major fears: loss of identity and devaluation.

This is a brief review of complex social, economic issues confronting health care providers. In essence, the health care professions have never been in a more paradoxical position where the potential for individual development of capabilities, talents, and interest in a health care career were more supported from a societal standpoint or more suspect by members of that society. Finally, there is the problem of competition for professional survival, which too has had the paradoxical effect of honing the boundaries of the health care careers and stimulating distrust and animosity between health care providers.

THE HEALER'S ROLE

Helping others and being needed by others offer important intrinsic rewards for all health-oriented professionals. Career satisfaction comes from numerous and various sources including self-actualization, exposure to a wide range of human experience, socially useful work, challenging intellectual pursuits, and usually a reliable income. In the past, society has granted professionals autonomy and the responsibility for their own conscience as being necessary for their work. The current societal attitude toward the health care field has, in numerous ways, questioned, if not eroded and undermined, that autonomy. The health care professional's assumption has been that he/she could work satisfactorily only if immune from ordinary social pressures and if free to innovate, to experiment, and to take risks without the usual social repercussions if there is failure. The escalating number of malpractice suits against health care professionals is ample evidence that if the health care professional functions in the traditional manner, he/she is at risk for a legal suit. The courts now decide whether or not the ultimate justification for any health care professional's action is that the action was done to the best of his/her judgment. In the past, colleagues might be consulted, but the decision was that of the health care provider, and if he/she erred, he/she would probably be defended by colleagues. Today the course is hazardous. Colleagues may defend and colleagues may attack or negate the health care professional's decision and behavior through peer review and court testimony.

Yet the most important factor in predicting the consumer's general satisfaction with his/her care is a perception of the adequacy of the provider's conduct. In turn, the professional's behavior will be sensitive and reactive to the problems encountered in his/her work. Anxiety and tension in the professional as well as in the patient/client impede the natural flow of communication. Anxiety and tension evoke coping mechanisms that may be personally destructive of the health care provider as well as damaging to the therapeutic or helping relationship. Obviously a stressed provider cannot listen empathically nor can he/she respond effectively. Constructive involvement in the problems of others requires concentration, energy, and peace of mind. The importance of the provider's behavior in the outcome of care has been well documented. If the provider is perceived as caring and friendly, the outcome is more likely to be successful. A patient's/client's compliance or willingness to follow a therapeutic regimen is a critical indicator of the patient's/client's satisfaction.

In essence, people's expectations of all health care and counseling providers depend on two critical variables: (1) a personal level of need gratification expressed through the provider/consumer relationship and (2) a social acceptance of the rights and privileges of the professional person. The first variable may be divided into four headings: the person's reasons for seeking assistance, the personality of the consumer and of the provider, the cultural and social status of the consumer, and the characteristics of the provider in his/her type of practice and physical setting. Interactions take place between these variables. In addition, there is always the possibility that one factor may be negated or modified by another.

The second variable focuses on the healer's role in the relationship. Becoming a consumer of health care or counseling requires a person to be dependent and trusting and willing to discuss intimate aspects of his/her life with another person. In one sense the health care provider combines the traditional stereotype of the protective, nurturing maternal role with the authoritative, omnipotent wisdom of the paternal role. Insofar as the symbolic dimensions of the parental figures are also assumed as valuable and perhaps valid personal attributes by the health care provider, the consumer will be reinforced to consider his/her perception as a correct basis for the interaction. Obviously, if the health care consumer desires, in varying degrees, these attributes and the health care provider does not agree, either for personal or for professional reasons, to provide that relationship, the relationship is endangered or frustrating for both persons.

As mentioned earlier, the conflict that can develop within the provider between the demands of the professional role and the need for personal gratification can ultimately lead to role strain and burnout. In a consideration of role strain, it is important to bear in mind that, to a large measure, a person constructs the meaning of his/her own stress. Individual differences in the capacity to cope with difficulty also exist and can make the difference between those who suffer deeply and are immobilized and those who are challenged and grow through the mastery of stressful experiences.

An eventual outcome of role strain can be burnout. Maslach and others have described burnout as a loss of concern for people, an emotional exhaustion that involves cynicism and the dehumanized perception of patients/clients (Maslach, 1976, 1978; Pines & Maslach, 1978). The basic causes lie in the disruptive emotional aspect of caring for people, including demanding and unreasonable patient/client behavior, types of illnesses that are difficult to treat, working long hours and with a large number of people, and denial of strong emotions produced in treating or caring for people. Educational institutions have been cited as encouraging fragmentation and dehumanized perceptions of clients/patients so that the providers are taught to split off their feelings and emotions from their intellectual approaches.

Almost 30 years ago Fox noted the "detached concern" in the provider (Fox, 1957). This concept is basic for understanding role strain and burnout. Fox pointed out that detached concern is idealized in educational settings;

it is part of the socialization process of the health care professional's formal education. On the other hand, detached concern can lead to discomfort because it involves creating arbitrary walls or compartments that are difficult to maintain under the pressure of patients' demands or the professional's personal needs. In fact, it may be seen as a prime prerequisite of professional behavior. Detached concern is different from empathy in which there is a projection of one's own consciousness into another person.

Another source of stressful tension has arisen in the evolving definition of each health care career: its education, professional functioning, and relationship to other health care professions. One example of this problem is the development of the new health care professions and new settings for their services (i.e., public health clinics, storefront clinics) (Glasscote et al., 1980). The health care providers who work within these settings have sometimes been titled indigenous experts. By definition, they are similar to their consumer in some critical features, that is, the providers may be reformed alcoholics or drug abusers. They may have had similar ethnic, racial, or economic status as the clientele. Since their sociocultural background and life experiences are similar to that of the consumers, their education and roles are directed toward a more meaningful relationship with the target population. They act as identifiers of persons in need of help, sources of knowledge of appropriate resources available, providers of care themselves, and interpreters to other professionals of the world of the consumer, which may be quite different from that of the providers. The provider who has a number of areas of shared experiences with the consumer is most able to react to the feelings and attitudes of his/her clientele, who often display apathy, depression, fear of the unknown, and distrust toward the more traditional individual provider, agencies, and institutions. This is particularly true for seriously disadvantaged persons who have deeply engrained attitudes and beliefs bordering on paranoia toward traditional sources of assistance.

Nevertheless, the special abilities and talents of indigenous providers have posed serious problems in definitions of role boundaries. In one sense, all the new health care and counseling providers are trained to be intermediary persons, fulfilling specific roles. Yet, by definition, they are between groups, that is, between the client or patient and the professional person who is trained to treat highly specialized diseases and illnesses or work with well-defined groups of people. Therefore, an intermediary provider may have a poignant problem. He/she may be between the group from which he originated, for example, a drug abuser or an ethnic minority group, and the one by which he/she was educated, for example, physician or psychologist. His/her role is akin to that of a chameleon who blends into but is not part of either group. He/she may vacillate in behavior that is indicative of either working within the consumers' setting or within the professional setting. The resultant tension and anxiety may lead to renunciation of the role or manipulation of both the clients and the professionals who are in charge of the provider. As a result, it will give him/her a sense of false control and power over both groups.

The role ambiguities and professional competition that are occurring because the concepts and ideals of health care and counseling are in transition require a continued reassessment of the education and training of the new types of providers and an awareness of these changes by all providers. Their education must achieve a delicate balance between the person's creative potential, which arises from his/her specific background and knowledge, and the knowledge and skills that are necessary to do a job. Finally, the educational process and the job itself must allow for continued growth in both the type of task performed and the degree of responsibility allowed. People perform with the highest degree of excellence and self-satisfaction when they perceive a congruence between job expectation and job reality.

The person's capacity to adapt to the requirement of changing life role is important for competence and self-esteem. The educational and job experiences should offer opportunities for growth through mastery of the demands of the situation. But the work may prove to be stressful because of either the particular demands of patients/clients, the fatiguing effect of working long hours, the unpleasant interpersonal relationships at work, or the personality characteristics of the provider. Every person must identify the sources of stress and find ways to terminate or ameliorate their effects.

PERSONALITY CHARACTERISTICS

Each person brings to a profession nuances in personality structure that reflect his/her family and cultural experiences, physical characteristics, and psychological makeup. The relationship between personal attributes, choice of helping profession, and morbidity and mortality with regard to cardiovascular disease, hypertension, depression, suicide, alcoholism, and drug abuse has long been a matter of research interest (Chodoff, 1972; Glass, 1977; Hirschfeld & Klerman, 1979; Modlin & Montes, 1964; Roeske, 1982a; Thomas, 1971; Vaillant et al., 1970, 1972). The research includes epidemiological studies of individual-occupational interaction, longitudinal lifespan development of individuals, and studies of individuals in a specific type of occupational milieu. Other researchers have assessed the prevalence of these problems in clergy and teachers. For example, King's epidemiological studies indicate that white Anglican and Lutheran clergy and undergraduate and university teachers have very low rates of the previously mentioned diseases and illnesses (King, 1971; King & Bailar, 1978; King et al, 1975). In studies contrasting the health status of these professions with other occupations, namely, physicians and lawyers/judges, King concludes that the value system of clergymen may be one factor responsible for their good health. A spiritual view of the world combined with less emphasis on competition, individuality, and materialism may promote better psychological adaptation. Nevertheless, it is important to note that King's studies occurred during the 1950s and 1960s, a period when there were few clergymen and teachers whose educational and professional life was focused on counseling. There is a need for research about the correlation between shifts in responsibility in these groups toward health counseling and types of morbidity and mortality.

Our understanding of the personality characteristics or patterns that are most frequently related to morbidity for the health care professional come mainly from studies of physicians. The personality characteristics include competitiveness, high expectations of self, rigidity, and excessive concern for details, which are professional assets in caring for others but can also become a significant contributor to the individual's downfall. The type A personality is a person who epitomizes these characteristics. Other types of personality structure that are found in persons who tolerate professional stress poorly include passive-aggressive, narcissistic, and dependent personalities (Roeske, 1982a; Thomas, 1971; Vaillant et al., 1970, 1972).

There have been two major longitudinal studies of the physician's personality and symptoms of distress that include marital problems, alcoholism, drug abuse, depression, and suicide (Thomas, 1971; Vaillant et al., 1970, 1972). Vaillant's study of Harvard men and Thomas' study of Johns Hopkins Medical School graduates clearly identified in persons who became ill a basic insecurity, dependency, depressive tendency, and vulnerability to stress and often a highly ambivalent attitude toward the profession, that is, loving it yet clearly resenting its continuing demands because it fails to meet the physician's own needs. These personality characteristics were present when the person entered the university and/or medical school. One example is Thomas' long-term studies of the psychological characteristics of medical students that are of predictive value in identifying physicians prone to mental illness or suicide. These researchers found that physicians who committed suicide had as medical students rated themselves on several types of psychological tests significantly higher than nonsuicidal physicians in the areas of thoughtfulness, anger, hostility, depression, negativism, suspiciousness, verbal expansiveness, dependency, and impulsivity.

Since depression is the most common psychological disorder in professional persons, the data from research about affective disorders are of heuristic importance. The studies of depression-prone people suggest that they are more likely to break down under stress, have less energy, are more insecure and sensitive, tend to worry more, are less socially adroit, and are more emotionally needy and more obsessional than other people (Chodoff, 1972; Hirschfeld & Klerman, 1979). They have an inordinate narcissistic need for direct and indirect support from other people to maintain their self-esteem. They have a low frustration tolerance and may employ various coping techniques—submissive, manipulative, coercive, piteous, demanding, and placating—in order to maintain needed relationships. The depression-prone person has a cognitive set of negative attitudes towards self, the world, and the future that establishes and reinforces negative social relationships.

Women health care professionals, in particular women physicians, have been the focus of study with regard to depression and suicide (Roeske, 1976, 1982a; Symonds, 1976). From the available data, women physicians apparently are one fourth as likely as male physicians to be alcohol or drug abusers and very rarely have sexual intercourse with patients (Kardener et al., 1976; Roeske, 1982a). Tragically, most data about the self-destructive behavior of female physicians, psychologists, chemists, and mathematicians is found in the epidemiological data about their suicides. Psychiatrists interested in this research point out that the crude death-by-suicide rate for women physicians is 40.7 per 100,000 deaths as compared to an overall death-by-suicide rate of 11.4 per 100,000 among white women over the age of 25. The data thus shows that women physicians between the ages of 25 and 55 are nearly four times more likely to kill themselves than most other women. The death-by-suicide rate of women psychologists and chemists is similar to that of women physicians. The crude death-by-suicide rate for men physicians is 38.1 per 100,000; hence it is similar to the rate of women physicians. However, the majority of male physicians who commit suicide kill themselves after reaching the age of 45 (68%), whereas the majority of women physicians do so before age 45 (58.6%). The researchers reporting these data have as a primary interest affective disorders. They believe that depressive disorders among physicians, particularly among women physicians, is unusually high. Such a conclusion is based primarily on suicide data. The reports fail to take into account personality characteristics, marital status, presence and number of children, and type and amount of professional involvement, although these factors have been noted to be of crucial importance in other reports about women physicians (Roeske, 1976, 1982a). Furthermore, the woman professional in a traditionally male profession who is single and in her 30s is different from other women of the same age, including other women in her profession. Marriage and children often mark a critical turning point in a woman's life. Their absence and a sense of loneliness and alienation can result in tragedy despite professional competence and social acclaim.

Basic personality characteristics determine how the individual will adapt to the health care career. Many tend in their early life-style to rely on defense mechanisms of repression, rationalization, denial, reaction formation, and the suppression and displacement of emotions, although not always maladaptively. Many are virtually phobic about seeking help for themselves whether their troubles are physical, professional, or psychological. Any request is seen as undermining the public's and health care provider's personal image of self-sufficiency.

The family background of individuals who become professionally and personally disabled has a characteristic pattern in which they are dominated and overprotected by parents who also have rejecting attitudes. They often fail to acknowledge and support their child's interests and successes. Excessive and continued dependency on the mother well into adulthood is an important variable. Fathers are neither steady, companionable, understanding, nor warm. The detachment from the father is contrasted with the often demanding, controlling, and even seductive mother, according to studies of professional men. Physical illness during childhood stimulates and supports the mother's behavior. It also focuses attention of the child on the importance of health and the anxiety-producing effects of illness for a sense of incompetence and inadequacy. A history of mental illness in the family, particularly depression, suicide, and alcoholism, and these disorders in the health care provider prior to his/her formal education are significant personal and family background experiences that correlate with later impairment.

CURRENT FAMILY-SOCIAL REFERENCE GROUPS

Childhood experiences are frequently recapitulated in current social relationships. In carrying over personality characteristics and interpersonal patterns of behavior into adulthood the person may have loaded the at-risk balance toward high vulnerability for impairment. Such a person often avoids a need for sharing his/her feelings and the feelings of his/her spouse and children through discussion and communication of uncertainties and humanness. The ambivalence in the relationships at work and at home may be heightened if the health care provider suppresses direct hostility toward his/her patients or clients and either develops a similar pattern of repression of hostility at home or expresses the displaced feelings of hostility from work onto significant social relationships. The critical role of the spouse and other intimates in fostering the health care provider's sense of omnipotence and their accepting a secondary role in his/her life cannot be underestimated in the development of impairment.

In conclusion, although the role of the provider may be a shield and a weapon in marital and parenting conflicts, the resultant effects are serious stressors for everyone involved.

THE HEALTH CARE CONSUMER AND PROVIDER RELATIONSHIP

Basically the same issues are involved in the origins and effects of stress in the person who seeks help as has been described for the provider. The quality of the early childhood experiences, dependency on parental figures, the support and encouragement for development of individuality and expression of special talents, the definition of goals set in adolescence and young adulthood with their ongoing assessment and attainment are all issues that pertain to the consumer as well as to the provider's health. How the consumer has integrated personality characteristics will be evidenced in symptoms and expressed in the consumer/provider relationship. The technical terms for this aspect of the relationship are transference and countertransference.

Transference means the distortion of a realistic client/counselor or patient/therapist relationship in which the client/patient puts feelings, behavior, and thoughts from past relationships that are now unconscious and repressed into the counselor/therapist. In addition to responding to the signals for expected behavior from the patient that arise from transference, the counselor/therapist likewise may perceive the patient as representative of some aspects or actual persons from his/her past. This phenomenon is called countertransference. As mentioned previously, when a person seeks professional help, he/she is placed emotionally in a childlike position of dependency with a concomitant necessity of trust in the wiser, experienced professional. The regression in the service of care or cure may simultaneously stimulate latent emotional conflicts within the patient/client. Sixty years ago Freud wrote that "every human being has acquired by the combined operation of inherent disposition and of external influences in childhood, a special individuality in the exercise of his capacity to love, that is, in the conditions which he sets up for loving, in the impulses he gratifies by it, and in the aims he sets out to achieve in it" (Freud, 1953). Thus, the patient/client and the provider who have not successfully mastered childhood developmental tasks and separated from primary parental figures and matured into adult love relationships are exceptionally vulnerable to pathological client/provider interactions.

Additional variables affecting the client/health care provider relationship include the impact of the current stress situation on self-esteem, the person's perception of future possibilities for reestablishing that self-esteem, and the personal meaning of the present stage of life, especially the meaning of adolescence, midlife, and dying. An erotic solution for the client and possibly the health care provider's inner stress when these variables and erotic transference/countertransference are prominent is a social pattern that is common and even openly displayed in contemporary society. The seeming social permissiveness for such behavior may seem to condone sexual behavior in the consumer/provider relationship. Hence, erotic behavior conveys a sense of social acceptability that belies its untherapeutic implications (Ginsberg et al., 1972; Kardener et al., 1976; Roeske & Blazer, 1983; Stoller, 1974).

The combined facts that more women than men are consumers of a wide variety of all types of care and that women have been socialized to use erotic behavior as a means for establishing and maintaining self-esteem and intimate relationships contribute to their seeking a fantasy cure through the healer's erotic self. Insofar as the provider is vulnerable by virtue of a lack of satisfaction with work, unhappiness in intimate relationships, or depression, he may allow or encourage the woman to prescribe the erotic solution or treatment. Furthermore, if the provider is middle-aged and becoming aware of a decrease in physical powers and sexual potency, an adolescentlike sexual sensitivity and interest may be fostered as the provider attempts to deny anxiety and fears about the aging process and eventual death.

Studies of men who are particularly prone to an extreme pathological midlife crisis reveal that they have failed to achieve an adequate separation from their mothers (Ginsberg et al., 1972; Roeske & Blazer, 1983; Stoller, 1974). They were often pampered as children and developed a façade of independence. Such men have conflicting desires for dependency and freedom, nurturance and autonomy, that are intensified by the recognition that they are aging. Their fear of dependency on their wife-mother may trigger a panic into separation, divorce, and affairs with other women, particularly younger women and especially women patient/clients. The younger women offer a sense of rejuvenation.

Women providers are confronted with the meaning of a return to dependency on a symbolic mother for the patient/client with all its attending joys of being comforted and anxieties about being controlled. A special problem for the female provider with a woman patient/client is the provider's conflict about the client surpassing the provider in achievements. The provider may wish the patient/client to achieve the health care provider's unfulfilled goals, but such a result can lead to restimulating feelings of degradation or humiliation that derive from an inner sense of being sex-role-stereotyped as a woman (Roeske, 1982b).

In conclusion, the nuances and complexities of the consumer/provider relationship with its inevitable potential for rekindling both earlier frustrating and supportive, satisfying relationships require that the provider be sensitively aware of and understand himself/herself. He/she must find personal and professional gratification in his/her work and a personal life-style that expresses and accepts intimate thoughts, feelings, and behavior if he/she is to avoid increasing an at-risk potential for illness.

REFERENCES

Chodoff, P. (1972). The depressive personality: A critical review. *International Journal of Psychiatry Medicine, 27*, 196–217.

Etzioni, A. (1969). *The semi professions and their organizations.* New York.: Free Press.

Fox, R. (1957). Training for uncertainty. In R.K. Merton, et al., (Eds.), *The student physician.* Cambridge, MA: Harvard University Press, pp. 207–241.

Freud, S. (1953). The dynamics of transference (1912). In *Collected Papers,* Vol II. London: Hogarth Press, pp. 312–322.

Ginsberg, G.L., Frosch, W.A., & Shapiro, T. (1972). The new impotence. *Archives of General Psychiatry, 26*, 218–222.

Glass, D.C. (1977). Stress, behavior patterns, and coronary disease. *American Scientist, 65*, 177–187.

Glasscote, R., Kohn, E., Beigel, A., Raber, M., Roeske, N., et al. (1980). Preventing mental illness—Efforts and attitudes. Joint Information Service, American Psychiatric Association.

Health Resources Statistics Reported from the National Center for Health Statistics, U.S. Department of Health, Education, and Welfare, Public Health Service, Office of Health Research, Statistics, and Technology, National Center for Health Statistics, PHS 79-1509, 1976–77 Edition.

Hirschfeld, R.M.A., & Klerman, G.L. (1979). Personality attributes and affective disorders. *American Journal of Psychiatry, 136*, 67–70.

Kardener, S.H., Fuller, M., & Mensh, I.N. (1976). Characteristics of "erotic" practitioners. *American Journal of Psychiatry, 133*, 1324–1325.

King, H. (1971). Clerical mortality patterns of the Anglican communion. *Social Biology, 18*, 164–177.

King, H., & Bailar, J.C. III (1978). Mortality among Lutheran clergymen. *Milbank Memorial Fund Quarterly, 46*, 527–548.

King, H., Zafros, G., & Hass, R. (1975). Further inquiry into Protestant clerical mortality patterns. *Journal of Biosocial Sciences, 7*, 243–254.

Maslach, C. (1976). Burned-out. *Human Behavior, 5*, 16–22.

Maslach, C. (1978). The client role in staff burn-out. *Journal of Social Issues, 34*, 111–124.

Modlin, H.C., & Montes, A. (1964). Narcotics addiction in physicians. *American Journal of Psychiatry, 121*, 358–365.

Pines, A., & Maslach, C. (1978). Characteristics of staff burnout in mental health settings. *Hospital and Community Psychiatry, 29*, 233–237.

Roeske, N.C.A. (1976). Women in psychiatry: A review. *American Journal of Psychiatry, 133*, 365–372.

Roeske, N.C.A. (1979a).Education of the paraprofessional. In J.D. Noshpitz (Ed.), *The basic handbook of child psychiatry, Vol. 4,* New York: Basic Books, pp. 511–519.

Roeske, N.C.A. (1979b). Issues involved in changing roles and role relationships. *Journal of American Medical Women's Association, 34*, 372–383.

Roeske, N.C.A. (1982a). Stress and the physician. *Journal of the Indiana State Medical Association, 75*(2), 108–119. (Reprinted from *Psychiatric Annals, 11*(7), 10–32, July 1981.)

Roeske, N.C.A. (1982b). Women and a changing society: Implications for transference/countertransference. *Canadian Journal of Psychiatry, 27*, 562–568.

Roeske, N.C.A. (1984). Introduction: Two cultures. *Psychiatric Annals, 14*(5), 316–320.

Roeske, N.C.A., & Blazer, D.G. (1983). Mid-life and later life. *Journal of Psychiatric Education, 7*(1), 56–70.

Starr, P. (1982). *The social transformation of American medicine.* New York: Basic Books.

Stoller, R.J. (1974). Symbiosis, anxiety and the development of masculinity. *Archives of General Psychiatry, 30,* 164–172.

Symonds, A. (1976). Neurotic dependency in successful women. *Journal of the American Academy of Psychoanalysis, 4,* 95–103.

Thomas, C.B. (1971). Suicide among us: II. Habits of nervous tension as potential predictors. *Johns Hopkins Medical Journal, 129,* 190–201.

Vaillant, G.E., Brighton, J.R., & McArthur, C. (1970). Physicians' use of mood-altering drugs. *New England Journal of Medicine, 282,* 365–370.

Vaillant, G.E., Sobowale, N.C., & McArthur, C. (1972). Some psychologic vulnerabilities of physicians. *New England Journal of Medicine, 287,* 372–375.

Chapter 5

A Case of Family Medicine: Sources of Stress in Residents and Physicians in Practice

Joann Hawk, Ph.D., and
Cynthia D. Scott, Ph.D. M.P.H.

Many factors have been linked to impairment in physicians. Among these factors are personality characteristics, coping styles, premorbid mental health, and environmental stresses that are a by-product of medical training and practice (Pfifferling, 1980; Vaillant et al., 1972). Health and stress are becoming increasingly understood as phenomena with interdependent physical, psychological, social, and environmental aspects (Chan, 1977). Physicians are of special interest because of their pivotal role as health care providers and because of the increasing manifestations of stress and impairment among these professionals.

The literature concerning stress reveals that there is no single agreed-upon definition of stress. In fact, there are several overlapping models of stress, i.e., physiological, life events, cognitive appraisal, and interactive. It seems that the most accurate indicator of stress might be the self-report of the individual who is experiencing the stress. In this view, individual differences, coping styles, and other mediators of stress can be accounted for without being delineated. This allows an overview of specific stressors that individuals within a particular situation encounter, which can then be seen as overall pressures that apply to most of those involved in that profession.

Another important concept to keep in mind when thinking about stress within a specific profession is that of career development. Cartwright (1979) suggests that the sources of stress in the profession of medicine be seen within a life span career development model (Crites, 1976). Each stage of a health career has specific tasks, problems, and rewards. As an individual progresses through life, career roles interact with other life roles (such as spouse, parent, etc.) sometimes leading to conflict, enrichment, harmony, and integrative complexity. In this process, transitions between stages can be problematic. Raskin (1972) refers to initiation periods as times of anxiety. This pattern can be seen throughout an individual's life cycle within the health professions. There are specific stages of career development in becoming a physician —premedical schooling, medical school, residency training, practice, and retirement. For the purpose of this chapter, only the first four stages will be discussed.

PREMEDICAL SCHOOLING

Prior to entering medical school, a student must work very hard academically to show him/herself worthy of medical school admission (Tuttelman, 1975). Not only is academic excellence required, but test scores, personality measures, and interviews are of great importance for admission to medical school. The student learns to be extremely competitive, to narrow goals and activities, and to focus only on getting into medical school. Consequently, this is the time that the student begins to internalize stress.

MEDICAL SCHOOL

Medical students and their learning environment have been studied extensively. The widespread prevalence of stress-induced anxiety and emotional disturbances has been well documented (Becker & Geer, 1958; Gough & Hall, 1973).

Gaensbauer and Mizner (1980) studied the developmental tasks of medical students at the Universisty of Colorado Medical Center. They were able to delineate developmental stresses and the adaptive and maladaptive responses of the students. The researchers found that emotional disturbance was related to both the developmental stresses and the adaptive capacity of the student, based on long-standing individual character structures. Other researchers (Bojar, 1971; Lief et al., 1960) found that the interaction between a student's adaptive capacity and the demands and stresses of the medical school environment is the most useful focus for understanding the nature of emotional disturbances in medical students.

Boyle and Coombs (1971) studied first-year medical students over a period of five years at the Bowman Gray School of Medicine. They administered the California Psychological Inventory and in-depth interviews to obtain personality profiles that related to emotional stress in the medical students. They found that students with low stress scores tended to be outgoing, sociable, helpful, cooperative, warm, talkative, and concerned with making a good impression. The low-stress students were also independent and resourceful. By contrast, the students with high stress scores were more socially distrustful, inhibited, moody, self-centered, cool and distant, conventional, and conforming. Sources of stress reported by these medical students were fear of their inability to absorb all the materials presented, fear of getting bad grades, fear of error of diagnosis or prescription, limited recreational and social outlets, loneliness, and death of a patient. Edwards and Zimet (1976) found that a lack of personal freedom, excessive academic pressures, and feelings of dehumanization were chief concerns of the medical students who participated in this study.

Medical school is a time when students start to internalize their professional role. This professional socialization process includes mastery of knowledge and learning to cope with the uncertainty of medical practice (Light, 1979). This is the process whereby the medical student transforms from the compliant student to the independent and aggressive professional (Burstein, et al., 1979).

RESIDENCY TRAINING

Once physicians graduate from medical school and complete an internship, they are eligible to be accepted into a residency training program within their specialty choice. It is at this time that the student becomes a "real doctor." These physicians are both students and professionals; they think of themselves as doctors and students because their training is to continue the mastery of medicine. There has been a trend in the past few years toward specialty certification, and almost all medical-school graduates now undertake some sort of residency training (Levit et al., 1974).

A number of studies have reported a higher rate of psychiatric illness, alcoholism, and drug abuse among residents. Russel and co-workers (1975) found that residents under 30 years of age were at a higher risk for psychiatric problems, and Valko and Clayton (1975) found that 30% of the residents they interviewed were depressed, with the depression beginning within one month of the start of the residency; 63% of these residents were working more than 100 hours per week.

The literature highlights a number of stress-related issues that occur as part of the residency training. The first of these is that the residency itself is a professional socialization process where the resident physician is engaged in a developmental process. A problematic by-product of this process is the identity crisis that many first-year residents experience (Burr, 1975; Kantner & Vastyan, 1978).

The second major issue is that during the course of residency training the physician becomes increasingly more responsible for the medical care of the patients, with the end product being that the resident can then function autonomously. Bosk (1980) outlined some of the problems that a physician must cope with regarding inpatient management. The major issue is uncertainty in diagnosis, which leads to problems in decision making. Although modern technology has elevated the current state of medical knowledge, there are still many limitations and uncertainties in the diagnostic process.

One of the biggest problems that residents have is fatigue from long hours of responsibility (24 hours in the hospital, two to five days a week) and psychological problems associated with sleep deprivation, such as difficulty in thinking, depression, irritability, depersonalization, inappropriate affect, and recent memory deficit (Friedman et al., 1973).

Nelson and Henry (1978) surveyed family practice residents and their spouses at the University of Minnesota Family Practice Training Program and found that the biggest problem reported by the residents was scarcity of time. This meant that the residents did not have enough time to spend with friends and relatives and in leisure activities. The researchers also found that the time problems decreased as the year of residency increased, and that time scarcity was more of a problem for married residents than for unmarried residents. This time scarcity also left the resident with little time to study and keep up with the medical literature. Another reported stressor was lack of self-confidence, which was highest in the first-year residents and resulted in reservations about continuing in family medicine.

PRACTICE

Considerably more attention has been paid to the early stages of career development than to the later stages involving establishment, maintenance, and retirement. Some of the stress of practice has been delineated (McCue,

1982), and these later stages have become important focuses for further research. The main explorations in this area with regard to stress emerge in the framework of the impaired physician (Doub et al., 1980). The rest of this chapter will highlight and discuss recent findings in the study of stress in family practice physicians.

THE STUDY OF STRESS IN FAMILY PRACTICE PHYSICIANS AND RESIDENTS

Hawk (1982) and Scott (1983) designed studies that addressed stresses that family practice physicians in practice and residents in training have reported. The first study (Hawk, 1982) included 61 family practice residents from three residency training programs in Northern California. The second (Scott, 1983) included 60 randomly selected family practice physicians who were practicing in five Northern California counties.

The respondents in both studies included 85 men and 36 women, ranging in age from 26 to 82. The mean age of the residents was 31 years, and the mean age of the practicing physicians was 44 years. The residents reported working an average of 80 hours per week, and the physicians in practice reported that they averaged 40 hours per week. Physicians reported being in practice from 0 to 22 years, and of these practicing physicians, 13% did not complete a residency.

Family Practice Residents

The residents in this study were asked to rate their level of stress. Overall, they rated their stress as moderately severe. They were then asked to specify their greatest source of stress. Their responses were grouped into seven categories. The first category was time pressures, which were best illustrated by the resident who said, "I have too much to do and not enough time to do everything." Another quipped that he "worked 36-hour days."

The second category is low self-confidence, or "feeling like I don't know enough about medicine to be doing what I am doing." The next category reported is the demands of the residency. These demands are from patients, family, other physicians, other residents, and from themselves. A different type of demand was reported by other residents who felt that the pressures of the program were the greatest stress. Program demands include the number of hours spent at work, number of nights on call, types of rotations, and the pressures to learn massive amounts of medical information. Another category of stress reported by the residents was that they perceived that the work in the hospital was endless; as soon as one task was completed or one patient was taken care of, three more appeared to take its place. One resident reported that he found that if he deliberately slowed his pace, he could control the amount of work that piled up, as other residents would "cover" for him. Unfortunately, this coping device created more problems than it solved, because he alienated himself from the support of his peers, was criticized by the faculty as being unmotivated, angered the nursing staff, and his self-esteem dropped radically. In short, he created more stress than he was originally handling.

Choosing family practice as a residency requires that the resident be willing to be a generalist, which was reported as a stress. One resident spoke about how wonderful it would be to be like a colleague in the hospital who was a neonatal hematologist. The resident was thrilled at the fantasy that he could "know every bit of the literature in his area." It is often frustrating to feel that you must know everything that there is to know about all areas of family medicine; this includes not only high-technology medicine, but family systems and psychological theories and techniques. In addition, family practice is a specialty involving high patient interaction, and the resident must learn to develop a working relationship with patients from all age levels and medical categories. Another problem that the residents in this study faced was that often physicians from other specialties "looked down on them" because they were generalists. The residents even spoke of pressure in medical school from professors, such as, "You are so bright, why would you want to go into family practice?" This question was asked in such a way that the student felt that only a fool would choose family medicine as a specialty area.

The residents were asked if they ever considered quitting the residency, and about two-thirds of the residents said that they had. The reasons that the residents gave for wanting to quit were problems with the program, loss of a feeling of personal well-being, long and excruciating work hours, the demise of any sort of life outside of being a resident, political pressures with being in family practice (see previous paragraph), and wanting to transfer to another specialty residency (two of the residents actually did transfer to other specialties: one to surgery and the other to anesthesiology). Those who decided to continue with the residency were asked what had stopped them from quitting. Most of them said that inertia stopped them, and others felt that a sense of perspective helped them to continue. There were those who felt that they had made a commitment to finishing what they had started, whereas others just did not want to move and felt that quitting the program would create some financial problems. Another group found that the residency became more satisfying after they had contemplated quitting, probably because it gave them some feeling of choice and control in their career.

For the most part, the profile of stress changes by year of residency. The second-year residents reported the highest levels of stress. That is the year in the programs that were surveyed when the residents work on their own for the first time. Although they have "backup," they are responsible for their own cases and work more independently than they did as either medical students or first-year residents. The first-year residents reported the next highest level of stress. This is the year when residents begin to acclimate to the residency and feel a sense of the emotional and physical demands of the residency. In addition, residents see that they have another two and one-half years left of ever-increasing responsibility. The third-year residents reported the lowest stress of all. That is the year when the residents are allowed to take more elective time, which many of the residents choose to do outside the program. Also, these residents are beginning to see "the light at the end of the tunnel," which makes them begin to think about what they will be doing after they graduate and how to terminate the patients that they have treated for the past three years. Another third-year resident responsibility is that of chief of service, which is a more administrative position, and supervisory/backup person for the first-year residents. They have learned to work more efficiently and to delegate responsibilities to auxiliary personnel. Third-year residents do not experience the rush and pressure of first- and second-year residents.

An important stress reported by all residents was that of trying to combine both a personal and a professional life while in the residency. The residents reported that the people in their personal lives (spouse, family, etc.) complained that they did not spend enough time with them, which made the residents feel guilty for "neglecting" their families. Paradoxically, the residents felt as though they received a great deal of support from their families and friends. In fact, it is notable that none of the residents reported receiving no support. Because of the demands of the residency, residents have little physical or emotional energy to devote to relationships outside the residency, which creates interpersonal problems and conflicts with those who are closest to the resident. In addition, the residents reported a feeling that they are not understood by their loved ones, which appears to be rooted in the same problem. For the most part, the residents are very close to their families, especially their spouses or significant others, and rely on them for support during the stressful time of the residency. Problems seem to appear when the resident does not have enough time to spend developing or maintaining relationships, which can lead to loss of valued friends or conflicts with their families. Some of the residents have compared the conflict between their personal and professional lives as a "three-year juggling act."

Practicing Physicians

When asked to rate their stress, the physicians in practice reported that the level of stress is moderate. This overall rating of stress can be misleading, since there was a wide fluctuation in the responses of this group. Some of the physicians reported that they experienced little or no stress whereas others reported high to severe stress; therefore, the moderate rating reflects the dispersion of the group. Other factors that contributed to the variation in responses, such as type of practice, age, and number of hours worked, will be discussed later in this section.

The demands and responsibilities of a practice was rated as the greatest cause of stress for these physicians. Difficult patients was another stress; as one of the doctors put it, "I get tired of trying to treat people who are hostile and defensive—people who want a medical solution to their nonmedical problem." Another stress is a problem that all physicians in practice in this age of constantly changing technology face and that is staying on top of the new innovations in the profession and keeping up with the pertinent literature. Physicians in family practice, because it is a general specialty, have a particularly difficult time with this aspect of practice and often find themselves having to refer a patient to a specialist, just because the family doctors feel that they do not know enough about the problem to treat the patient adequately.

Physicians in practice are also stressed by their relationship with the community. They reported that there are a lot of "politics" involved in being a family doctor. The final stress reported was the financial pressures of practicing medicine. The doctors interviewed were very unhappy about the high cost of malpractice insurance and the expensive overhead of running an office. They could see that they brought in a lot of money for the services they rendered, but that most of the money went for overhead, and that made them feel resentful. They also spoke of being told in medical school that they were the "elite," which would bring them financial security and respect. In recent years, that has not been the case, because of rising costs of practice and other professions surpassing physicians in income and esteem.

Like the residents, the physicians in practice rated the stress of combining a personal and a professional life higher than any of the other stresses. They listed in descending order the ways that their personal lives suffer because of their professional lives. Their relationships with others is first on the list, followed by not enough time to do all the things they feel need to be done, so that interests outside of medicine get ignored, and personal well-being becomes affected. Approximately one third of the respondents said that their personal life does not suffer because of their professional life. Most likely those individuals have set up a practice that is not as demanding on them for time and energy to keep the practice going.

The physicians were asked how their relationships with family and friends were affected by being a family practice physician. Most of the doctors felt that their profession had a positive influence on their relationships with others. They spoke of the respect, admiration, and family pride that others had in their profession. Yet, others felt that they were treated differently, which they did not perceive as positive. For instance, one of the doctors said, "Outside people don't know how stressful it is and are not interested in hearing any differently." Others talk about being "wed" to the role of family doctor and how that distances them from others. Family life suffers from lack of time spent with their families and the family's uncertainty about the physician's presence at a gathering when they are on call. One doctor talked about going out on social occasions and being "beeped" by his service and having to leave a party just after he arrived, which left his wife feeling frustrated and angry and left him feeling guilty for spoiling her evening. The time pressures also create the probability of less contact with family and friends and an accompanying feeling of isolation. Again, the paradox of this situation is that these physicians report that they receive a great deal of support from family and friends, both in and out of medicine.

Physicians were asked an open-ended question about what their greatest source of stress was, and the following categories of response were listed, in descending order: demands from patients, personal expectations, work versus family choices, political pressure, the kind of practice they were in, and financial pressures. The broad array of stresses listed points to the complexity of identifying sources of stress in the practice of family medicine and the difficulty in finding consensus among practitioners. Not only are the demands for technical skill and expertise vital, but the ability to work with patients, community, and colleagues is equally important. In addition, the support of the physician's personal network of family and friends is critical. There is no clear set of stressors in family medicine, but it appears that there are both structural and personal stressors, with no one source being clearly identified by this sample as an overwhelmingly big problem. Instead what is seen is a scattered field of difficulties that might be anticipated to change with the situation over time.

Caution must be exercised in interpreting the data from this group of family physicians, because only 32 of the physicians who participated in the study worked in solo private practice. The others were employed in clinics, HMOs, teaching, and emergency rooms. The solo private practice group was the largest, with physicians practicing as part of a group practice as the second largest group. The practicing-physicians group was much older (mean age of 44) than the residents group, mostly (65%) married, and worked fewer hours (mean: 40 hours per week). This would tend to skew the information to the more positive–less stressed end of the spectrum.

Sex Differences

Overall, in both studies, the women reported higher levels of stress on all measures than the men. All participants were asked whether their practice/training experience was different because of their sex. Sixty-eight percent of the male residents and 88% of the female residents responded that their training experience was different because of their sex. When asked how it was different, they spoke of sexist attitudes of attendings and staff. Many times women residents reported that they were treated as if they were not as competent as men residents, and that some of the attendings and staff gave preferential treatment to men residents. Another problem is patient selection. There is a feeling by some that many patients, particularly older male patients, do not want a woman caring for them and that the women residents had most of the women patients and the obstetrical and gynecological cases. Both the men and the women residents said that the women must be more professional. One woman resident summed it up by saying, "A woman has to be gold to pass for silver." Another difference involves outside support. The women residents said that they need a "wife," that is, someone to help them at home, shopping, doing the laundry, etc., and missed that sort of support. The men said that having a wife or significant other helped them to focus on the residency without having to worry about their home.

Although there were only 12 women in the practicing-physician group, most of them felt that their practice was different because they were women. A majority of the men felt that their practice was different because they were men. The reason cited by both groups was that there were different levels of acceptance for men and women in family practice. Some felt that there was more and/or less support for women in practice, depending on whether the woman was married, which assumed that married women had more support. Both groups spoke about a general feeling that things were different but found themselves unable to define exactly what it was. A term that was often used to describe this feeling was "subtle sexism." Some of the older male physicians found it difficult to adjust to women in what they had always considered to be an all-male profession. A typical example is that traditionally there is only one locker room or lounge for doctors to use to change clothes or sleep, and in some hospitals the women physicians must use the nurses' quarters to change clothes.

Positive Aspects

When a study focuses on stress, there is a temptation to look only for the negative aspects. These studies tried to balance the negative with the positive. We found that all the participants in both studies felt very good about themselves as family practice physicians. Overall they rated themselves as somewhat better than other physicians that they knew. They reported feeling a high level of personal accomplishment, which helps to mediate some of the stress. When asked about the best thing about being in family practice, both residents and those in practice agreed on the variety of experience that being in family practice affords. It is very difficult to get bored when you see such a wide variety of medical cases. Another positive factor is the kind of patients who come to family doctors. This group of residents and practitioners enjoyed their patient population. Many commented on the satisfaction that they experienced in working with whole families and "being around" for all major family events (births, deaths, etc.). All participants in this study found family medicine to be very challenging, and they reported that they were very satisfied by having that kind of practice. Finally, they spoke about the kind of personal care that they feel they gave their patients. Since they developed relationships that lasted over long periods of time, they could be more involved in the patient's care.

Both groups were asked how they coped with the stress of practice/residency. Most of the residents reported that they coped by expressing their emotions either through crying, anger, or feeling depressed. Others said that they "adapted" to the stress, which they reported to be a self-adjustment of their attitudes and feelings toward stressors. Some reported that the strategic use of time was an important coping mechanism. Some residents said that they coped best by being able to talk over their problems with other people, either other residents, friends, faculty, or, in some cases, their psychotherapist. Catching up on sleep and asking for help from others when they need it were the two least-described ways of coping.

Physicians in practice, since they could exercise more control over their lives, described some different coping strategies. These strategies were broken into six major categories: (1) rearrange schedule, e.g., change appointments, schedule fewer patients, work longer on some days so that other days can be taken off; (2) express emotions—cry, get angry, yell, feel upset; (3) increase activities, for instance, take part in activities outside of the daily routine, see a movie, go hiking, get away; (4) get help—talk to someone like friends, colleagues, psychotherapist, spouse; (5) readjust their expectations, e.g., decrease the amount of work that they expect from themselves, don't get so involved in patient's problems, be less comprehensive; (6) not very well, that is, these doctors said that they do not cope well, they do not know what to do and feel unsure of what kinds of coping behaviors will help.

DISCUSSION

Overall, the two groups of physicians who participated in these two studies appeared to range from severely stressed to not stressed at all. The noticeable difference is the number of years that a physician has been involved in medicine. Stress appears to decrease slowly from the time that a person is in the third year of residency to 20 years down the career path. But how does this affect impairment? That question requires further research, but one aspect that emerges from these two studies is that if a physician can make it through the residency and the first number of years of practice, he/she stands a better chance of not being impaired than those who become overwhelmed with the stress of these early years.

Residency has its own specific set of stressors, but some of them carry over after graduation. Those that seem most evident are the time pressures, the difficulty of combining a personal and a professional life, and the problems that women in family medicine face.

One of the practicing physicians who was interviewed talked about the carryover of the time pressures: "You may be able to get out of the residency, but it's real hard to get the residency out of you." It seems logical that if large corporations train their administrative personnel in time management, something along those lines could be instituted for physicians, either in the residency or in continuing education for those already in practice. Residents graduate from most residency training programs with little knowledge about how to run a practice. If some training in that area could be instituted, residents might not feel it so necessary to "break their backs" in the early years of practice, which could lead to a more balanced practice schedule.

Another consistent problem that both practicing physicians and residents have in common is trying to balance both a professional and a personal life. In fact, trying to have both a career and a family life is the most outstanding stress of all the stresses that were mentioned. This is a consistent problem for both men and women whether or not they are in a residency or practicing in the community. Other professionals who work long hours sometimes report experiencing the waning of family life, but physicians are unique. As a group, physicians have been singled out as being the "cream of the crop," and all through their career, they are challenged to remain in this esteemed position. Consequently, this requires them to put work first, often to the detriment of personal relationships. Physicians have a unique responsibility that no other profession has; that is, they can save lives. This is a large burden that they have been trained to carry. Therefore, the patient and his needs must always come first.

Physicians who have learned to set up their priorities so that they can spend time pursuing personal interests and relationships do better than those who allow themselves to acquiesce to the demands of medical practice. Self-renewal and self-care are important concepts for physicians who want to remain healthy. Course work in techniques of self-care would be very valuable for all physicians whether they be residents, medical students, or practicing physicians. Since a physician's professional socialization begins in medical school, this would be an ideal time to institute some of these concepts. Therefore, the physician-to-be would have the idea of his own health as a main concern, one that has been integrated and reinforced all the way along the educational process.

The women physicians in both studies reported higher levels of stress than their male counterparts. A great deal of the problem stems from the fact that, historically, medicine has been a male-only profession. Prejudice and sexism is still prevalent in today's medical settings. As more and more women choose medicine as a career, these problems will change. Until then, the women in practice and in residency still have a hard time because they are not a part of the "good old boys network." A suggestion for these women would be to institute a "good old girls network," where women help other women to cope with the rigors of medical training and practice.

Women who choose medicine also face other problems. They experience a great deal of ambivalence when faced with decisions that concern the conflict between their loyalties to their practice and their families. These women have a dual role to play, which is not an easy shift to make, because of the seeming discrepancy of the two roles. Unmarried women in medicine have a particularly difficult time finding suitable men to date. They report that many men are intimidated by their status, intelligence, and education. Their male colleagues show little interest in them, and men from other professions are "scared" of dating a woman who is also a doctor. It is also difficult for these women to meet eligible men, because of their position in the community and the long hours that are required by their profession. Therefore, it might be helpful to understand the special stresses that women physicians experience in order to encourage organized changes such as flexible residency programs and shared practice models. This would help to reduce role strain and potentially increase professional participation by women.

As we have discussed, family physicians' experience of stress in their training and practice provides a reference point to examine some of the organizational, situational, and personal factors that contribute to the overall strain in the practice of medicine. This in-depth exploration of stress from one specialties' viewpoint provides the encouragement to understand other specialties' experiences. The goal is to continue the dialogue between physicians and a continued focus on individual and environmental interaction in the alleviation of stress and impairment.

REFERENCES

Becker, H. S., & Geer, B. (1958). The fate of idealism in medical school. *American Sociological Review, 23*, 50–56.

Bojar, S. (1971). Psychiatric problems of medical students. In G.B. Blaine, Jr., & C. C. McArthur (Eds.), *Emotional problems of the student*. New York: Appleton-Century-Crofts.

Bosk, C. L. (1980). Occupational rituals in patient management. *New England Journal of Medicine, 303*, 71–76.

Boyle, B. P., & Coombs, R. H. (1971). Personality profiles related to emotional stress in initial year of medical training. *Journal of Medical Education, 46*, 882–888.

Burr, B. D. (1975). The first-year family practice resident: An identity crisis. *Journal of Family Practice, 2*, 111–114.

Burstein, A. G. Loucks, S., Kobos, J. C., & Stanton, B. (1979). Psychological characteristics of medical students and residents. *Journal of Medical Education, 54*, 56–58.

Cartwright, L.K. (1979). Sources and effects of stress in health careers. In G.C. Stone, F. Cohen, & N.E. Adler (Eds.), *Health Psychology*. San Francisco: Jossey-Bass.

Chan, K.B. (1977). Individual differences in reactions to stress and their personality and situational determinants: Some implications for community mental health. *Social Science and Medicine, 2*, 89–103.

Crites, J. O. (1976). A comprehensive model of career development in early adulthood. *Journal of Vocational Behavior, 9*, 105–118.

Doub, N. H., Warschawski, P., & Kessler, I. I. (1980). Summary of the epidemiologic research on the impaired physician. First International Research Symposium on the Impaired Physician, Baltimore.

Edwards, M.T., & Zimet, C.N. (1976). Problems and concerns among medical students. *Journal of Medical Education, 51*, 619–625.

Friedman, R. C., Kornfeld, D. S., & Bigger, T. J. (1973). Psychological problems associated with sleep deprivation in interns. *Journal of Medical Education, 48*, 436–441.

Gaensbauer, T. J., & Mizner, G. L. (1980). Developmental stresses in medical education. *Psychiatry, 43*, 60–70.

Gough, H. G., & Hall, W. B. (1973). A prospective study of personality changes in students in medicine, dentistry and nursing. *Research in Higher Education, 1*, 127–140.

Hawk, J. E. (1982). Sources and levels of stress in family practice residents: A descriptive study (Doctoral dissertation, California School of Professional Psychology, Berkeley, 1982). *Dissertation Abstracts International, 43*, 3720B.

Kantner, T.R., & Vastyan, E.A. (1978). Coping with stress in family practice residency training. *Journal of Family Practice, 7*, 599–600.

Levit, E. J., Shavshin, M., & Mueller, C. B. (1974). Trends in graduate medical education and specialty certification. *New England Journal of Medicine, 290*, 545–549.

Lief, H. I., Young, K., Spruiell, V., Lancaster, R., & Lief, V. F. (1960). A psychodynamic study of medical students and their adaptational problems: A preliminary report. *Journal of Medical Education, 35*, 696–704.

Light, D. (1979). Uncertainty and control in professional training. *Journal of Health and Social Behavior, 20*, 310–322.

McCue, J. D. (1982). The effects of stress on physicians and their medical practice. *New England Journal of Medicine, 306*, 458–463.

Nelson, E. G., & Henry, W. F. (1978). Psychosocial factors seen as problems by family practice residents and their spouses. *Journal of Family Practice, 6*, 581–589.

Pfifferling, J. H. (1980). *The impaired physician: An overview*. Chapel Hill, N.C.: Health Sciences Consortium.

Raskin, M. (1972). Psychiatric crisis of medical students and the implications for subsequent adjustments. *Journal of Medical Education, 47*, 210–215.

Russell, A.T., Pasnau, R.O., & Taintor, Z.C. (1975). Emotional problems of residents in psychiatry. *American Journal of Psychiatry, 132*, 263–267.

Scott, C. D. (1983). Sources and levels of stress: An exploratory study among family practice physicians. Unpublished doctoral dissertation, The Fielding Institute, Santa Barbara, California.

Tuttelman, C. (1975). Fear and loathing in organic chemistry or A look at premedical student culture. Unpublished manuscript.

Vaillant, G., Sabowale, N., & McArthur, C. (1972). Some psychologic vulnerabilities of physicians. *New England Journal of Medicine, 287,* 372–375.

Valko, F. J., & Clayton, P. J. (1975). Depression in the internship. *Diseases of the Nervous System, 36,* 26–29.

Chapter 6

Role Conflict for Women Physicians

Dalia G. Ducker, Ph.D.

Medicine has traditionally been a male-dominated profession. Not only are the majority of physicians men, but males also hold most of the positions of power and authority in the medical profession (Braslow & Heins, 1981; Nadelson & Notman, 1983; Walsh, 1977). In recent years, however, an increasing number of women have entered the field. Thus, although women constituted 8.9% of the practicing physicians in 1970 (Bureau of the Census, 1970), by 1982 they accounted for 14.8% of the employed physicians in the United States (Bureau of the Census, 1983). These figures gain further meaning when we know that in 1982–83, 26.8% of graduating medical students were women, and in 1983–84, 33.6% of the total medical student body and 33% of the first-year medical student enrollment were women (K. Turner, personal communication, 1984).

These figures are important for several reasons. First, they reflect a broader trend toward an increased representation of women in the working world (Bureau of the Census, 1983). However, it is not the greater numbers per se that are of importance here, but rather the changed attitudes and values that they may reflect. Thus, one aspect of this trend may be a shift in related societal norms about the relative importance of work and home for women and the decreased primacy of the homemaking role (Avery, 1981; Elliott, 1981; Gray, 1983; Heckman et al., 1977; Johnson & Johnson, 1976; Kotkin, 1983; Mandelbaum, 1981; Skinner, 1980; Weisman et al., 1980).

Second, it has also been suggested that this increased representation of women may have broad implications for the nature of medical practice in the United States. Some commentators have predicted, for example, major shifts in patterns of work and specialty distribution (Bowman & Gehlbach, 1980; Dimond, 1983; Leserman, 1980; Relman, 1980; Weisman et al., 1980). Others are cautious about these suggestions. They predict that it will take approximately 40 years for women to make up 25% of the physicians in the United States, and therefore "it is unlikely that any dramatic changes in the practice of medicine in the forseeable future can realistically be attributed to the contribution of women" (Braslow & Heins, 1981, p. 132).

Whatever its larger significance for society and the medical profession, this phenomenon of the increased entry of women into medicine is especially relevant to a discussion of stress because it is expected to have implications for the context in which women physicians work. It is possible that changes in the representation of women in the medical profession will be accompanied by changes in conditions, both outside and inside the profession, that produce stress for women physicians (Southgate, 1975), and, therefore, they must be considered in any discussion of the topic. Unfortunately, questions about the effects of changes are *not* addressed directly in the literature reviewed, owing to a variety of methodological limitations, including the fact that no longitudinal studies on this topic have been conducted. Some information can be inferred by looking at the studies conducted at different periods with different samples and measures. However, conclusions about the effects of change are limited in such an approach. Thus, this issue will not be the primary focus of this discussion but is offered as the broader context in which the evidence reviewed should be evaluated.

In past years, medicine has been considered a stressful field for women (Nadelson & Notman, 1983; Notman & Nadelson, 1973). The questions are whether this is *still* so and, if so, why? As Nadelson and Notman (1983) point out, in any discussion of stress among women physicians it is important to ask whether the stresses encountered by this group are different—both in degree and in content—from those facing their male colleagues. The thesis of this discussion is that there are two major differences between the situations of male and female physicians and that these lead to different kinds and amounts of stress for the two groups. Although the two sources are similar in that they both involve the beliefs of others (which may also be internalized), they differ in regard to who holds these beliefs and in their specific content. The first difference lies in societal norms about the proper relationship between women's professional and family lives; the second involves the attitudes of their professional colleagues about the suitability of their professional involvement. It is argued that both of these affect not only the amount of strain women physicians feel but also their professional performance. These will be discussed in the terms of role theory, specifically as sources of role conflict and strain.

SOURCES OF ROLE CONFLICT

Role conflict is a complex concept and has been defined to include several types. The type of interest here is interrole conflict, which refers to the situation that arises when the expectations held by two or more people or groups regarding several positions are incompatible with each other (Shaw & Costanzo, 1970). Role strain has been defined by Goode (1960) as the felt difficulty in fulfilling role demands.

Nonprofessional Demands

One way in which the experience of women physicians differs from that of men in the field involves the nature of their nonprofessional responsibilities and the societal norms regarding their relative priority. Most professions are very demanding, requiring a high level of commitment of time and energy (Bailyn, 1964; Epstein, 1970; Holmstrom, 1972; Rossi, 1965). This means that in order to be successful one must be prepared to give these commitments top priority. However, marriage and motherhood also include obligations that are rigorously demanding as well as constant and repetitive (Darley, 1976; Epstein, 1970). Thus, professional women who marry and have children acquire additional roles, with many added demands on their time and energy. In her analysis of the situation, Epstein (1970) concludes that the American conjugal family system heavily weights the obligations of women's roles in the family so that they are assumed to be primary for women in our society. Coser and Rokoff (1971) describe the resulting conflict as one of normative priorities. Women professionals experience conflict not only because they participate in two different activity systems with incompatible time demands, but also because the underlying values clash: "Professional women are expected to be committed to their work, 'just like men' at the same time as they are normatively required to give priority to their family" (p. 535). Traditionally, women have assumed the majority of the responsibility with regard to family roles, and it has been considered appropriate that they do so (Heckman et al., 1977; Johnson & Johnson, 1976; Kotkin, 1983; Skinner, 1980). Even when they are part of a dual-career couple, women have been found to do most of the work in caring for home and family (Beckman & Houser, 1979; Bryson et al., 1976; Eisenberg, 1983; Elliott, 1981; Johnson & Johnson, 1977).

What is the evidence for such role conflict among women physicians? Most of it comes from personal accounts and anecdotal reports by women physicians describing the conflicts arising from their various roles. Rinke (1981b), for example, concludes that the social pressures on women, combined with the career demands of medicine, make it very hard for them to maintain the multiple roles of wife, mother, and physician. Angell (1981) concludes that the average woman in medicine must make major compromises in her professional and/or family life in order to attend to these two sets of competing responsibilities. She states succinctly that "women trade career advancement for time to raise their families" (Angell, 1982, p. 64). But, beyond that, she finds that they believe that this is how it *has to be*, that juggling responsibilities is the inevitable price they must pay for having both a career and a family life. In elaborating on this theme, she describes how women physicians seem to accept this situation as inevitable and thus absorb the burdens of having two jobs (Angell, 1982).

Although there is suggestive evidence that the norms may be changing (Lorber, 1982), it is clear that men's careers still take precedence over those of their wives (Eisenberg, 1983). Heins (1983) discusses the demands of the parenting role and its incompatibility with full professional participation for women physicians. She concludes that a woman who decides to have children must either play a "superwoman" role or modify the demands of her work life and move over to a slower career track, with the resulting professional handicaps.

In one of the few systematic studies on this issue, Heins and co-workers (1976) found that a majority of the women doctors in their sample did almost all their own housework. Similarly, Nadelson and co-workers (1979) reported that among their sample the major child-care responsibilities inevitably fell to the women.

Attitudes of Colleagues

Another way in which women's experience of being a physician differs from that of men involves the attitudes of their colleagues about the appropriateness of their interest in medicine. According to role theory, role conflict arises here from beliefs and expectations on the part of male professionals about the fit between stereotyped feminine characteristics and the characteristics of competent professionals. These cultural norms define women as outsiders in professions considered unsuitable for them. Goode (1957) has defined professions as communities that try to control the behavior of their members. In male-dominated fields women's sex status becomes salient. As a result, male colleagues expect their behavior to be unpredictable and feel

that they cannot be trusted. Because they do not expect women to conform
to the norms of the profession, men create a professional context that makes
women's participation difficult. They achieve this not only through deliberate
discrimination, but also through more subtle efforts to exclude women from
access to many of the informal channels of information exchange and networks of communciation (Epstein, 1968, 1970).

Looking at the medical profession, evidence suggests that some male physicians still hold attitudes that may create an unpleasant atmosphere for
female colleagues and possibly result in discrimination, although it has also
been suggested that such attitudes are changing (Mandelbaum, 1981). These
attitudes have been discussed in anecdotal reports (American Academy of
Pediatrics, 1983; Howard, 1983) and studied in a variety of samples using
several measures. Results indicate that male physicians hold more conserv-
ative views than female physicians on issues related to women's full professional participation (Heins et al., 1979).

Evidence that this trend is likely to continue comes from a study of medical
students by Leserman (1980). She found that women more readily acknowledged and were more sensitive to issues concerning prejudicial treatment of
women physicians than men, who seemed to be unaware of and uninterested
in these problems. Other recent studies of medical students and physicians
have found men to show less favorable attitudes toward women in academic
medicine and to be less sensitive to their problems than women (Ruhe &
Salladay, 1983; Scadron et al., 1982).

Looking at a specific aspect of attitudes, beliefs about the appropriateness
of medical specialties for women, Ducker (1978) found that male physicians
on a medical-school faculty, regardless of their own field, recommended the
various medical specialties differently for women and men physicians. The
field most highly recommended for women was child psychiatry, followed
by pediatrics, psychiatry, and anesthesiology. The field least recommended
was urology, followed by orthopedics, neurosurgery, and general surgery.
These recommendations appear to reflect certain latent assumptions. The
recommended specialties are those that offer opportunities for limited time
commitments and that are believed to call for qualities and aptitudes commonly attributed to women. These same themes are detectable in the types
of factors seen by the raters as advantages and disadvantages of selected fields
for women. To the extent that these beliefs are based on stereotypes about
women, they suggest that women will encounter negative attitudes from their
male colleagues and thus experience role conflict.

CONSEQUENCES

Because of combined internal and external pressures, these sources of role
conflict have a variety of consequences for women physicians. The closeness

and strength of the connections vary, however. The link is sometimes direct and obvious, as in measures of felt role strain. At other times the relationship is less direct, but still clear, as in the reasons women give for cutting down their hours or interrupting their practices. And in still other cases, a larger inferential leap must be made, as when examining practice patterns or the relationship between family status and career attainment. These consequences also vary in severity, but in most cases do not lead to incapacitating reactions. The following discussion will elaborate on the basis for these inferences and focus on relevant research findings.

In looking at these consequences, it should be kept in mind, however, that they are multidetermined and that the intent of this discussion is not to suggest that role conflict is their only antecedent. Rather, it is believed that the social norms and collegial attitudes that impinge on women physicians' lives are so potent, through the influences they exert both on them and on their peers, that they affect these women's feelings and behaviors (Darley, 1976). A word must also be inserted as to the limits of the evidence to be presented. The literature involves systematic studies of both probability and nonprobability samples as well as anecdotal reports and reflection on personal experience. It should also be kept in mind that, whenever possible, only the more recent studies will be included in this review.*

Role Strain

If the situation facing women physicians results in role conflict, it is expected that they will report experiencing strain. There have been few studies in which women physicians have been asked directly about the level of discomfort they experience in combining their various roles. Those that do exist have found that a majority of women physicians *do* report experiencing some form of role strain. This includes reports of feeling that there were too many demands on their time and energy (Heins et al., 1976) and that family responsibilities interfere with careers (Callan & Klipstein, 1981). Cartwright (1978) found that a majority of her sample experienced at least intermittent strain and that the level of strain was positively related to the number of children involved.

In a survey of women physicians in four specialties, Ducker (1980) found that a majority of the sample reported that their personal lives suffered because of their professional lives. However, 10 years later, the proportion experiencing strain was lower (Ducker, 1983c). The aspect seen as being

---

*Previous reviews should be consulted for information on older studies. There is also an extensive literature on medical students and physicians in training, which, for the most part, has not been included here.

affected most frequently was social life. This decrease may be related to the fact that at the time of the retest, fewer of the women still had children at home.

It also appears that in comparative studies women report more strain than men related to marriage and family responsibilities (Nadelson et al., 1979). Ducker (1983a) found that woman were less likely than men to feel that their practices suffered because of their personal lives, but they were more likely to feel that they had to give up other professional opportunities because of their personal commitments. Conversely, women were more likely than men to say their personal lives suffered because of their professional lives. They did not differ, however, with regard to the amount of actual strain they reported experiencing.

Satisfaction

Another feeling that may be used as a measure of the reaction of women physicians to role conflict is satisfaction with various life domains (Nadelson & Notman, 1983; Yogev & Harris, 1983). The findings in this area are more limited but suggest a high level of overall life satisfaction among women physicians (Ducker, 1982). Women physicians also indicate high levels of satisfaction with their personal lives and careers (Cartwright, 1978; Ducker, 1982). In comparison to male physicians, female physicians' levels of satisfaction have been found to be similar or higher (Ducker, 1983a; Goldstein et al., 1981).

It should be remembered, however, that the relationship between role strain and satisfaction is somewhat ambiguous. Looking at career satisfaction, Cartwright (1978) found these two feelings to be independent. Ducker (1982) examined overall life satisfaction and found the two feelings to be significantly negatively correlated.

Psychiatric Illness

Psychiatric illness is obviously the result of many complex causes. However, evidence of different rates between male and female physicians may be taken as another indicator of reactions to differential levels of role conflict in the two groups (Mausner & Steppacher, 1973; Rothblum, 1981). The evidence to date, although not extensive, does seem to suggest that women have a disproportionately high incidence of these types of disorders.

Thus, Welner and co-workers (1979) report that a higher percent of the women physicians in their sample than a comparison group of women Ph.D.s were clinically depressed. Furthermore, they found that women physicians had a significantly greater number of depressive episodes. These authors caution, however, that their system of diagnostic criteria allowed for the inclusion of subjects with mild or moderate affective disorders, a vast majority of whom had never been hospitalized. Evidence of the problems involved in defining depression is provided by the findings of Clayton and co-workers (1980). They reexamined the data used by Welner et al. and found that significantly fewer physicians and Ph.D.s met their criteria for a lifetime major depressive disorder.

Suicide

Another type of behavior that has been examined as an indicator of high levels of role conflict among women physicians is suicide rate. Suicide, too, is a response to many internal and external pressures. However, role conflict, in the most extreme cases, has been proposed as one of its antecedents (Carlson & Miller, 1981; Cartwright, 1979; Eisenberg, 1983). The literature on incidence of suicide is especially difficult to interpret owing to several methodological and conceptual problems; however, it appears to suggest that women physicians have an unexpectedly high suicide rate.

In 1968, Craig and Pitts reported evidence of a slightly higher rate of suicide in female than in male physicians and concluded that this rate was about four times as high as that for the general female population of the same age. (The rate for male physicians did not differ from that of the general male population.) On the basis of these rates, they also concluded that there is a high rate of affective disorders among these women.

In 1974, Steppacher and Mausner reported finding that both the male and female suicide rates were lower than those reported by Craig and Pitts. However, the rate for male physicians was still only 1.15 times greater than that of the overall male population, whereas the rate for female physicians was three times that of the female population. Moreover, more suicides among the women than among the men occurred during training. Also, a higher rate was found among single women. (Similarly, in 1981, Pepitone-Arreola-Rockwell and co-workers found that the annual suicide rate among women medical students was significantly higher than for men medical students and for their agemates in the national population.)

Pitts and co-workers concluded in 1979 that the suicide rate was higher for women physicians than for men physicians and about four times that of all white American women of the same age. They again inferred a high rate of primary affective disorders among women physicians.

In a study of a small number of psychiatric inpatients, Jones (1977) found a higher percentage of suicide attempts among female than male physicians.

He concluded that younger married women physicians were especially vulnerable to suicide. Rose and Rosow (1973) reported that in their sample, there were no significant differences in the suicide rates of men and women, although this finding may be due to the small number of female suicides in their study.

This literature on differential rates of suicide has stirred considerable controversy in the "Letters to the Editor" sections of several journals over the years. The conclusions most often challenged are those inferring a high rate of affective disorders among women physicians on the basis of the data on suicide rates. Carlson and Miller (1981) have provided a systematic methodological critique of this literature. They believe that the relationship between affective disorder and suicide is only a partial explanation of the higher risk of suicide among women physicians and that many factors are involved, including role conflict. It is noteworthy, however, that recently in a study of residents, Janus and co-workers (1983) found that a greater percent of women than men indicated that suicide seems at times "welcome" or "conceivable."

Professional Participation

More evidence of role conflict for women physicians comes from research findings on several types of professional behaviors that are indicators of levels of professional participation. This conclusion is based on the assumption that given roughly equivalent levels of ability and motivation in women and men physicians, gross differences in levels of professional participation and attainment must, to some extent, be related to differences in the professional environment, specifically to the two types of role conflict described previously (Cohen & Korper, 1976; Ducker, 1974). Over the years, there has been considerable evidence of greater professional involvement and achievement of success by male physicians than by female physicians (Dykman & Stalnaker, 1957; Kosa & Coker, 1965; Powers et al., 1969; Rosenlund & Oski, 1968; Scher, 1973). Some authors have concluded that the gap is narrowing, but the findings of even the recent studies suggest that differentials still remain (Eisenberg, 1983; Heins et al., 1976; Mandelbaum, 1978).

One of the most frequently used indicators of professional participation has been the number of hours worked. Thus, the claim has been made that working part time is a common way for women to adjust their work to their family life, giving them more time to attend to their home commitments (Elliott, 1981; Mandelbaum, 1978). This is also an area in which sex differences have been found consistently, even though the gap may be decreasing (Williams, 1978).

Heins and co-workers (1977) report that a majority of their women physicians were working full time at the time of their study, including those with young children. However, more women than men worked part time or did not work at all. Furthermore, fewer women than men were found to belong to professional organizations, and those who did belong were less active than their male colleagues. Similarly, Bobula (1980) found that the female physicians in his sample worked fewer hours per week and fewer weeks per year than the male physicians. Comparing his results to those of an earlier study, he concluded that the difference is decreasing because women are working more.

Looking at related variables, Cohen and Korper (1976) found that working full time was more common among women who were single, did not have children, or had fewer than two children. They concluded that reducing the workload was a compromise response to conflicts arising from the dual responsibilities of career and family demands. An indication that this trend is likely to continue comes from the results of a recent study in which women medical students reported that they planned to work professionally significantly fewer hours than men (Rosen et al., 1981).

Ducker (1983a) found that the men in her sample worked more hours per week than the women at both points in time studied. Nevertheless, looking at other indices of professional involvement, she found that the two groups did not differ significantly at either time with regard to number of hospital admitting privileges held, professional conventions per year attended, journals read regularly, professional memberships held, days per week spent without work, and days per year of vacation time. This speaks to the value of a broader definition of professional participation and suggests that not all aspects are affected equally by role conflict.

Another aspect of professional participation that may be related to role conflict is the type of practice chosen. This connection is based on the assumption that women choose jobs with regular and limited hours in response to conflict (Angell, 1981; Elliott, 1981; Mandelbaum, 1978). In this area as well, evidence of differences between women and men is found repeatedly. Specifically, although there are differences among the samples, women continue to take salaried positions with limited and predictable demands that they regard as being more compatible with family obligations more often than men (Bobula, 1980; Ducker, 1974, 1983a; Heins et al., 1977). There is also evidence that some women physicians have changed their career direction and that these changes have been necessitated because of difficulties in managing both families and careers, e.g., the need for keeping regular hours while the children were young (Callan & Klipstein, 1981).

Another relevant aspect of professional participation is career interruptions (Cartwright, 1977; Elliott, 1981; Mandelbaum, 1981). It is believed that women sometimes take time off from their careers to attend to the needs of their family lives—needs that cannot be accommodated by a profession whose structure is determined by men's career patterns. Continuing evidence is found for a high rate of interruptions, especially among married women (Cartwright, 1977; Cohen & Korper, 1976; Mandelbaum, 1979a). Furthermore, a greater proportion of women than men physicians interrupt their careers, and these interruptions last for a longer time and are most likely to be instigated by family concerns such as pregnancy and childbearing (Heins & Braslow, 1981; Heins et al., 1977; Ducker, 1983a). It must be noted, however, that a majority of women who interrupt their careers do so for short periods, often less than two years (Cartwright, 1977; Cohen & Korper, 1976; Heins & Braslow, 1981; Ducker, 1983a).

Professional Success

Professional success is another variable expected to be affected by the sources of role conflict discussed previously (Ducker, 1974). This conflict is expected to influence women's ability to participate fully in their careers by limiting both the time they have to commit to their professional lives and their opportunities for rewards and advancement. It is especially difficult to measure, and a variety of indices have been used; however, results continue to furnish evidence of problems for women. Using a composite measure of professional attainment, Lorber and Ecker (1983) found that female physicians were significantly less likely to have a high level of attainment than male colleagues at the middle stage of their careers. Using a path analyses model, they found that family responsibility had a significant negative effect on professional attainment for women and a nonsignificant positive effect for men.

Also using a composite measure, Ducker (1979) found that men and women in her sample did not differ in their levels of professional success. However, male physicians *felt* significantly more successful than their female colleagues. Ten years later there were still no differences in actual achievements, but the women's ratings of their abilities had come up to the level of the men's (Ducker, 1983a). It was interesting to note that the women's self-ratings were unrelated to actual accomplishments (Ducker, 1983b).

Another index of professional attainment in medicine is achievement of board certification. Kehrer (1974) found that a significantly greater percent of the men than of the women in her sample had attained board certification. Slightly higher rates were found by Cohen and Korper (1976) and Callan and Klipstein (1981) looking at women only. Heins et al. (1977) reported a similar sex difference, although the percentages were also higher.

An additional means of gauging women's levels of achievement in the medical profession is by examining their representation in the various levels of academic medicine. This criterion has become especially important in recent years as the number of women medical students has increased and there has been greater emphasis on the need for mentors and role models (American Academy of Pediatrics, 1983; Eisenberg, 1983; Farrell et al., 1979; Heins, 1983; Nadelson & Notman, 1983; Rinke, 1981a; Roeske & Lake, 1977; Scheiber & Doyle, 1983). In her analysis, Rinke (1981a) concludes that women physicians have had major difficulties in achieving positions of academic leadership in medical schools and that the situation has not improved perceptibly over the years. Scadron (1980) describes the situation graphically when she states that "women have been moving at a glacial pace in penetrating the upper echelons of medical school administration and the higher professional ranks" (p. 299). She concludes that women have been and still are clustered in the lower untenured faculty positions, in traditional "nurturant" specialties, and in administrative posts dealing with student and minority affairs.

These conclusions are illustrated by the figures showing that, although the proportion of women faculty members in medical schools has increased, especially in recent years, distribution across the various departments in medical schools has remained about the same, with the greatest number in psychiatry and pediatrics (Eisenberg, 1983; Higgins, 1982). The percentage of women assistant and associate professors has increased, but women have remained underrepresented in full professorial ranks (Braslow & Heins, 1981; Heins, 1983; Jolly, 1981). In a study of promotion policies at three medical schools, Wallis and co-workers (1981) found that women faculty members are promoted more slowly than men at all levels of the academic ladder, so that as rank rises, the proportion of women at that rank declines.

Heins (1983) recounts the most recent achievements of women in academics. In 1982, the first woman dean of a coeducational medical school was appointed. In the same year there were also 60 women associate deans and 58 women department chairs or acting chairs, more than 9% and 2% respectively, of the total numbers.

Specialty Choice

Choice of specialty has also been viewed as being at least partly determined by a desire in women to minimize role conflict (Ducker, 1974; Mandelbaum, 1981; Matteson & Smith, 1977). Thus, they have been overrepresented in specialties that already have high proportions of women in them, that are believed to be receptive to women, that supposedly call for aptitudes and interests characteristic of women, and that allow for limited and regular work hours (American Academy of Pediatrics, 1983; Angell, 1981; Ducker, 1978; Elliott, 1981; Nadelson & Notman, 1978). This is another area in which there is some indication that change has occurred in the last few years (Williams, 1978). The most recent evidence suggests that although the distributions of women and men across specialties are becoming more similar, differences still remain (American Academy of Pediatrics, 1983; Geyman, 1980; Mandelbaum, 1978; Weisman et al., 1980). An increasing number of women have begun to choose the fields of family medicine, internal medicine, and obstetrics-gynecology (Braslow & Heins, 1981). Nevertheless, they are still overrepresented in pediatrics, pediatric subspecialties, psychiatry, neurology, and hospital-based specialties. They are underrepresented in surgery, the surgical subspecialties, and family medicine (Barondess, 1981; Weisman et al., 1980), although an increased percentage of women in certain surgical specialties has been noted (Eisenberg, 1983). This trend is likely to continue because as of 1982, the specialties with the largest percentages of women residents were pediatrics, child psychiatry, psychiatry, dermatology, and obstetrics-gynecology. The smallest percentages were still in the surgical subspecialties (Crowley, 1983).

Marital and Family Status

Another source of evidence about the consequences of role conflict is the data on the marital and family status of women physicians. Goode (1960) conceptualized the management of multiple roles as involving role bargains and selection among alternative roles and suggested several possible strategies for dealing with strain. One specific mechanism that he proposed was the elimination of certain roles, e.g., wife and mother, from the role set. Epstein (1970) found this to be true among the women lawyers whom she studied. It is also possible that women physicians use this mechanism, in the form of eliminating marital and/or family status, as a means of preventing or reducing strain (Ducker, 1974; Eisenberg, 1983; Kaplan, 1982; Mandelbaum, 1981).

Over the years, including the most recent studies, fewer women than men physicians have been found to be married, although the gap may be narrowing (Heins et al., 1976; Lorber & Ecker, 1983; Mandelbaum, 1978; Nadelson et al., 1979). Similar rates have been found in studies on women physicians only (Callan & Klipstein, 1981; Cartwright, 1977; Cohen & Korper, 1976). Divorce is another possible consequence of role incompatibility (Mawardi,

1979; Nadelson & Notman, 1983). In a large-scale study focusing on divorce rates among physicians, Rose and Rosow (1972) found that women physicians have a higher divorce rate than men. Similar results have been found in more recent studies looking at smaller samples (Heins et al., 1977; Lorber & Ecker, 1983; Nadelson et al., 1979).

Consistent data are also found indicating that a smaller percentage of women than men physicians have children (Nadelson et al., 1979; Heins & Braslow, 1981; Lorber & Ecker, 1983). Furthermore, among physicians with children, men have a greater number than women (Nadelson et al., 1979; Heins et al., 1977; Lorber & Ecker, 1983). Similar but somewhat lower rates were found in the studies of women physicians only (Callan & Klipstein, 1981; Cartwright, 1977).

SOCIAL SUPPORT

Thus, the situations facing women and men physicians seem to differ, and these differences appear to have consequences for women's emotional and behavioral reactions. In trying to understand women's responses, it is helpful to look at evidence on mitigating or exacerbating factors that have been found to be related to the various outcomes. Several variables have been investigated, although none have been studied systematically or in great detail. One of these, social support, will be discussed here because of its direct relevance to the types of pressures discussed previously. The research in this area is sparse and fragmentary, but suggestive of its importance as a factor mitigating the effects of role conflict for women.

Social support is a general term that includes many types of relationships, varying not only in degree of closeness or intimacy but also in amount and type of help provided. Its presence implies underlying attitudes of acceptance and encouragement, and its absence implies attitudes of disapproval and possibly even prejudice. It can be found (or not found) in the two spheres discussed in relation to the two sources of role conflict, that is, in both the larger society and the professional world.

One source of support that has been studied extensively is attitude of spouse. In research on professional women in general, it has been found consistently that a husband's attitude toward his wife's work is an important factor in her ability to pursue a career (Baruch & Barnett, 1980; Birnbaum, 1975; Gray, 1983; Holmstrom, 1972; Johnson & Johnson, 1976). This relationship has also been found among women physicians (Lopate, 1968). Recently, Ducker (1982) found not only that a majority of the women physicians in her sample reported that their spouses were supportive, but also that there was a significant positive relationship between emotional support from spouse and overall life satisfaction and a negative relationship between support and feelings of role strain. Lorber (1982) studied couples in which both partners were physicians and also found that a majority of the women felt that their husbands were supportive of their careers. In addition, she found that such couples greatly influenced each others' career decisions, including choice of location of postgraduate training, choice of specialty, and choice of career type. Kaplan (1982) found that among women medical students over 30, those who received less support from spouses experienced more strain.

Heins and co-workers (1982) have found that extrafamilial support is important in the career choice of physicians, and it has been suggested that it is also an important factor in women physicians' ability to manage multiple roles (Lippitt, 1982; Scher et al., 1976). Although no systematic research has been done on this issue among women physicians, there are reports of the success of discussion and support groups set up specially to help women medical students deal with work-related psychological stresses (Davidson, 1978; Goldstein, 1975; Hilberman et al., 1975; Konanc, 1979; Nadelson & Notman, 1983; Scheiber & Doyle, 1983).

Support can also be more broadly conceptualized as including the larger network of professional colleagues who provide not only help in attaining specific goals such as jobs, promotions, and referrals, but also access to the wider professional community (Lorber, 1982). Rinke (1981b) discusses the process of professional socialization and describes the obstacles that interfere with this process among women physicians, including their exclusion from the informal network of contacts and information exchanges necessary for success (and which have been found so prevalent among men doctors). She contends that such support is important for the development of a strong occupational identity that is crucial for an inner sense of competence and a productive career, and that women physicians are often deprived of those benefits.

In an empirical test of these ideas, Lorber (1981) interviewed a sample of male and female internists. On the basis of her findings, she concluded that women physicians benefited from sponsorship during postgraduate training, but were less likely to receive active help from colleagues in setting up their practices or in obtaining positions of leadership in the medical community. In academics, such sponsorship was more likely to help men than women gain administrative positions. Lorber described the subtle ways in which women are excluded from high-level positions and concluded that their male peers seem unable to perceive them as leaders: "Without active sponsorship for high positions by men whose word is trusted by their male colleagues, women physicians have a visibility and credibility gap that their very real professional attainments do not seem able to fill" (p. 333). Looking at office practices, she found a similar pattern. Men were more likely than women to have active sponsors who gave them referrals, taught them how to run a practice, and helped them get hospital affiliations. Similarly, Goldstein et al. (1981) found that among their sample of psychiatrists, both the women and men agreed that women received less support than men from male psychiatrists.

SUMMARY, CONCLUSIONS, AND RECOMMENDATIONS

In summary, women physicians have been found to experience greater role conflict than their male colleagues. As discussed previously, it is difficult to draw conclusions about changes over time because of methodological limitations of the data; nevertheless, it appears that despite the increased percentage of women in medicine, these sources of conflict remain in the early 1980s. It has also been inferred that this conflict, at least in part, contributes to the differences between men and women physicians in various feelings and behaviors assumed to be indicators of stress.

There is still much to be understood about stress for women physicians, and other aspects of the problem have not been discussed here. In this review the focus has been on external determinants of conflict in the social environment. Other authors have put greater emphasis on intrapsychic concepts in looking at both antecedants and consequences of conflict. They discuss the internally experienced conflict between the qualities associated with achievement, e.g., aggression, rationality, and independence, and those associated with the feminine role, e.g., nurturance, emotionality, and social responsiveness (Brown & Klein, 1982; Crovitz, 1980; Mandelbaum, 1979a, 1981; Nadelson & Notman, 1983; Notman & Nadelson, 1973), that result from the socialization of women according to prevailing sex role stereotypes. Rinke (1981b) describes this as an identity crisis that arises for women who attempt to adapt womanhood to a male professional model emphasizing masculine character traits.

Furthermore, the consequences examined here have dealt with a limited range of feelings and behaviors. Other reactions may be less readily identifiable but may also be affected by these sources of conflict (Nadelson & Notman, 1983). McCue (1982), for example, describes some of the patterns of behavior that he believes reflect stress among physicians. Among these are emotional and social withdrawal from family, friends, and colleagues. To date, these have never been examined systematically among women. Another area that needs further exploration among women physicians is the phenomenon known as burnout. Muldary (1983) describes burnout among health professionals and speculates that, as a consequence of women's attitudes toward work and the role conflict they encounter, they are likely to experience a high level of burnout.

Another area of inquiry has involved studies of factors related to responses to conflict. Several researchers have investigated personality, background, and demographic characteristics related to various adaptations. Cartwright (1977, 1978) reports the characteristics she found related to satisfaction with work, role harmony, and career continuity. Similarly, Mandelbaum (1979a, 1979b, 1981) has conducted a longitudinal study of women physicians who are career persisters and nonpersisters and has described the profiles of women who chose each of these career paths.

Still another perspective on role conflict in women professionals emphasizes the actual mechanics of daily functioning, describing a variety of coping mechanisms employed (Gray, 1983; Hall, 1972). Few systematic studies have focused on the coping mechanisms of women physicians, but suggestions have been made as to effective strategies (Angell, 1982; Cartwright, 1978; Dimond, 1983; Ducker, 1980; Heins, 1983; Lippitt, 1982; Romm, 1982). These include setting priorities, learning to delegate responsibilities, using support systems, eliminating nonessential commitments, and trying to change the attitudes and expectations of significant others. This is another area in which more study is needed.

Greater attention also needs to be paid to several groups of women physicians with special problems. Thus, there has been some discussion of the problems of women who have entered medicine relatively late in life. Kaplan (1982), for example, found that women medical students over 30 face certain institutional and personal barriers that are different from those of younger women. Minority women physicians may also have unique career issues related to their ethnic and cultural backgrounds (American Academy of Pediatrics, 1983). Lovelace (1983) studied a sample of black women physicians and found them to have high levels of career satisfaction, role harmony, and role integration, which she related to certain traditions within their culture.

It should also be noted that this review has not considered differences due to age and/or life stage. The stresses inherent in the medical profession differ depending on the stage of the woman's medical career (Cartwright, 1979). Furthermore, the demands of family life also change, depending on the stage of family development (Barnett & Baruch, 1978). It would be useful to consider women physicians' specific life stage when investigating the presence and consequences of role conflict. Perun and Bielby (1981) advocate the developmental approach. Such a model should consider the interaction of age and gender roles and women's need to synchronize work and family cycles throughout adulthood.

Finally, it has sometimes been argued that combining family and work lives need not always have a negative effect on women. Barnett and Baruch (1978) contend that much of the research on women and work has been limited by the assumption that, for women who are married and have children, the work role is almost inevitably a source of conflict and, as a result, the positive aspects of combining roles have been ignored. In fact, in a study of working women, they found positive correlations between commitment to work and role pattern satisfaction and self-esteem (Baruch & Barnett, 1980). Applying this finding to women physicians suggests that although those who are married and have children and work are most likely to feel strain (Ducker, 1980), they may also experience the most satisfaction or have the highest level of well-being, feelings that derive from having both affective and instrumental needs met as well as from having proved themselves competent to handle these challenges.

Barnett and Baruch (1983) go on to argue that in examining role conflict the emphasis should not be on the number of roles, but on the quality of experience within the particular roles occupied. They interpret the findings of their study of a large sample of working women to mean that the role of parent, rather than that of worker, is the major source of stress for women, and that this parental role, rather than the work role, is likely to have a negative effect on a woman's well-being. Research is needed on this question among woman physicians.

In conclusion, the findings reviewed are believed to have implications both for individuals and for the medical profession as a whole. For individual women physicians, these findings suggest the need to be aware first of the potential sources of conflict in their environment and second of the options for ways of dealing with those that exist. It is important for them to understand that conflict arises from attitudes that reflect underlying values and priorities, ideals of what constitutes an adequate spouse, parent, or physician. These are not reflections of how things necessarily must be, but rather of how some people think they ought to be. Each women can evaluate her own options and choose the best path for herself. Each woman cannot act alone, however, unaffected by the society and the profession of which she is a part. Real constraints accompany these beliefs, which in turn restrict the choices that she can make.

The professional world in general, and medicine in particular, have been structured to be compatible with the needs of males (Angell, 1981; Heins, 1983; Nadelson & Notman, 1978), and until today women have had to struggle to try to fit their lives into this model. A variety of writers have suggested changes that might help women physicians, such as increased availability of part-time work, easily accessible day-care facilities, and programs for making more leadership positions available to women (Angell, 1981; Braslow & Heins, 1981; Cohen & Korper, 1976; Heins, 1983; Rinke, 1981a; Yogev & Harris, 1983). Arguments have also been made for the importance of more social support, especially from spouses, as well as for more role models (Angell, 1982; Davidson, 1978; Heins, 1983; Kaplan, 1982; Nadelson & Notman, 1983; Rinke, 1981b; Roeske & Lake, 1977).

Unfortunately, none of these are enough in themselves. Mumford (1983) has described the dangers of the current ethos in medicine in which a life of stress and deprivation is seen as inevitable and, to some extent, desirable. As has been discussed, certain conditions may be especially problematic for women physicians, but they are harmful for their male colleagues and the general public as well, and thus should be reevaluated and, whenever possible, modified.

REFERENCES

American Academy of Pediatrics (1983). Women in pediatrics. *Pediatrics, 71*(4, part 2), 679–719.

Angell, M. (1981). Women in medicine: Beyond prejudice. *New England Journal of Medicine, 304*(19), 1161–1163.

Angell, M. (1982). Juggling the personal and professional life. *Journal of the American Women's Association, 36*(2), 79–81.

Avery, M. E. (1981). Women in medicine, 1979: What are the issues? *Journal of the American Medical Women's Association, 36*(2), 79–81.

Bailyn, L. (1964). Notes on the role of choice in the psychology of professional women. *Daedalus, 93,* 700–710.

Barnett, R. C., & Baruch, G. K. (1978). Women in the middle years: A critique of research and theory. *Psychology of Women Quarterly, 3,* 187–197.

Barnett, R. C., & Baruch, G. K. (1983). *Women's involvement in multiple roles, role strain and psychological distress.* Unpublished manuscript. Wellesley College, Center for Research on Women.

Barondess, J. A. (1981). Are women different? Some trends in the assimilation of women in medicine. *Journal of the American Women's Association, 36*(3), 95–104.

Baruch, G. K., & Barnett, R. C. (1980). On the well-being of adult women. In L. A. Bond & J. C. Rosen (Eds.), *Competence and coping in adulthood.* Hanover, N. H.: University Press of New England.

Beckman, L. J., & Houser, B. B. (1979). The more you have, the more you do: The relationship between wife's employment, sex-role attitudes, and household behavior. *Psychology of Women Quarterly, 4*(2), 160–174.

Birnbaum, J. A. (1975). Life patterns and self-esteem in gifted family-oriented and career-committed women. In M. T. S. Mednick, S. S. Tangri, & L. W. Hoffman (Eds.), *Women and achievement.* New York: Wiley.

Bobula, J. D. (1980). Work patterns, practice characteristics, and incomes of male and female physicians. *Journal of Medical Education, 55,* 827–833.

Bowman, M. W., & Gehlbach, J. H. (1980). Sex of physician as a determinant of psychosocial problem recognition. *Journal of Family Practice, 10*(4), 655–659.

Braslow, J. D., & Heins, M. (1981). Women in medical education: A decade of change. *New England Journal of Medicine, 304*(19), 1129–1135.

Brown, S. L., & Klein, R. H. (1982). Woman—Power in the medical hierarchy. *Journal of the American Medical Women's Association, 37*(6), 155–164.

Bryson, R. B., Bryson, J. B., Licht, M. H., & Licht, B. G. (1976). The professional pair: Husband and wife psychologists. *American Psychologist, 31,* 10–16.

Bureau of the Census. (1970). *Census of population.*

Bureau of the Census (1983). *Statistical Abstract of the United States: 1984.* Washington, D.C.: U.S. Department of Commerce.

Callan, C., & Klipstein, E. (1981). Women physicians in Connecticut: A survey. *Connecticut Medicine, 45*(8), 494–496.

Carlson, G. A., & Miller, D. C. (1981). Suicide, affective disorder, and women physicians. *American Journal of Psychiatry, 38*(10), 1330–1335.

Cartwright, L. K. (1977). Continuity and noncontinuity in the careers of a sample of young women physicians. *Journal of the American Medical Women's Association, 32*(9), 316–321.

Cartwright, L. K. (1978). Career satisfaction and role harmony in a sample of young women physicians. *Journal of Vocational Behavior, 12,* 184–196.

Cartwright, L. K. (1979). Sources and effects of stress in health careers. In G. C. Stone, F. Cohen, & N. E. Adler (Eds.), *Health psychology: A handbook* (pp. 419–445). San Francisco: Jossey Bass

Clayton, P., Marten, S., Davis, M. A., et al. (1980). Mood disorder in women professionals. *Journal of Affective Disorders, 2,* 37–46.

Cohen, E. D., & Korper, S. P. (1976). Women in medicine: A survey of professional activities, career interruptions, and conflict resolutions. *Connecticut Medicine, 40*(3), 195–200.

Coser, R. L., & Rokoff, G. (1971). Women in the occupational world: Social disruption and conflict. *Social Problems, 18,* 535–554.

Craig, A. G., & Pitts, F. N. (1968). Suicide by physicians. *Diseases of the Nervous System, 29,* 763–772.

Crovitz, E. (1980). Women entering medical school: The challenge continues. *Journal of the American Medical Association, 35*(12), 291–298.

Crowley, A. E. (1983). Graduate medical education in the United States. *Journal of the American Medical Association, 250*(212), 1545–1547.

Darley, S. A. (1976). Big-time careers for the little woman: A dual-role dilemma. *Journal of Social Issues, 32*(3), 85–96.

Davidson, V. A. (1978). Coping styles of women medical students. *Journal of Medical Education, 53,* 902–907.

Dimond, E. G. (1983). The future of women physicians. *Journal of the American Medical Association, 249*(2), 207–208.

Ducker, D. G. (1974). *The effects of two sources of role strain on women physicians.* Unpublished dissertation, the City University of New York.

Ducker, D. G. (1978). Believed suitability of medical specialties for women physicians. *Journal of the American Medical Women's Association, 33*(1), 25–32.

Ducker, D. G. (1979). *Role strain and professional participation of women and men physicians.* Unpublished paper.

Ducker, D. G. (1980). The effects of two sources of role strain on women physicians. *Sex Roles, 6*(4), 549–559.

Ducker, D. G. (1982). *Life satisfaction in women physicians.* Paper presented at the meeting of the American Psychological Association, Montreal, Canada.

Ducker, D. G. (1983a). *The career patterns of midlife women and men physicians: A longitudinal examination.* Paper presented at the meeting of the American Psychological Association, Anaheim, Calif.

Ducker, D. G. (1983b). *A longitudinal study of female physicians: Changes in perceived competence over time.* Paper presented at the meeting of the California State Psychological Association, San Francisco.

Ducker, D. G. (1983c). *Role strain in women physicians: A longitudinal study.* Paper presented at the meeting of the Western Psychological Association, San Francisco.

Dykman, R. A., & Stalnaker, J. M. (1957). Survey of women physicians graduating from medical school, 1925–1940. *Journal of Medical Education, 32,* 3–38.

Eisenberg, C. (1983). Women as physicians. *Journal of Medical Education, 58,* 534–541.

Elliott, C. M. (1981). Women physicians as workers. *Journal of the American Medical Women's Association, 36,* 105–108.

Epstein, C. F. (1968). Women and professional careers: The case of the woman lawyer. Unpublished doctoral dissertation, Columbia University.

Epstein, C. F. (1970). *Woman's place.* Berkeley: University of California Press.

Farrell, K., Witte, M. H., Holguin, M., & Lopez, S. (1979). Women physicians in medical academia: A national statistical survey. *Journal of the American Medical Association, 241*(26), 2808–2812.

Geyman, J. P. (1980). Increasing number of women in family practice: An overdue trend. *Journal of Family Practice, 10*(2), 207–208.

Goldstein, M. Z. (1975). Preventive mental health efforts for women medical students. *Journal of Medical Education, 50,* 289–291.

Goldstein, M. Z., Bromet, E. J., Hanusa, B. H., & Lasell, R. L. (1981). Psychiatrists' life and work patterns: A statewide comparison of women and men. *American Journal of Psychiatry, 138*(7), 919–924.

Goode, W. (1957). Community within a community: The professionals. *American Sociological Review, 22,* 195–200.

Goode, W. (1960). A theory of role strain. *American Sociological Review, 25,* 483–496.

Gray, J. D. (1983). The married professional woman: An examination of her role conflicts and coping strategies. *Psychology of Women Quarterly, 7*(3), 235–243.

Hall, D. T. (1972). A model of coping with role conflict: The role behavior of college-educated women. *Administrative Science Quarterly, 17,* 471–486.

Heckman, N. A., Bryson, R. B., & Bryson, J. B. (1977). Problems of professional couples: A content analysis. *Journal of Marriage and the Family, 39*(2), 323–330.

Heins, M. (1983). Medicine and motherhood. *Journal of the American Medical Association, 249*(2), 209–210.

Heins, M., & Braslow, J. (1981). Women doctors: Productivity in Great Britain and the United States. *Medical Education, 15,* 53–56.

Heins, M., Smock, S., Jacobs, J., & Stein, M. (1976). Productivity of women physicians. *Journal of the American Medical Association, 236*(17), 1961–1964.

Heins, M., Smock, S., Martindale, L., Jacobs, J., & Stein, M. (1977). Comparison of the productivity of women and men physicians. *Journal of the American Medical Association, 237*(23), 2514–2517.

Heins, M., Hendricks, J., Martindale, L., Smock, S., Stein, M., & Jacobs, J. (1979). Attitudes of women and men physicians. *American Journal of Public Health, 69*(11), 1132–1138.

Heins, M., Hendricks, J., & Martindale, L. (1982). The importance of extrafamily support on career choices of women. *Personnel and Guidance Journal, 60*(8), 455–459.

Higgins, E. (1982). Women faculty members at U.S. medical schools. *Journal of Medical Education, 57,* 202–203.

Hilberman, E., Konanc, J., Perez-Reyes, M., Hunter, R., Scagnelli, J., & Sanders, S. (1975). Support groups for women in medical school: A first-year program. *Journal of Medical Education, 50,* 867–875.

Holmstrom, L. L. (1972). *The two-career family.* Cambridge, MA: Schenkman.

Howard, R. B. (1983). Watch out, guys: The women are here. *Postgraduate Medicine, 73*(4), 13–19.

Janus, C. L., Janus, S. S., Price, S., & Adler, D. (1983). Residents: The pressure's on the women. *Journal of the American Medical Women's Association, 38*(1), 18–21.

Johnson, C. L., & Johnson, F. A. (1977). Attitudes toward parenting in dual-career families. *American Journal of Psychiatry, 134*(4), 391–395.

Johnson, F. A., & Johnson, C. L. (1976). Role strain in high-commitment career women. *Journal of the American Academy of Psychoanalysis, 4*(1), 13–26.

Jolly, P. (1981). Women physicians on U.S. medical school faculties. *Journal of Medical Education, 56,* 151–153.

Jones, R. E. (1977). A study of 100 physician psychiatric inpatients. *American Journal of Psychiatry, 134*(10), 1110–1123.

Kaplan, S. R. (1982). Medical school and women over 30. *Journal of the American Medical Women's Association, 37*(2), 39–50.

Kehrer, H. (1974). Professional and practice characteristics of men and women physicians. In J. Warner & P. Aherne (Eds.), *Profile of medical practice.* Chicago: American Medical Association.

Konanc, J. (1979). What support groups for women medical students do: A retrospective inquiry. *Journal of the American Medical Women's Association, 34*(7), 275–283.

Kosa, J., & Coker, R. E. (1965). The female physician in public health, conflict and reconciliation of the sex and professional roles. *Sociology and Social Research, 49,* 294–305.

Kotkin, M. (1983). Sex roles among married and unmarried couples. *Sex Roles, 9*(9), 975–985.

Leserman, J. (1980). Sex differences in the professional orientation of first-year medical students. *Sex Roles, 6*(4), 645–660.

Lippitt, R. (1982). MSMS conference to focus on two challenges to committed professional women. *Michigan Medicine, 81*(18), 198.

Lopate, C. (1968). *Women in medicine.* Baltimore: Johns Hopkins Press.

Lorber, J. A. (1981). The limits of sponsorship for women physicians. *Journal of the American Medical Women's Association, 36*(11), 329–338.

Lorber, J. A. (1982). How physician spouses influence each other's careers. *Journal of the American Women's Association, 37*(1), 21–26.

Lorber, J. A., & Ecker, M. (1983). Career development of female and male physicians. *Journal of Medical Education, 58,* 447–456.

Lovelace, J. C. (1983). *Role conflict, role integration, and career satisfaction in Afro-American physicians.* Unpublished dissertation, California School of Professional Psychology, Berkeley.

Mandelbaum, D. R. (1978). Women in medicine. *Signs, 4*(1), 136–145.

Mandelbaum, D. R. (1979a). Personality variables related to the career persistence of women physicians. *Journal of the American Medical Women's Association, 34*(6), 255–259.

Mandelbaum, D. R. (1979b). Education, medical training, and practice variables related to the career persistence of women physicians. *Journal of the American Medical Women's Association, 34*(10), 384–391.

Mandelbaum, D. R. (1981). *Work, marriage, and motherhood: The career persistence of female physicians.* New York: Praeger.

Matteson, M. T., & Smith, S. V. (1977). Selection of medical specialties: Preferences versus choices. *Journal of Medical Education, 52,* 548–554.

Mausner, J. S., & Steppacher, R. C. (1973). Suicide in professionals: A study of male and female psychologists. *American Journal of Epidemiology, 98*(6), 436–445.

Mawardi, B. H. (1979). Satisfactions, dissatisfactions, and causes of stress in medical practice. *Journal of the American Medical Association, 241*(14), 1483–1486.

McCue, J. D. (1982). The effects of stress on physicians and their medical practice. *New England Journal of Medicine, 306*(8), 458–463.

Muldary, T. W. (1983). *Burnout and health professionals: Manifestations and management.* Norwalk, Conn.: Appleton-Century-Crofts.

Mumford, E. (1983). Stress in the medical center. *Journal of Medical Education, 58*(5), 436–437.

Nadelson, C. C., & Notman, M. T. (1978). *Physician stress and impairment: Special concerns for women.* Paper presented at the meeting of the American Psychiatric Association, Atlanta, Ga.

Nadelson, C. C., & Notman, M. T. (1983). What is different for women physicians? In S. C. Scheiber & B. B. Doyle (Eds.), *The impaired physician* (pp. 11–25). New York: Plenum.

Nadelson, C. C., Notman, M. T., & Lowenstein, P. (1979). The practice patterns, life styles, and stresses of women and men entering medicine: A follow-up study of Harvard Medical School graduates from 1967–1977. *Journal of the American Medical Women's Association, 34*(11), 400–408.

Notman, M. T., & Nadelson, C. C. (1973). Medicine: A career conflict for women. *American Journal of Psychiatry, 130,* 1123–1127.

Pepitone-Arreola-Rockwell, F., Rockwell, D., & Core, N. (1981). Fifty-two medical student suicides. *American Journal of Psychiatry, 138*(2), 198–201.

Perun, P. J., & Bielby, D. D. (1981). Towards a model of female occupational behavior: A human development approach. *Psychology of Women Quarterly, 6*(2), 234–252.

Pitts, F. N., Schuller, A. B., Rich, C. L., & Pitts, A. F. (1979). Suicide among U. S. women physicians, 1967–1972. *American Journal of Psychiatry, 136*(5), 694–696.

Powers, L., Parmalee, R. D., & Weisenfelder, H. (1969). Practice patterns of women and men physicians. *Journal of Medical Education, 44*, 481–491.

Relman, A. S. (1980). Here come the women. *New England Journal of Medicine, 302*(22), 1252–1253.

Rinke, C. M. (1981a). The economic and academic status of women physicians. *Journal of the American Medical Association, 245*(2), 2305–2306.

Rinke, C. M. (1981b). The professional identities of women physicians. *Journal of the American Medical Association, 245*(23), 2419–2420.

Roeske, N. A., & Lake, K. (1977). Role models for women medical students. *Journal of Medical Education, 52*, 459–466.

Romm, S. (1982). Woman doctor in search of a job. *Journal of the American Medical Women's Association, 37*(1), 11–15.

Rose, K. D., & Rosow, I. (1972). Marital stability among physicians. *California Medicine, 116*, 95–99.

Rose, K. D., & Rosow, I. (1973). Physicians who kill themselves. *Archives of General Psychiatry, 29*, 800–805.

Rosen, R. H., Heins, M., & Martindale, L. J. (1981). Practice plans of today's medical students. *Journal of Medical Education, 56*, 57–59.

Rosenlund, M. L., & Oski, F. A. (1968). Women in medicine. *Annals of Internal Medicine, 66*, 1008–1012.

Rossi, A. (1965). Barriers to the career choice of engineering, medicine, or science among American women. In J. A. Mattfeld and C. G. Van Aken (Eds.), *Women and the scientific professions* (pp. 31–127). Cambridge, Mass.: M. I. T. Press.

Rothblum, E. D. (1981). Depression among women in medicine. *Connecticut Medicine, 45*(8), 501–503.

Ruhe, P., & Salladay, S. (1983). Changing views of women in medicine. *Nebraska Medical Journal, 68*(8), 250–253.

Scadron, A. (1980). AMWA's experiment in planned change: A report on the "women in Medical Academia" project. *Journal of the American Medical Women's Association, 35*(12), 299–301.

Scadron, A., Witte, M. H., Axelrod, M., Greenberg, E. A., Arem, C., & Meitz, J. E. (1982). Attitudes toward women physicians in medical academia. *Journal of the American Medical Association, 247*(20), 2803–2807.

Scheiber, S. C., & Doyle, B. B. (1983). Conclusions and recommendations. In S. C. Scheiber & B. B. Doyle (Eds.), *The impaired physician* (pp. 169–172). New York: Plenum.

Scher, M. (1973). Women in psychiatry. *American Journal of Psychiatry, 130*(10), 1118–1122.

Scher, M., Benedek, E., Candy, A., Carey, K., Mules, J., & Sachs, B. (1976). Psychiatrist-wife-mother: Some aspects of role integration. *American Journal of Psychiatry, 133*(7), 830–834.

Shaw, M. E., & Costanzo, P. R. (1970). *Theories of social psychology*. New York: McGraw-Hill.

Skinner, D. A. (1980). Dual-career family stress and coping: A literature review. *Family Relations, 29*, 473–480.

Southgate, M. T. (1975). Remembrance of things (hopefully) past. *Journal of the American Medical Association, 232*(13), 1331–1332.

Steppacher, R. C., & Mausner, J. S. (1974). Suicide in male and female physicians. *Journal of the American Medical Association, 228*(3), 323–328.

Wallis, L. A., Gilder, H., & Thaler, H. (1981). Advancement of men and women in medical academia. *Journal of the American Medical Association, 246*(20), 2350–2353.

Walsh, M. R. (1977). *Doctors wanted: No women need apply.* New Haven: Yale University Press.

Weisman, C. S., Levine, D. M., Steinwachs, D. M., & Chase, G. A. (1980). Male and female physician career patterns: Specialty choices and graduate training. *Journal of Medical Education, 55,* 813–825.

Welner, A., Marten, S., Wochnick, E., Davis, M. A., Fishman, R., & Clayton, P. J. (1979). Psychiatric disorders among professional women. *Archives of General Psychiatry, 36,* 169–173.

Williams, P. B. (1978). Recent trends in the productivity of women and men physicians. *Journal of Medical Education, 53,* 420–422.

Yogev, S., & Harris, S. (1983). Women physicians during residency years: Workload, work satisfaction and self concept. *Social Science & Medicine, 7*(12), 837–841.

Chapter 7

Physicians, Stress, and Family Life: A Systemic View

Shae Graham Kosch, Ph.D.

What's good about medicine is that there's always something to do, so you don't have to think about your problems; what's bad about medicine is that there's always something to do so that you don't have time to think about your problems enough.—Haseltine & Yaw, *Woman Doctor*, 1976, p. 70

THE SYSTEMS VIEW—DEVELOPMENT AND MAINTENANCE OF FAMILY DYSFUNCTION

From general systems theory and family systems theory, it can be postulated that an individual's stressors are related to the sociocultural environment, intrapersonal processes, interpersonal processes, and the physical environment. A person does not exist in a vacuum, rather in a whorl of complex and interconnected relationships that exert pressures for movement in certain directions, be they behavioral or affective. According to general systems theory, events are conceptualized in terms of systems or "sets of units or elements standing in some consistent relationship or interactional stance with each other" (von Bertalanffy, 1968, p. 38). In the case of an

110

overly stressed physician, there are many elements that create and maintain the conditions for the stressed state. Homeostasis within the system is maintained by a balance and interplay between all elements, and the level of stress is one such aspect that is encouraged to remain static. Change one part of the system and it will have ramifications among the other elements. Homeostasis of the system is maintained in a dysfunctional family by the symptomatic member remaining symptomatic (Minuchin et al., 1978; Watzlawick et al., 1967). One of the basic emphases of both general systems theory and family systems theory is on mutual or circular causality, that is, on how the different elements of the system interact with each other to create a certain state of equilibrium. It is noted that any phenomenon that occurs in the system is one of multicausality, and one of the best methods to identify avenues of change or morphogenesis within the system is to look at the contributing aspects of each element.

According to Brody and Sobel's (1979) interpretation of general systems theory, health is the "ability of a system (for example, cell, organism, family, society) to respond adaptively to a wide variety of environmental challenges (for example, physical, chemical, infectious, psychological, social)" (p. 93). Health is seen as a positive, active process and includes a consideration of the broader environmental, sociocultural, and behavioral determinants of health, as well as somatic well-being. Health is also seen as a dynamically changing state in which environmental forces can precipitate a lower level of health, a restoration of equilibrium, or a growth-enhancing reaction. In Brody and Sobel's framework, disease is the failure of a living system to react adaptively to environmental challenges or internal changes. As all levels or elements in a living system are interconnected, both health and disease result from the interplay of the various factions. In looking at the phenomenon of physician stress and its disruptive effect on family life, then, it is crucial to consider the interplay of various elements and their contribution to the development and maintenance of family dysfunction.

It is also crucial when designing rehabilitation programs involving impaired physicians that the results of change on other sectors of the system be considered, and not just the influence of a program on the physician. For instance, a current trend among hospital staffs includes encouraging the physician to attend to his/her physical fitness. Physicians are encouraged to participate in weight-reduction programs or cardiac-conditioning programs, with the assumption that a physically healthy physician will be more immune to impairment. If a physician with a busy clinical schedule starts spending two hours a day in a physical-conditioning program, however, that is two hours less that he/she will have available for family interaction. While trying to strengthen part of the system to reduce the risk of impairment, then, the program may actively increase dysfunction in the family sphere.

ELEMENTS THAT CREATE THE "M.D. IN A PRESSURE COOKER" ENVIRONMENT

The major elements that contribute to an excessive level of stress in the physician's life include societal elements, medical system contributions, family contributions, and self-contributions of the physician. Before each of these elements is discussed, it is important to put in context the influence of societal sources and the interplay of family and societal sectors. As Ransom and Massad (1978) note, "Societal sources include the effects on the family of external influences such as industrialization, urbanization, changing technology, economic recessions, mass media and evolving images of what it means to be a person or a family" (p. 27). Furthermore, Ransom and Massad contend that each family and its functions are regulated through exchanges with societal units and thus serve an external set of purposes, as well as their internal functions as a living system. The authors note that one interchange between the economy and the family includes the family allocating a certain amount of time or performance capacity from at least one member in order to obtain monetary reimbursement, goods, or services. It is also important to note that certain members of the family, or certain units combined as subsystems of the family system, may not always agree as to how this interchange between the family unit and society should be managed. The crux of the systems perspective on the family and society can be described in the following manner:

> In families, each subsystem participates simultaneously in other systems and is continuously involved in efforts to maintain sufficient constancy with them so that the relevant relationships may survive. The "strategies" that result often produce unforeseen and unintended consequences that create conflict or disorder at some nodal point in the total process. Of importance . . . is the ecologic law . . . that any adaptive change in one part of the family, if uncorrected by some change in the others, will always jeopardize the relationship between them. (Ransom & Massad, 1978, p. 30)

It is important to remember this contextual perspective as we isolate various factors and subsystems to look at each of their contributions to the phenomenon of overly stressed physicians.

Although we do not have empirical data on the variables related to family dysfunction among physicians, behavioral scientists have turned their attention to the elements or factors that create this situation clinically. One of the most interesting projects was that of Lane Gerber (1983b), a clinical psychologist, who performed "anthropological studies" of physicians in their natural environment. According to Gerber, he actually "lived with the physicians" by going to rounds with them in the morning, the conferences they attended, home to dinner with them, and back to the hospital while they were on call. One of Gerber's major conclusions was that society supports work as a first priority and values the family only insofar as it supports the worker to do his/her important work. When the worker is at the top of the occupational hierarchy, as is the physician, the pressure on the family to support work and the worker must be even more accentuated than for persons in less prestigious or demanding careers.

Societal Contributions

Image and expectations

A physician in our culture is seen as a "special person" (Gerber, 1983a), with special responsibilities, privileges, prestige, and social standing. In the United States culture, in fact, the physician is at the top of the hierarchy in terms of job prestige, above other health professionals, scientists, and business persons. In many other countries, being a physician is not at the top of the hierarchy, which is probably related to the value that a culture places on health and such factors as the sex distribution of persons engaging in various professions. In the United States, however, attaining the rank of M.D. is one means by which to actualize the myth and cultural ideal that hard work and devotion will reap individual rewards. The physician, then, can be seen as one variant of an American "go-getter" (Boorstin, 1974), a person who attains a badge of prestige by "making it" against great odds, similar to the accomplishments of a pioneer in the unknown and dangerous Old West.

Another cultural change that may contribute to the meaning of the physician's position is that of the societal salience of religious beliefs. In the 1800s in the United States, persons looked to their spiritual leaders, their ministers, for guidance through this life and guidance toward the afterlife. As America became increasingly secularized, and lost its collective emphasis on the hereafter, the focus of people on preserving their "life on earth" became accentuated. With this focus came greater expectations and demands on physicians to preserve and enhance "life on earth." One way to view the hero worship of the contemporary physician by the American populus, then, is to understand that the physician has acquired roles once held by explorers and the clergy. He/she is now looked to as the "court of last resort" to heal wounds, both physical and spiritual, to preserve life, and to help patients through difficult periods. This hero worship is a two-edged sword, however, and although it imbues the physician with extraordinary power that can be used as a placebo effect for healing, it also makes people intolerant of failures or mistakes on the part of a physician and likely to be disgruntled by the physician's deficits. The increase in the frequency and monetary demand of malpractice suits is related to many variables, but one aspect is certainly patient demand for "life-or-death perfection" among physicians, in which their hero is omniscient and omnipotent and should know the etiology and course of disease and have an appropriate cure. The public expects and demands that medicine be an exact science, not an art, and patients have become increasingly dissatisfied with physician ignorance, not just incompetence or negligence.

Looking at the system again, it is true that physicians who have ongoing continuous relationships with patients are the least likely to be sued, even if a mistake appears to be blatant, because patients are less likely to sue physicians whom they perceive as friends and/or social colleagues. Strangers, which are what most highly technical specialists are to their patients, are more likely to be the target of a malpractice suit. Again, then, from a systems' perspective, the trend toward increasing specialization in medicine has changed the relationship between the subsystems of patients and practitioners. Each subsystem has a different alliance with each other than previously, and an adversarial interaction occurs with more frequency.

Patients also demand availability from their physicians, and literally want them to be on call 24 hours a day, seven days a week, to respond to their questions or demands for service. In fact, physician availability is the area of greatest concern or dissatisfaction to patients. In addition, societal elements now expect physicians to be "healthy" themselves and not fall prey to impairment. Citizens, through legislatures and courts, are becoming more active in pressuring organized medicine to "police its own" or laws may be enacted without medicine's input.

Financial aspects and work aspects

Another important element in the United States society contributing to a "pressure cooker environment" for physicians is that of earning an "hourly wage," rather than being in a flat-salary position. It is true for most physicians that time is money, that the number of hours spent in patient care is directly related to their income level. Physicians are tempted to "work overtime" much as are factory workers, to reap the financial benefit of extended time. In fact, many physicians feel like they are trapped in a life "in the hospital factory" and experience the same kind of pressures and stressors that hourly workers do. They do not have a union to work for them for better working conditions and more humane hours. As the financial distribution factor in this society has varied and some occupational groups have actually earned funds up to the level of physicians, there have been morale problems among physicians and a desire to maintain their financial advantage.

Young physicians also feel that they must make a substantial income in their early years of practice because of the expense they incurred during their medical training. Even within the last decade, the cost of medical education has increased dramatically, and students find that they are $40,000 or $80,000 in debt at the completion of their training. They then choose a specialty that will give them a high level of reimbursement, which may also be one that demands long hours.

A systemic compromise

In the last few years, family practice residency faculty have noticed that many graduates are choosing HMOs, urgent-care centers, or emergency rooms for their first postgraduate position. This trend seems to be a direct response to the need to have a determined income level when beginning practice and the unwillingness to borrow yet more money to establish a practice or join a partnership. One other reason that physicians cite for choosing these types of practice situations is that they will have fixed hours, with a light call schedule, and will be able to "have a reasonable schedule" after completing the grueling years of residency training. It does appear that this trend may allow these new graduate physicians to have a more humane schedule and be able to tend to family needs in a more thorough manner than physicians who enter a busy private practice with unspecified hours and a heavy call schedule. The medical system has responded to the demand by one subsystem—patients—for physician availability and the need of the other subsystem—physicians—to not always be available. The proliferation of free-standing emergency rooms and urgent-treatment centers is a development that evolved out of the differing needs of societal subsystems. This development should enable patients to receive services while allowing physicians to have some control over their work schedule.

The Medical System Contribution

Medical system "parents"

For the person matriculating at a medical school, most of the educational role models are physicians who work excessively hard. Students select role models whom they admire and with whom they identify. These are frequently the physicians who work long hours, are most current in the literature in their field, and seem to have time, also, to listen to their students' concerns. It is not possible that these "super docs" have adequate time with their families, if they have them. Another aspect to consider is that the teacher role models may be at a different family–life cycle stage than medical students or residents and thus they may have more time to devote to their career without cheating family life. For instance, they may have already worked out mechanisms by which they and their spouses solve problems, or they may have already raised their children. All the student sees, however, is that the physician is routinely at work 12 or 14 hours a day, and the medical student assumes that he/she must fit into this mold. The younger trainee, however, may have small children at home or is in a marriage at an earlier stage of the family–life cycle, one that needs more attention and work to negotiate a successful relationship. One's peers and colleagues throughout medical training and progression through residency and into practice also reinforce the "workaholic" as a "super doc." In fact, one of the most negative descriptions of any colleague is that he/she seems not to be "really committed" to the practice of medicine.

One crucial aspect of the medical system's contribution to the level of stress among its trainees is the expectation that each trainee must go through the "rite of passage" of internship and residency. Faculty members frequently have the attitude that "they had to work very hard" and thus expect that the younger trainees need to be subjected to a certain amount of hard work and sleepless nights. Povar and Belz (1980) state that the "stress test of one's emotional capacity for punishment takes place during residency where personality, professional obligations, and personal expectations clash with particular force" (p. 632). These authors also note that the lack of sleep occurring during residency often leads to irritability, a state of heightened sensitivity, and depression. They cite a 1975 project that reported that up to 70% of interns were clinically depressed in the first part of their internship year. If a trainee becomes extremely depressed and cannot complete training, the faculty's attitude is often that it is fortunate that this happened then instead of further along in the career, as this is bona fide evidence that the person was not "cut out to be a physician" in the first place.

Scientism

Another contributing factor in the medical system is the ascendancy of science and the scientific mode over earlier cultural values. Scientism is directly related to overwork, partly because of the proliferation of knowledge in all areas but also because of the belief that scientists should take all variables into account and test hypotheses carefully. Medical decision making is, in reality, an educated art at best and cannot follow a scientific protocol that will prevent errors. There are both societal pressures and medical system pressures to view medicine as a science, which places the burden of being exact on physicians when they are diagnosing or treating. Many medical students decide to subspecialize in an area of internal medicine in order to acquire a specific, attainable knowledge base. Most students are horrified at the thought of becoming a family physician, for instance, because the broad array of diverse patients and diseases with which they would deal seems overwhelming. Even the most diligent student or physician makes errors, but the fear of these or of being humiliated by mistakes is enough to cause physicians to read one more article or go back and look at the results of one more laboratory test, when they are stumped by a patient diagnosis. In reality, the dilemma is that even when one "knows everything," it is never quite enough, and the trainees can literally talk themselves into an inferiority complex by realizing the amount of material that they do not know.

The Contribution of Family-of-Origin

The family-of-origin contributes to the phenomenon of "my son, the doctor" in several important ways. One frequently encountered pattern is a family in which one parent, at this point in our culture usually the father, is a physician and the message is conveyed (at least implicitly) that no other occupational choice on the part of the child will be acceptable to the parents. Again, since physicians are at the top of the occupational hierarchy, the family covertly states to the person that no other endeavor will be worthy of him/her. Because of a tendency for intelligence to "regress toward the mean," a child may not have the innate intellectual capacity of his/her parents. Thus, a child may have the desire and family pressure to become a physician, but may entirely lack the intellectual capability to do so. Even when an offspring has clearly superior intelligence, because of the intense competition for slots, the applicant may not be accepted by any medical schools. I suspect that there are strong family-of-origin contributions when United States citizens avail themselves of medical training at the off-shore Caribbean schools. When family-of-origin contributions are not as strong, upon failing admission to medical school, a student may simply decide on graduate training in biology, chemistry, psychology, or some other field that piques his/her interest. When families will not tolerate any other choice, however, the student decides to achieve medical training at all costs, even that of going to a Caribbean school. As the very astute family therapist Jay Haley contends, a scientist can find more evidence that "being a doctor" is inherited than that "being a schizophrenic" is genetically linked.

Self-Contributions

In terms of the person or personality of the physician and the contributions that the self makes to an overly stressed state, the major thing that can be stated is that the physician is a high-achieving person. It is important to recognize the similarities between all high achievers, regardless of their ultimate choice of field or vocation, and to realize that physicians have more similarities than differences to Ph.D.s in biology, physics, or psychology. It is also crucial to note that physicians are not a homogenous group, and individuals vary along many dimensions. The few generalizations that are included, then, in terms of self-contributions must be seen as generalizations which do not apply to many individual cases. It must furthermore be noted that the individual traits of the physician do not exist without the contributions of the context in which they are placed. This discussion is based on the observations, research, and statements of health care professionals about their colleagues.

Povar and Belz (1980), in reviewing the literature on physicians and illness, noted that physicians as a whole are "excessively obedient, quite dependent, and given to passivity and feelings of self-doubt. Poor self-image and a sense of inferiority are common. Reaction formation, a favorite defense, leads physicians to deny these traits and to overcompensate for them" (p. 632). In addition, these authors stated that physicians may develop an authoritarian style, which encourages others to be dependent on them, and may engage in intellectually competitive games to mask their extreme fear of failure. They also stated that physicians do not know how to ask for or give support to others, and that their isolation is one of the major problems that causes them not to seek assistance when under stress.

Bressler (1976), in reiterating the kind of self-contributions described by Povar and Belz, contended that the "altruistic, service-oriented work of a physician can serve deep emotional needs, and for some it can also heal childhood wounds" (p. 172). On the other hand, although physicians "need to be needed," the extreme dependency of patients on them can cause emotional conflicts rather than healing them. Bressler stated that many physicians who were addicted to drugs or alcohol stated that their patients' dependency needs were so emotionally taxing to them that the physicians "had no incentive left for seeking renewal by satifactory relations with spouse, children, friends; by recreation; or by interest in community affairs" (p. 172). In the most severe case, physician suicide is seen as the result of depression caused by this tendency to accept great pressure in one's life.

Bressler contended that most people attempt to achieve both financial and emotional independence through their occupations; physicians, on the other hand, through a type of reaction formation, try to deny their intense dependency needs by overwork. One way for a physician to not feel dependent on his/her spouse, for instance, is to be so busy at the office that there is not enough time for the spouse to feel excessively leaned upon. An extreme analysis of the physician's individual or self-contributions to overwork is the following quote by Mawardi (1976):

> Today many believe that the physician . . . who is completely overwhelmed by the time factor is so because of his own ego. The physician's narcissism keeps him from ever saying "no" or believing that his patients can get along for a day without him. (p. 1486)

MEDICINE AND THE FAMILY-OF-ADULTHOOD*

Medical Marriages

It is a "chicken-or-the-egg" problem to figure out whether physicians have poor marriages because they overwork or overwork because they have poor marriages. It is also impossible to evaluate the relative contributions of personal factors or personality traits in the selection of mates by physicians from the problems that develop as a result of their being influenced by the medical system. One hypothesis might be that physicians (who have certain personality traits such as counterdependency and fear of intimacy) develop marriages low in communication and interaction, which are also encouraged by the medical system, which further along this feedback loop exacerbates the poor marital relationship. Vaillant and Brighton (1970) examined several facets of successful physicians' lives whom they determined to be psychologically healthy. They found that almost half these physicians had poor marital relationships and that 40% were divorced, compared with 14% of the nonphysician control group. These authors contended that the divorces were not caused by hard work or long hours, rather that the physicians accepted long hours as a response to their unhappy marriages.

Communication and Interaction

Gerber's (1983b) contention that physicians and spouses do not have time for the important work of couple interaction, such as working out fighting, sexuality, or issues about child rearing, is very significant. Physicians do not

---

*Family-of-adulthood is used rather than family-of-procreation in deference to couples who do not have children.

have the time or psychological space in which to perform this important couple work with their spouses. Physician couples tend to have low communication and low interaction. Systems theorists have proposed that the role of angry interactions between spouses can stabilize a dysfunctional system (Lederer & Jackson, 1978). An interesting corollary to this can be proposed: Detached partner situations wherein the spouses have low contact and no angry exchanges may lead to system instability. Physicians and their spouses frequently do not "have time for" angry exchanges and neglect the important work of couple interaction, disagreement, and resolution. They frequently rigidify into a particular pattern revolving around role issues (Glick & Borus, 1984). They are especially likely to divorce during transitional stages, such as at the completion of medical school, the end of internship, or the end of a residency, which indicates that the couples are not able to work out new ways of dividing responsibilities between professional and family tasks.

In the Perlow and Mullins (1976) study of medical student marriages, there was a strong association between degree of communication between marital partners and marital satisfaction. Also, there was a correlation between degree of communication and the congruence of expected and performed roles among marital partners. The authors concluded that effective communication in medical student marriages is a crucial variable in creating a satisfactory relationship. One way to increase communication would be to undertake marital counseling during medical school. Perlow and Mullins reported that 38% of physician spouses indicated that their marriages could have profited from counseling, although most were satisfied with their marriages.

Equality

Another important element has to do with the perceived equality of power between physicians and their spouses. It appears that "for marriages to work or for discord to abate, there has to be a perceived equality of power. . . . This equality . . . refers mainly to the level of compromise between wishes such that both spouses' subjective worlds are appreciated to an equal extent" (Seagraves, 1982, p. 247). One of Gerber's (1983b) major points is that physicians and their spouses need to have a relationship that contains this perceived equality. Gerber suggested that it is important for the physicians' spouses to have careers or daily activities that are significant to them, which balances the importance of the physicians' career. Although this appears to be an excellent suggestion that might lead to less marital discord, it does not account for the fact that the expectations for physicians' practices were based on a model in which physicians had spouse-supporters at home maintaining the household while they worked. As Glick and Borus (1984) pointed out, male physicians have frequently selected a marital partner who will abandon her career needs to meet the needs of her husband's profession and will "mind the home store" while the husband devotes his energies to medicine. One way to understand the idea of career equality among physicians and spouses and the demands of medicine is that our expectations for marital equality and balanced relationships have changed, but have not been paralleled by changing expectations about the time and energy that physicians devote to their career. In other words, the expectations within the family system have changed in one direction, but the family system's relationship to the economy or the outside societal forces has not. Physicians who have equal marriages, then, may be extremely stressed in their careers because the type of spouse support that the medical system expects cannot be maintained when the spouses have busy careers.

Real-Ideal Discrepancies

One way persons get dissatisfied with their marital relationships is by having a large ideal versus real discrepancy, that is, a discrepancy between their relationships as they actually perceive them and their desired or expected relationships. I propose that the greater the ideal versus real discrepancy, the greater the level of dissatisfaction. One phenomenon that occurs in physician families is "waiting for someday" (Gerber, 1983a), in which family members think that they will have more time together or a better relationship when medical school is completed, when residency is completed, or after a certain number of years in practice. What most of those families discover at some point is that "someday" never comes, and that the physician continues to maintain the same amount of time away from the family as he/she did early in the career. At some point, then, the physician or the spouse realizes that the discrepancy between their real relationship and the one that they desire is always going to be maintained at the current level, and their dissatisfaction with this arrangement becomes more pronounced, to the point that separation or divorce is considered. As some of Gerber's interviewees explained, it appears that a division of time and labor develops early in the marital relationships and medical careers of the families, which tends to be maintained during later stages of career and family development. Members of the family should not expect that tomorrow will bring a significant change and need to work during early stages of career development to get time for family matters.

Burr (1971) contends that role discrepancy is inversely related to marital satisfaction. When one's spouse expects certain roles to be performed by the other and the actual performance of these roles meets the expected performance, harmonious marital interaction results. If, however, various points of conflict arise, each marital partner is likely to rate the marriage as unsatisfactory. Discrepancies may occur in several target areas of marital roles and responsibilities: financial considerations, marital relationship activities, sexual activities, recreational activities, child rearing, relationships to family-of-origin, and various aspects of social behavior outside the marriage.

Physician Stress During Divorce

One of the most insightful discoveries of family systems theory is that a seemingly "weak" partner may actually maintain more strength in the couples' balance of power than the apparently "strong" partner (Sluzki, 1978). Thus, a physician may be thought by the couple to be the "strong" one because of the prestige and importance of the career position, and it may be incorrectly assumed that the physician will fare best if the couple decides to divorce. Interestingly, this is frequently not the case, as the physician dissolves into helplessness and despair, while the spouse sets about creating a new life. In the physician's world there is an incredible amount of hidden dependency—there is always someone to answer the telephone, balance the books, make appointments, or prepare patients for examinations. Often at home, family life is organized around the M.D.'s timetable and career, and the needs of the physician are met "on demand." When this is no longer the case during the transition of divorce, physicians may be ill equipped to handle the enforced independency that is thrust on them.

PARENT-CHILD RELATIONSHIPS

The "E and D Syndrome"

When one parent is overly involved in his/her career outside the household, or other extrafamilial activities, a common pattern emerges in which the children or a particular child will be overly involved, or enmeshed, with the parent who is at home and relatively disengaged from the parent who is outside the home. This phenomenon can be referred to as the "e and d syndrome." Family therapists usually designate this as an enmeshed family with a peripheral parent, but I think it is essential to stress that there is both enmeshment and disengagement occurring simultaneously in the family milieu from the child's perspective.

When one parent in the family is a physician, there are many societal, organizational, collegial, and intrapersonal forces that lead to a situation of an extremely imbalanced bond between children and parents. The systemic forces exerted on a physician are likely to result in a dysfunctional family structure. In fact, it is important to note that the physician must exert an incredible amount of energy to resist this natural trend and to counter the variables that lead to family dysfunction. He/she must stand against educational ideas, societal expectations, and his/her own conscience to devote a balanced amount of time and energy to family life. It cannot be emphasized too strongly that it is a "no-win" situation; in almost all instances, the physician who devotes an adequate amount of time to family for healthy family functioning is seen as negligent in his/her clinical or professional duties. To win in this situation, a physician must be able to garner sufficient feelings of self-esteem and competence from "involved parenting" and be able to feel adequate in professional duties, despite medical colleagues not being as laudatory as one would wish.

The "D and D Syndrome"

The disengagement and disengagement syndrome occurs when both physician and spouse are overly engaged outside the household and thus disengaged from the children. When the societal sector demands full-time employment of persons in the work force, and both parents work, the child or children seem to get a lesser share of parental time and energy. Although this phenomenon can certainly occur just as easily when Papa is a police officer and Mama is an administrative secretary, there seems to be a greater pull when both parents are health professionals. When "doctor marries doctor" (Magee & Magee, 1983), the children are at least more prone to guilt if they request that parents take time off for family activities than when the parents' occupations do not require care giving to other people. Although this pattern in which the parents are both involved outside the family in careers is healthier in the sense of providing parental balance, it may be more taxing or stressful than for the children in the previously described "e and d syndrome." The child's resentment about lack of parental involvement will be more evenly distributed between parents, however, and an unhealthy state of triangulation may be less likely. With strong extended-family ties, or a live-in caretaker with children, the effect of overly busy parents might be less stressful. If someone is at home to care for the children on an ongoing basis, a healthy family milieu can exist with parents who are overly stressed in the workplace. It is also important to underscore that the family–life cycle stage is a variable in this situation, and when parents are both busy outside the household during children's infancy or in the very later stages of child rearing, this may be less stressful to children than during the crucial middle years.

Career Success and Self-Esteem

One of the difficulties in this situation for physicians is that they are very oriented toward concrete facts and quantitative data. It is easy to quantify one's "success" in terms of number of patients seen, number of obscure illnesses diagnosed, number of successful surgeries performed, or any other criterion of professional life. It is much more difficult to feel competent as a spouse or as a parent if a person is oriented toward facts and data. What would the physician do: Count the number of times spouse or children make appreciative remarks? Look for the results of good parenting in successful child behavior? Count the number of laughs by each family member that would indicate their happiness? It is very difficult for persons to feel successful at family interactions, as they always involve ambivalent feelings and actions and cannot be calibrated. It is very seductive for a successful professional (again, it must be emphasized that this is not unique to physicians) to be lured into focusing more and more on his/her career because of the ability to set goals and successfully meet them in the professional arena as compared to the family sphere.

I have observed middle-aged parents where the physician-father, who had delegated all child-care responsibilities to the mother, felt very exasperated when the child ran into difficulty. He sincerely believed that as parents, neither he nor his wife had been successful, whereas he had been very successful in bringing home money and furthering his career for the betterment of the family. The path to success in academic medicine is clear: One must develop skills as an excellent clinical teacher, one must perform some service commitments, and one must research, research, research. As long as one is academically capable, is careful to select an appropriate area of research, and has enough social skills to be promoted to committee assignments, he/she can attain the desired status of tenured and promoted full professor. There certainly are some variables, extraneous to competence, that impinge on the success of one's career, such as procuring grants through contacts with persons across the nation, but these seem manageable to the academician. To be a successful parent, however, involves many extraneous variables not in the control of the physician. Peer group influences, media exposure, the illicit drug trade are all variables that may make the best of parenting attempts unlikely to create the kind of child that one desired. It is a natural, instinctive human tendency to move toward certain success rather than nebulous success or failure. And that, unfortunately, is the choice of many physicians. Likewise, in terms of success at being a spouse, with divorce being as prevalent as it is, many persons—certainly not just physicians—question their ability to successfully matriculate the curriculum of marriage and create a viable relationship over a long period of time. Again, when stressors occur, it is easier to be lured into overwork with immediate rewards and tangible indicators of progress than to stay at home and battle out a relationship to see if "success" might be obtained.

Medical Roles and Sex Roles

Being a wife-mother-doctor is different from being a husband-father-doctor. For women physicians who also marry and have children, the task of keeping their stress level within reasonable limits may be more difficult than for many of their male colleagues. Societal expectations of wife and mother are that she will spend a considerable portion of time or energy on family activities, and she is considered negligent if she does not. A wife-mother-doctor is literally in the "hot seat" of conflicting roles and finds that she cannot meet her own, her spouse's, her in-laws, or society's expectations of achievement in any one of the roles. Unlike her male counterpart, if she succeeds at her professional role better than her other roles, she is frequently seen as being selfish or self-centered, and not being a good wife or mother. Similarly, if she also outshines her husband in the professional sphere, she may be accused of not devoting enough time and energy to support her husband in his career. These kinds of expectations are never leveled against a man: If he succeeds in his professional life, he may not be lauded as being an exemplary husband or father, but neither will he be often criticized. The importance of a man's success in the professional sphere has been enculturated so completely that it is the only area in which success is crucial to other's perceptions or a man's own self-esteem. For a woman, the prevailing attitude is still: "Be a good wife and mother, and if you have time beyond that to be professionally successful, then more power to you. But if you succeed at the cost of wifery and motherhood, then you have gained nothing and will lose self-esteem and the esteem of others." There is no way to adequately emphasize the amount of guilt that professional women feel in trying to balance roles of wife/mother and career professional. When the sitter drops the child off after a workday, it is usually the wife, not the husband, who makes apologies for the mess in the living room, the dirty dishes in the sink, or the garbage smelling in the kitchen. Even if one or more of those tasks are clearly the husband's responsibility, it is still the wife who often feels the public shame for failing at important expectations concerning household tasks.

If a woman becomes pregnant during internship or residency, she experiences both overt and covert censure by her colleagues, male and female alike. The fact that she will disrupt part of her training, be unavailable for some of the call schedule, and alter other trainees' schedules is enough for them to think (at least fleetingly) that medicine would be better off by not admitting women. There will even be jokes to this effect, and the woman is expected to laugh good-naturedly at comments such as, "That's why we shouldn't let women in medicine; they're always going to be off having babies." The only "happy baby" stories I have heard in the family-practice residencies in which I have worked are when a third-year resident becomes pregnant during the latter part of the third year, and the baby is obviously going to be due after the end of her training. Then the trainees seem to be able unequivocally to share her joy. There does not seem to be the same ambivalence when one of the male trainees is expecting a new baby in his household before training ends, and the teasing is not of the same nature.

There is, in fact, no "good time" for a woman trainee to have a baby either during medical school, internship, residency, fellowship, or early practice. A number of trainees delay childbearing until completion of their residencies, but as one third-year resident (who is in her midthirties) said to me recently, she does not see how she will be able to manage a child with her new practice responsibilities after graduation and feels that she is indeed too old to raise a child at this point. With the recent change in medical-education standards, so that older persons are accepted into medical school and residencies, one pattern that has seemed to work well for women is to have children before medical school and residency training, as it does seem more possible with older children to combine a strenuous schedule and parenting. Another model, that of having a househusband, who would take care of the household responsibilities while the physician trained and practiced, is used by some persons, but certainly has more social censure for both the woman physician and her spouse than does the sex-reversed pattern. There is always the choice of not marrying and not having children, which does reduce role strain in many ways. However, as reported in several studies, single younger women physicians are at great risk for depression and suicide; so this does not necessarily lead to better emotional health.

It is easy to determine and perceive the essential conflicts between roles for women in medicine. One interesting observation is that the "essential harmony between 'feminine' role expectations and the caretaking activities of medicine is often ignored" (Notman & Nadelson, 1973, p. 1126). In one sense, women providing health care as physicians is an extension of their frequent role in families, that of a family health specialist. Individuals consult physicians for about one of seven illnesses and have the remainder treated in their family situation, usually by women. In this light, the nurturing, caretaking role of women and that of providing professional health care is complementary, not conflicting. One problem is that organized medicine demands so much time and energy of its practitioners that it is difficult for them to balance caretaking in their own families and in their professional lives. As a seasoned woman pediatrician reported to me recently, she was unaware that one of her children had pneumonia for a week, as her conviction was that anyone ill in her family just had a mild virus, as she was going off to the hospital to care for the "really sick people."

Although the Glick and Borus (1984) article details many crucial dilemmas regarding role conflicts and status and power issues, the entire focus is on *male* physicians and their spouses. In fact, the authors imply that the cultural changes in male-female relationships may lead to increased marital dissatisfaction:

> With so many young physicians' wives not accepting the notion that they should devote themselves to family matters at the expense of their own careers, there is often no one at home "minding the family store" while the young physician is heavily engaged in his training or early practice. (Glick & Borus, 1984, p. 1856)

For women physicians, it is even less likely that there will be someone at home "minding the family store" while they are involved in their professional duties.

Some academic disciplines have accounted for this societal or historical change in regard to families and have encouraged fathers to take "paternity leave" at the time of the birth of their children and to be involved in child rearing in the early stages. In fact, the whole interest of bonding between parents and children, including fathers, and the role of fathering in child development became a popular topic in psychology in the 1970s. From anecdotal reports, men in psychology were encouraged by their colleagues to develop an active role in the family and home life, whereas men in medicine have not been subjected to the same attitude by the system in which they live and work. In fact, medical colleagues, again from anecdotal reports, tend to show a pitying attitude toward a male colleague who is overstressed or overworked and spending a substantial amount of time on home and family tasks. The prevailing attitude still seems to be "Poor Joe, he would have the misfortune to have married Susan, a devoted career woman, so that he simply has too much to do at home and cannot fulfill his professional obligations adequately."

As Dr. John Nackashi (1984), a pediatrician specializing in developmental pediatrics, stated, "A male can be gone for 36 hours and people say that's alright because he's taking care of people, he's doing something good. But if a female doctor is gone for 36 hours, people think it's terrible that she is neglecting her family. There is a definite dichotomy." Nackashi, who considers himself a very involved family man, has said that he experiences disapproval from his medical colleagues about his priority on family responsibilities. It is probable that this attitude—traditional versus nontraditional—is somewhat regionally based, and physicians training and practicing in more progressive areas of the country would find the attitudes of their colleagues to be more supportive of their attentions being split between medicine and home and family.

One possible way to conceptualize the current dynamic is that the expectations and roles of males in families is in flux as far as the societal or historical contribution, and yet the expectations of the medical system have not kept pace with the developments about family responsibility in the societal sector. Societal expectations include, then, that a male physician both put in his 70- or 80-hour work week in his office and hospital setting and also demand a full 20 hours of time allocated to the home environment. Male physicians, then, are for the first time embroiled in the type of role conflict that female physicians have always known. The way adjustments and compromises will be made between various sectors and their expectations will be interesting to note in the coming decades.

PREVENTION OF FAMILY DYSFUNCTION AMONG PHYSICIAN FAMILIES

The Life of Physicians: The Great Balancing Act

A strategy to prevent family dysfunction among physicians and their "significant others" would involve methods to prevent disengagement, the phenomenon of a peripheral parent, and excessive stress. The strategy would also offer leisure/relaxation time during training and appropriate role models of physicians who balance career and family. Educational programs that address physicians and stress are crucial. One aspect that needs attention are methods of studying time and energy limits and avoiding the trap of trying to be "superhuman" at all activities. Another important phenomenon involves the idea that it is difficult to feel successful as a parent or spouse in the same manner that one can feel accomplished at work tasks. Physicians can quantitatively measure their success at work, but cannot assess their competency at home. Trying to sensitize physicians-in-training to ways of assessing competence in their personal sphere is crucial. Balancing time commitments, emotional energy, and work energy between home, career, and time for oneself is a very delicate and difficult procedure. Although the dilemma of this balancing act is not unique to people who practice medicine, but must be undertaken by all persons in demanding job situations, the seductiveness of medicine may be more powerful than that of other career callings, and the system of medicine encourages the physician to "forget home and self for the sake of the profession."

Parent-Child Subsystem Interaction

Parental-child hierarchy

Parents should keep the parental-child hierarchy clear, partly by joining in decision making and rule setting. All major decisions or rules should be clearly presented as those of both parents as a unit, and if one parent is absent when a major decision must be made, the decision should be delayed until the other parent has input, by telephone call or actual presence. It is crucial for children to feel that the parental hierarchy is acting as a unit, and that the parents will together structure the child's privileges, restrictions, and responsibilities. The danger in the physician's family is that the other parent gets relegated most of the child-rearing responsibilities, with the physician becoming a peripheral and noninvolved member.

Family time

Plan family together time on a daily basis, even if it is a very short period of time. Children need predictable "together time" with both parents. This could be a mealtime, a bedtime story, some activity in morning, afternoon, or evening; there must be some "special" time for the child with each parent. Plan a special activity separate from this daily contact on a weekly basis for all children. This kind of regularly scheduled family activity should help to prevent disengagement of the family members from the physician and the physician from the family members.

Children's concerns

Families should also devote a time to listen to the children's concerns on a regular basis, through some kind of family forum or weekly or monthly session. At this time, children can be listened to and take an active part in deciding how to solve some of the problems that parents and children have between them.

Children's "specialness"

Gerber stated that each physician spouse should have a strong interest of his/her own, such as a career, to maintain proper balance between spouses.

I think it is also crucial in maintaining proper balance in the entire family system, for *each child* to have a special interest or activity that is shared in the family on a regular basis. One way for the child not to feel that the physician-parent is the only "special" one in the family would be to have sufficient attention directed to the interest, activities, or achievements of other family members. One way to accomplish this would be to have a sharing time each week in which family members discuss what has been most significant for them during the week, and this gets recognized by the other family members.

Spouse Subsystem Needs

Intimacy needs

It is essential that marital partners' intimacy needs be met by planning "special" time on a daily basis and a weekly basis with one's spouse. Again, the amount of time or the activity needs to be determined by each individual couple or family, but the necessity for some contact on a regular basis is essential to healthy family functioning.

Communication

Plan some time for problem solving and trouble shooting. It is best not to let all problem solving occur during high-intensity, highly emotional periods in which a problem is at its apex. Regularly scheduled sessions designed for problem-solving allow difficulties to be confronted, discussed, and resolved in a more appropriate fashion. It is Gerber's (1983b) contention that medical marriages lack the "little bits of time" essential for couple conflict negotiation and resolution.

Autonomy needs

It is frequently helpful for both members of a couple to confront directly one partner's high need for autonomy and the other partner's comfort with the level of autonomy required by the partner. At least in regard to time, physicians need a high amount of separate time and thus autonomy. Often, however, the nonphysician spouse can be comfortable with or tolerate a higher degree of autonomy if certain rituals are put into the daily routine. Frequently just remembering to say a special "good-bye" in the morning or being certain there is one phone call to give some prediction as to the time that the physician will return can allay the anxieties of the person who is experiencing some separation anxiety. The most destructive pattern is for the physician to not only require and demand the high level of autonomy, but then blame the other spouse for excessive dependency when he/she is not comfortable with this arrangement. Again, this occurs in a context in which the physician does not recognize his/her own dependency because others in the medical system are always there for support. Reassurance and some positive statements appreciating the value of the other partner can go a long way in creating a healthy milieu in which long periods of separation are required. One couple with whom I worked solved part of this problem by having the husband write a note to the wife each morning on a 3 × 5 card that he regularly used to write up case presentation notes. The note would frequently say, "I shall think of you at 12 o'clock and send you loving thoughts." These kinds of strategies, although props at best, can help persons develop comfort with the realities of their situation.

Encourage appropriate autonomy by planning some recreational or other "alone time." Although individuals vary in their need for recreational time that includes others and that which is solely the province of one alone, persons should attend to their own needs and desires and be certain that they have some "alone time" that is relaxing and stress reducing to them. Again, the amount of time available for this will be somewhat dependent on career state and family life-cycle stage, and during early years of training or practice and early years of childbearing, "alone time" may need to be excluded in deference to other needs.

Sharing responsibility

Physicians and their spouse should share parental and family responsibilities to prevent imbalance. Being certain that the physician/parent has a daily predictable "interaction" or "duty" role with children is essential to prevent an imbalance. This interaction time or activity could be driving the children to school, fixing their breakfast, reading their bedtime story, bathing them, or whatever arrangement is comfortable for both spouses. Not only will this improve the sense of equality and sharing between the spouses who are overly busy in the outside world, but it will also send the message to all family members that the physician is crucial to family maintenance. Having home responsibilities also makes the physician feel needed and wanted at home, much as he/she is needed at the office or the hospital. Physicians often report that they feel like a "stranger" at home—an extra wheel—whereas they feel that they are an essential part of their "office family" or their "hospital family." Having essential responsibilities at home prevents this pattern of imbalance.

Self-Needs

In terms of their personal contribution to preventing impairment, physicians should watch certain life-style variables such as their exercise, drug use, or other health-related activities. Physicians could solicit support for maintaining their use at a low level or decreasing their use or could encourage family members to participate in a group exercise program. Physicians also need to set realistic goals that include time for all essential activities in their lives. They may need to do some self-evaluation or counseling around their excessive need for accomplishment or success and need to get their expectations for achievement whittled down to human size. They also might profitably avail themselves of stress-management techniques and discuss with one of their colleagues or a mental health professional how to handle life stressors.

A recent development in the medical field has been an emphasis on the role of exercise and the reduction of negative health behaviors such as smoking, overeating, and alcohol use in producing a healthier state for both patients and health care providers. There has been increasing emphasis on physicians using the program that they have established in hospitals for cardiac rehabilitation as a preventive measure, to maintain a state of health that is seen as good for them as well as an appropriate role model for their patients. Physicians who still smoke are looked at askance by their colleagues, and the percentage of physicians who smoke has decreased significantly over the last few decades. The notion of the impaired physician has become popular, and many programs have been developed to address this pressing need of the health care system. These movements have legitimized the necessity for a physician to take care of himself/herself and have brought into question the idea that the physician should run at full speed until he/she collapses.

Let it be hoped that a comprehensive program, as outlined here, might be able to prevent drug and alcohol abuse, depression, and suicide where the following "premorbid signs have been noted: A rushed existence under continuous pressure, doubts as to one's professional competence, endless doctoring, and the apparent inability to relax and recharge the battery through interpersonal relationships" (Bressler, 1976, p. 173).

REFERENCES

Boorstin, D. J. (1974). *The Americans: The democratic experience*. New York: Vintage.
Bressler, B. (1976). Suicide and drug abuse in the medical community. *Suicide and Life-Threatening Behavior, 6,* 169–178.
Brody, H., & Sobel, D. S. (1979). A systems view of health and disease. In D. S. Sobel (Ed.), *Ways of health*. New York: Harcourt, Brace, and Jovanovich.

Burr, W. R. (1971). An expansion and test of a role theory of marital satisfaction. *Journal of Marriage and the Family, 33*, 368–378.

Gerber, L. A. (1983a). *Married to their careers: Career and family dilemmas in doctor's lives.* New York: Tavistock.

Gerber, L. A. (1983b). Medical marriages: Healthy and dysfunctional families. Presented at Society for Teachers of Family Medicine Conference on Working with Families IV, March 11, 1983, Newport Beach, California.

Glick, I. D., & Borus, J. F. (1984). Marital and family therapy for troubled physicians and their families: A bridge over troubled waters. *Journal of the American Medical Association, 251*(14), 1855–1858.

Haseltine, F., & Yaw, Y. (1976). *Woman doctor.* New York: Ballantine.

Kanter, R. M. (1977). *Men and women of the corporation.* New York: Basic Books.

Lederer, W. J., & Jackson, D. D. (1978). *The mirages of marriage.* New York: Norton.

Magee, M. C., & Magee, J. E. (1983). Stress in the dual career marriage: When doctor marries doctor. Presented at 16th Annual Spring Conference of Society for Teachers of Family Medicine, May 8, 1983, Boston, Massachusetts.

Mawardi, B. H. (1976). Satisfactions, dissatisfactions, and causes of stress in medical practice. *Journal of the American Medical Association, 241*, 1483–1486.

Minuchin, S., Rosman, B. L., & Baker, L. (1978). *Psychosomatic families: Anorexia nervosa in context.* Cambridge: Harvard University Press.

Nackashi, J. (1984). Male consciousness-raising and the fathering movement. Presented at Conference on sexual exploitation: Origins, consequences, and strategies for change, May 17, 1984, Gainesville, Fla.

Notman, M. T., & Nadelson, C. C. (1973). Medicine: A career conflict for women. *American Journal of Psychiatry, 130*, 1123–1126.

Perlow, A. D., Mullins, S. C. (1976). Marital satisfaction as perceived by the medical student's spouse. *Journal of Medical Education, 51*, 726–734.

Povar, G. J. & Belz, M. (1980). Helping ourselves. *Journal of Medical Education, 55*, 632–634.

Ransom, D. C., & Massad, R. J. (1978). Family structure and function. In R. E. Rakel & H. F. Conn (Eds.), *Family practice* (2nd ed.). Philadelphia: W. B. Saunders.

Seagraves, R. T. (1982). *Marital therapy: A combined psychodynamic-behavioral approach.* New York: Plenum.

Sluzki, C. E. (1978). Marital therapy from a systems perspective. In T. J. Paolino, Jr., & B. S. McCrady (Eds.), *Marriage and marital therapy.* New York: Brunner/Mazel.

Vaillant, G. E., & Brighton, J. R. (1970). Physicians' use of mood-altering drugs: A 20-year follow-up report. *New England Journal of Medicine, 282*, 365–370.

von Bertalanffy, L. (1968). *General systems theory.* New York: Braziller.

Watzlawick, P., Beavin, J., & Jackson, D. D. (1967). *Pragmatics of human communication.* New York: Norton.

Chapter 8

Physicians in Transition: Crisis and Change in Life and Work

Dennis T. Jaffe, Ph.D.,
Michael S. Goldstein, Ph.D.,
and Josie Wilson, M.A.

In recent years, increasing attention has been focused on personal change throughout adult life (Gould, 1978; Levinson, 1978). Adults almost predictably experience significant changes in work, marriage, and family, and what is important to them. Although such changes affect those in every occupation and profession, physicians have been increasingly prone to such shifts. New patterns of medical practice, new health care settings and institutions, the rise of new techniques, and increasing variability in physician work styles have led to drastic changes in the nature of medical work. The traditional path of a stable practice, like the traditional personal developmental path of marriage, family, and children, can no longer be assumed to fit the career of many physicians. The contemporary physician can expect to face crises, changes, and shifts both in his/her personal life and values and in his/her way of practicing medicine.

In many situations, changes in personal life and career are strongly connected. This chapter deals with a special group of physicians who have experienced change in both their work and personal lives. Its aim is to show that under certain circumstances burnout may lead to a positive outcome. In at least some instances, personal crisis and dissatisfaction with medicine can lead to a new perspective on medicine, style of practice, and way of living.

In 1982, we interviewed 40 physicians who were members of a support group called "Physicians in Transition." The group met weekly, with continually changing membership, in Los Angeles during the years 1978 to 1983. Most physicians joined the group because they were experiencing some dissatisfaction in their medical work, or because certain personal changes or shifts had led them to look for ways to change professionally.

This group offers an interesting vantage point on the issue of burnout, values, and career satisfaction. There has been much concern about the phenomenon of "burnout" in the health professions (Freudenberger, 1980; Pines et al., 1981). Burnout has been defined as a state of extreme dissatisfaction with one's work, distancing from patients, impaired performance, low energy, and many related signs of impairment and depression. Using these criteria, many of the physicians in this group exhibited signs of burnout. But Physicians in Transition provided them with a social support group that redefined the frustrations and locus of their problems and directed them to nontraditional solutions.

Physicians came to this group because they perceived themselves as changing, often in both their personal and professional lives. Often these changes involved exploring new ideas and practices in medicine. Our interviews sought their perceptions of the process of change, its origins, and the effects of the change process on their medical work and their personal lives. The physicians we studied ranged in age from 33 to 64, were in both private and salaried practice positions (60% and 40%, respectively), and represented a range of specialties, with practices appropriate to their training. On the surface, and to the medical community, they appeared to be conventional physicians (see Goldstein and co-workers, 1985, for details of the study and its findings).

Yet during the period in which they belonged to the group, their way of seeing medicine and many aspects of their work changed profoundly. A number of the physicians saw the addition of a new "holistic" orientation to their work as a solution to both their personal/existential crisis and their professional burnout/dissatisfaction. This chapter summarizes some of the themes and processes that accompanied these transitions. Echoing Cherniss (1980), our suggestion is that for some health professionals, burnout can be seen as a response to certain structural problems and professional expectations concerning medical practice. Our study builds on this idea and identifies several ways in which burnout can lead to a positive resolution and to further personal and professional development.

THE HOLISTIC ORIENTATION: AN ALTERNATIVE

The group was identified with an orientation to health, healing, and illness that has been called holistic (Hastings et al., 1981), and about two thirds of the physicians we interviewed identified themselves with this perspective. Although holistic health/medicine is often linked in the popular mind with a range of specific techniques (e.g., Oriental medicine, homeopathy), it is more properly understood as an approach to understanding the nature of health, healing, and the practice of medicine. Although there is no clear definition of holistic health/medicine, the following characteristics are often associated with it:

1. An understanding of health, disease, and healing is based on the integration of the individual's physical, psychological, and spiritual dimensions.
2. Spirituality is seen as particularly crucial to healing.
3. Stress is seen as a general underlying issue in creating illness.
4. Life-style changes are included as part of treatment, to reduce risk factors in diet, activity, and stress response patterns.
5. The positive value of non-Western and nonempirically validated healing techniques is emphasized.
6. The individual is actively included in the treatment process and is seen as sharing responsibility for creating and maintaining health.
7. The social distance between patients and healers is minimized.
8. Medicine is seen more as an interactive educational process than as a series of active, often invasive interventions on a passive, uninvolved patient.

STAGES AND DETERMINANTS OF CHANGE

Four aspects of the transition process were common in the histories of our respondents. Although these themes often followed each other in sequence, in many respondents the themes were intertwined, and different themes or progressions were observed. However, we believe that these four stages, in whatever order, represent a model of the life/work transition process:

1. *Dissatisfaction* with medicine in general and one's own personal expectations of what being a physician would be like.

2. The *possibility of a new way* to practice and relate to medicine, which the physician learned about through books, articles, seminars, and conversations with other changing practitioners.
3. A *personal crisis or change period*, frequently a psychological or family crisis, perhaps a divorce, or a personal experience of illness. The crisis came commonly as a result of experiences (personal therapy, workshops, readings) in the new medicine, or the personal or marital crisis in some way led the physician to seek new ways and possibilities.
4. The outcome, which took the form of *a new approach to medical practice*.

Stage 1: Dissatisfaction and Burnout

Cherniss (1980) relates professional burnout generally to the frustration of idealistic expectations, the difficulty of feeling competent in one's work, and the lack of professional support and interaction. Our respondents generally met these criteria. For example, one physician talked about growing more unhappy with his busy office practice and about what he learned from three years of psychotherapy:

> In those three years I really got in touch with a lot of my feelings. I had gone through medical school, and I was trained in a certain way, and I was really a robot of the medical system. I was just carrying out what had been rigidly taught to me. In retrospect I see why I was uncomfortable. I was taught in a rigid way that things have to be done this way, investigated in such and such a way, and in the ensuing three years I found out it doesn't have to be, that there are alternatives, other ways. That's really been exciting. On the other hand, I feel angry at the fact that the system I went through is so narrow.

This physician, like several others, mentioned the difficulty of reconciling the heavy demands of medical practice with personal and family lives, the mechanistic and limited focus of medical practice with palliation of symptoms, the inability to really "cure" many ailments that were presented, the focus on making money and the consequent rush through patient visits, and the lack of spirituality and concern with the suffering of the whole person. The medical practices and settings these physicians worked in were perceived by them to lack sufficient care, to be devoid of personal support for their work, and did not seem to address what they felt were the more central questions of life, death, and healing that they wanted to explore.

These dissatisfactions grew in intensity, leading most of our respondents to certain physical and emotional symptoms of professional burnout—depression, physical illness, cynicism, detachment, alienation, extreme tiredness, and emotional withdrawal. One physician reports:

> I was married, and I slowly noticed that I was going crazy and doing crazy things. Self-destructive. I had to reassess my life. There were a number of interests and feelings that I had completely discounted for a number of years, such as that I had a lot of creative energy that was completely untapped in my medical work. There were whole areas in me that were capable of being in touch with forces in the universe, sources in myself, emotions, shutoff grief, and a lot of stuff. It was the unhappiness of the total trap I had forced myself into—I was going to be a surgeon, I was in an unhappy marriage, and I began to crack and then began to shift.

Stage 2: A New Way

At some time, these physicians became aware of the fact that others were experiencing the same problems and were proposing some novel responses. They learned of this from a variety of sources. They read popular and professional books, they heard of innovative medical practices and approaches from the popular media, they attended lectures and workshops by a variety of professional organizations, and many met a teacher or professional mentor who exemplified the new perspective and taught it to other physicians. Several such mentors had been associated with the Center for Healing Arts that initiated the transition group. It is possible that the presence of many such resources in California is an impetus to more physicians becoming involved in holistic medicine.

A typical reaction to these resources was the following:

> All of a sudden I noticed, as I started reading and going to these workshops, that everything started to be interconnected in a way. There was a group of people, literature, that seemed to be pointing in a similar direction, that was giving me security and trust in what I was doing. Instead of feeling alone and confused, I found not only did other people share my views, but there were other people who were even more involved in this, who had been doing it for a number of years. I felt validated. I think the validation was a tremendous springboard for me.

The presence of resources and support shifts a confused and tentative dissatisfaction to a clearer direction.

Of particular importance to these changing physicians was locating a professional support network that supported them in their exploration of new ideas. Many of our respondents reported initially feeling isolated, weird, irresponsible, and having negative confrontations with other physicians in their community. For example, one physician was surprised to meet one of his colleagues at a holistic conference, as neither had spoken openly of this exploration, and another reported intense criticism when he wrote that he "prayed" with a patient in the hospital chart.

After an experience of confrontation, or aloneness and isolation, the relief and validation resulting from locating a group of like-minded colleagues, who shared information and offered support, was often a critical juncture in crystallizing incipient change:

> I went off for three months with my family after my residency. I was in the midst of a virtual paradise where I had nothing to do and I discovered I was as adept at being depressed there as anywhere else. The depression was an experience that comes from the inside, and I learned that in the face of the void of not working, the unconscious mind will create whatever is necessary to fill up the void, and sometimes that's a physical disease. I knew I had to come back to the city and establish a practice.
>
> I went into practice with a friend who is a minister. So here you have this rebel psychiatrist and rebel minister who is a psychologist, and what we discovered was that in his training he had learned nothing about God, and in my medical training I had learned nothing about healing. So we started exploring what our training hadn't taught us, and we started exploring the interface between the physical body, emotions, and the spiritual. What became the most profound part of our growth was our relationship. Not only ours but the relationship with my family.

Stage 3: Personal Crisis

In our interviews, we found three major pathways through the four stages that we are proposing. Three case examples will each illustrate one of these routes. About a third of our respondents took each route.

The gradual route was taken by physicians who had always had a spiritual perspective in their work, and who came to see holistic medicine as an appropriate framework for expressing these long-standing beliefs. Dr. Ellen S. was a psychiatrist who married another psychiatrist during her residency. They trained together, developed practices, and had a child. She reports that she was always religious and always restless with what was being held up to her as good clinical practice. She felt that there was something wrong with the general medical orientation, which emphasized distance and deemphasized the importance of spirituality. Her husband did not share her feelings, and she did not pursue them. After a few years of practice, she began to attend workshops and seminars in holistic medicine, where she received support for the perspective she had put aside. In part because their differences in style and values could no longer be reconciled, they divorced. She continued to develop her expertise in holistic medicine, gradually modifying her practice, which she began to do at home, to fit her developing style. She feels that she always had these values, and that it simply took her a while to find out that they could fit into medicine. Her path, typical of those respondents who emphasized the connection between holistic medicine and spiritual and religious practices, was a gradual evolution.

Women seemed overrepresented among those who said they always held a holistic perspective, perhaps suggesting that the traditionally female way of seeing the world, emphasizing connection and wholes, has an affinity with holistic medicine. Remen (1979), a holistic physician, has written that holistic health represents the feminine principle in medicine.

The second and third routes into holistic medicine are transitions marked by crisis, often found among those physicians who exhibited the most extreme patterns of burnout. One set of crises involved intimate personal experience with illness. For example, Dr. Frank F. had a successful practice in an eastern city, a happy marriage, children, and all the trappings of medical success. Suddenly, within a period of two months, both he and his wife developed life-threatening diseases, necessitating long convalescences. During this period, he rested and began to rethink his priorities, to explore his inner needs and feelings, and meditated in a spontaneous fashion. "Getting started was part of a sudden awakening in me," he says. "I found I was living a dead life, living in my left brain, and I began to open up."

He sold his practice and moved west, taking an academic/teaching position. He entered personal psychotherapy and began to experiment with new techniques such as acupuncture and laying on of hands. His goal was "not to change medicine, but to change the way I practice it. The way I'm doing it personally now is by being able, through my own personal growth, to face patients eye to eye. I'm no archetypal superior being, but another human being who has expertise in a field. By doing that I'm able to relate on a personal basis to the patient without the awesome sense of being personally responsible for his physical life." He also has broadened his own life to contain "the full spectrum of what human beings are," including reading of world literature, participation in a religious community, and spending more time alone and with his family. He is also active as a teacher to medical residents, helping them learn to be more aware of their own feelings and the feelings of their patients. He typifies a group of our respondents whose change began as a result of a personal illness.

Several physicians remarked that when they were seriously ill, their personal concerns, their pain, and the feeling of being treated as a patient profoundly affected their sense of what was important for them to do as physicians:

> The most important influence on my change process was the life-threatening chronic disease that I developed, that nearly killed me, and that even now is very much part of my life. I had an internalized experience of the health/disease process. Instead of dealing with it out there, for somebody else as a patient, I had to turn the process inward, to deal with those issues in myself. I learned what was really important in healing. Fortunately or unfortunately, I've had to deal with it for myself in some unfortunate ways, creating for myself some situations that got my attention during these two periods of crisis (in his marriage and his illness).

The final path, exemplified by Dr. William T., focused on marital and family crisis. Dr. T. went through medical school with the financial and emotional help of his wife, Karen. She worked as a nurse until their first child was born, and Dr. T. entered residency. He entered emergency medicine because he wanted to work where "I was really needed as a physician." His first job was as an ER physician in a large hospital near a black ghetto. The impact of poverty and life-style on health became clear to him. In addition, he attended the "crazies," people who went from hospital to hospital for attention and medication. He often felt inadequate with those patients because he did not know how to have a positive impact on them.

Dr. T and his wife bought a home in the country and developed the life-style of a medical family. Karen, at home, became isolated and depressed. She was confused because she could not understand why she was depressed when they had everything they had wanted. As her depression and confusion grew, William withdrew, spending more and more time in the hospital where he felt more in control. He had an affair with one of the nurses at the hospital. Karen found out and threatened to leave unless they entered counseling.

The counselor helped them explore their feelings, communicate better, and begin to explore their goals and values, both individually and as a family. The therapeutic process was deeply meaningful to William, and he began reading the works of humanistic therapists, relating their ideas to his medical work. He started listening to his patients differently and began to talk to them about changes they could make in their own lives. He knew he was enjoying himself more and felt more helpful to his patients. He became known in the community as a humanistically oriented physician and was often sought by other professionals for consultations. As his practice changed, he began to discuss and write about the nature of medicine and the goals of treatment. Karen and he composed guidelines for patients and developed an assessment instrument to evaluate the full range of a patient's life-style. He began to meet with other holistically oriented professionals in the area and to plan a new type of whole-person health center. He opened the center, cut down on his hospital practice, and reported he felt much more integrated and satisfied in his work and his family life.

The path that Dr. T. took involves personal and family crisis, often including intensive involvement in personal psychotherapy. The therapy experience, often with a nontraditional therapist, is a model of a new kind of change and involvement. It leads physicians to look into themselves, to explore their personal needs and feelings, and to ask themselves what they want from life. At times, a confrontation with a spouse, or the spouse's involvement in holistic activities, initiated the change. A number of respondents reported that attending holistic conferences, which often include meditations and personal psychotherapeutic experiences, increased the value differences between spouses. About a third of our physicians experienced a marital separation during their transition period. What is most interesting is the close connection between the exploration of personal themes in psychotherapy and the practice of holistic medicine. Many of the psychological practices that were adopted by the physicians as their practices changed derived from their personal psychotherapeutic experiences. Therapy often provides a holistic model of personal relationship, and the psychotherapeutic model is one that can usually be applied to medical practice.

Stage 4: New Practice

As we have seen, the outcome of the change process is a new personal orientation, and a shift of perspective in practice. In future papers, we will describe the specific techniques and characteristics of the holistic medical perspective as it is practiced by these physicians and their peers. We are completing a study of the entire membership (approximately 465 physicians) of the American Holistic Medical Association, a five-year-old national organization, to explore these themes both more broadly and in greater detail.

Most of the physicians in our group continued their practices, although about a third took leaves of absence or changed to new practices or types of medical work. Very few of the physicians see their personal change processes as complete. Rather they see change as an ongoing process. We are probably looking at only a snapshot of their careers.

However, the respondents did report several consistent and enduring types of change. First, the majority report that they have become more sensitive to their own personal needs and have arranged their practice to give them more time for themselves. Self-care is an important theme in the holistic perspective, and many of the physicians report that leading a balanced life with more space for their personal needs and interests is an important outcome for themselves. For example, one of the physicians works half time in a salaried position and has time to pursue acting, which had been one of his earlier aspirations he felt he had to give up for medicine.

The physicians explored and utilized a wide variety of new techniques and practices in their work. These included acupuncture, relaxation, guided imagery, massage, and biofeedback. Structurally, they try to spend more time with patients and to inquire into a wider spectrum of the patients' lives. They do a lot of counseling in their practice and also teach spiritual practices such as meditation and self-healing. They report having a more mutual, sharing relationship with some of their patients.

However, most of our physicians continue to perform the traditional activities of medicine and treat many of their patients in the conventional manner. However, they feel that they have a different attitude toward the doctor-patient relationship. They do not see such a sharp split between their old and new professional selves. Many offered comments similar to this one from a 40-year-old internist:

> Now, I'm more or less comfortable with the blend [between traditional and spiritual medicine]. This is OK. It may not be where I'll be forever, but right now it feels good. Earlier it felt like I was being split right down the middle—the image I've often had is one of standing on two floats on a pond and feeling them floating off in opposite directions. Not so acute now. I have some anxiety, but I guess we all do now that medicine is in such a state of flux.

Most important, for purposes of this discussion, is that these doctors report much greater satisfaction in the practice of medicine and, in many cases, a rekindling of the flame of their initial commitment to the higher ideals of medicine. By practicing in a somewhat different way, they have helped resolve much that was in conflict about their personal and professional crisis.

We are continuing our study of a much broader group of holistic physicians and looking more deeply at these themes. The response to professional burnout and dissatisfaction in medicine by making deep changes in values, style, and philosophy of medicine may not be uncommon. The exact number of physicians who have been touched by this new philosophy is uncounted, and probably uncountable. But, our research suggests that the effect of these changes on medicine is becoming greater, and that we should look empirically at these new physicians, what they do, how they change, and what they believe.

REFERENCES

Cherniss, C. (1980). *Professional burnout in human service organizations.* New York: Praeger.
Freudenberger, H. (1980). *Burnout.* New York: Bantam.
Goldstein, M., Jaffe, D., Garell, D. & Berke, R., (1985). Holistic doctors: Becoming a non-traditional medical practitioner. *Urban Life, 14.*
Gould, R. (1978). *Transformations.* New York: Simon & Schuster.
Hastings, A., Gordon, J., & Fadiman, J. (1981). *Health for the whole person.* New York: Bantam.
Levinson, D. (1978). *The seasons of a man's life.* New York: Knopf.
Pines, A., Aronson, E., & Kafry, D. (1981). *Burnout: From tedium to personal growth.* New York: Free Press.
Remen, N. (1979). *The human patient.* New York: Doubleday.

II
Interventions for Prevention

Chapter 9

Faculty Interventions: How Far Should You Go?

Gerald Bennett, Ph.D., R.N.

The success of prevention and early intervention strategies to promote student well-being depends in large part on faculty commitment and involvement. Faculty roles in prevention are discussed in the Emergent Strategies section. This chapter focuses on the extent and limits of faculty involvement in advising, mentoring, or counseling the troubled student in the health professions. The fact that faculty in the health field are often both teachers and clinicians presents special benefits and complications not experienced in the traditional academic setting. Although this special situation is a source of conflict for many faculty and students, it also has the potential to foster an exceptional educational environment for health promotion and early intervention.

Faculty are themselves subject to burnout syndromes (Lenhart, 1980; Ray, 1984). An assumption made in the discussion to follow is that the overburdened and disillusioned educator is an unlikely source of support and guidance for the troubled student. Similarly, educators who view students as essentially outside the gates of the profession until graduation may view distress and strain as part of an initiation process and the need for intervention a character weakness (Reidbord, 1983; Welch, 1980). Faculty who practice

147

self-care and view the student as a worthy member of the professional community are more likely to embrace the roles of advisor, mentor, or counselor.

STUDENT PROBLEMS

If faculty are to intervene in a positive way with impaired students, an awareness of the problems faced by these students is crucial. Students are persons first and therefore may experience any of the misfortunes or ills of the human condition. However, the training years in the health professions are associated with some special, if not unique, problems. The so-called impairment problems are the focus of this book. These are problems that have a behavioral component that impairs the competent and caring practice of the chosen health profession or, in this case, the student role in that profession. Stress reactions and early manifestations of burnout, depression, and substance use disorders are the most common types of impairment seen in the student population.

A recent study found that medical, pharmacy, nursing, allied health, and graduate students in various health sciences shared the same spectrum of perceived problems (Bjorksten et al., 1983). The most commonly perceived problems were related to time management, in terms of both meeting school demands and finding breaks for leisure. Feeling powerless in the educational system was also a major concern. Medical students, compared to all other health sciences students as a group, reported their concerns as significantly more severe. These findings are consistent with an earlier study of problems among medical students which found that lack of time for recreation, lack of time for family or intimate friends, and being unable to learn everything were the most common concerns (Edwards & Zimet, 1976).

These problems, viewed in isolation, do not appear remarkable by modern standards. That is, one might reasonably argue that many people in contemporary society experience time pressures and unrealistic demands. Faculty may hasten to add that this is the real world and the sooner students learn to cope, the better. However, other factors interacting with these demands in the educational setting are student idealism, a need to achieve, a busy faculty, and the bitter realities of sickness care in university medical centers (Pfifferling, 1984).

What happens to students in such a system? At best, without guided or self-directed efforts to reduce stressful events, learn new coping strategies, and mobilize a support system, training in the health sciences is often a "process of disillusionment" (Schwartz et al., 1978). At worst, those students at high risk for depression, other psychopathology, or substance use disorders become seriously impaired. It is useful to maintain a clear conceptual distinction between the early manifestations of burnout, depression, and substance use disorders, even though there is often overlap. There are both theoretical and practical reasons for this. First, basic research shows a strong relationship between stress and burnout. But the direct relationships found between stress and depression and between stress and addictions are consistently weak. Second, the early manifestations of burnout are rarely life-threatening, whereas depression and addiction pose serious suicide or overdose risks. Furthermore, the effective approaches to helping students with the early manifestations of burnout, depression, or substance-use disorders are usually quite different.

Early Manifestations of Burnout

Brill (1984) proposed a "restricted" definition of burnout:

> An expectationally mediated, job-related, dysphoric and dysfunctional state in an individual without major psychopathology who has (1) functioned for a time at adequate performance and affectual levels in the same job situation and who (2) will not recover to previous levels without outside help or environmental rearrangement. (p. 15)

I endorse this "narrowly defined" concept of burnout. Its application to students in the health professions should be made carefully because students are not truly "on the job" until graduation. Harris (1984) characterizes neophyte professionals as free of burnout; they ". . . enter their first positions with incredible enthusiasm and intend to become a shining example of the ideal physician, lawyer, nurse, teacher, social worker, etc." (p. 33). But much of what we know about the well-being of medical and nursing students contradicts this image.

By the fourth year of medical school, students typically report concerns about career choice and some negative feelings about the work setting (Bjorksten et al., 1983; Bojar, 1971; Edwards & Zimet, 1976). One study revealed a steady decline in health habits as medical students progressed toward graduation (Kay et al., 1980). Senior nursing students are already aware of conflicts between their education and what they will encounter in practice (Kramer, 1974). Thus faculty should be alert to some of the early manifestations of burnout in their students. Signs and symptoms of burnout are summarized elsewhere in this volume.

Depression

A study of medical students seen at a large university counseling service revealed that 38% of these clients presented a problem of depression secondary to academic pressures and disillusionment (Weinstein, 1983). In other words, the primary problem was early burnout. Nevertheless, students are susceptible to primary depressions that are best understood and treated outside the context of burnout. Because of the risk of suicide, the prompt referral and treatment of depressed students cannot be overemphasized (Pepitone-Arreola-Rockwell et al., 1981).

Substance Use Disorders

As with depression, alcohol and drug problems may be secondary to early burnout. Furthermore, alcohol and drug problems may be secondary to depression. These secondary substance use disorders are best termed "substance abuse." Substance abuse implies dysfunction associated with alcohol or other drug use. On the other hand, addiction, which implies compulsive use, loss of control over amount and time of use, and continued use despite consequences, is a primary illness requiring specialized treatment.

Students in health careers are at high risk for alcohol and drug abuse because of their needs for stress reduction (Bjorksten et al., 1983; Kay et al., 1980; Tweed, 1979) and their access to controlled medications. For those students who are addiction-prone because of family history or other predisposing factors, progression from abuse to addiction can be rapid in this environment.

ETHICAL AND LEGAL CONSIDERATIONS

How far should faculty go in the identification and assistance of impaired students? This is essentially an ethical question with important academic, personal, and legal implications. The "Joint Statement on Rights and Freedoms of Students" (American Association of University Professors, 1968) and the "American Personnel and Guidance Association (APGA)* Ethical Standards" (APGA, 1981) provide clear guidance to faculty on matters related to the impaired student. From the legal perspective, the Family Educational Rights and Privacy Act of 1974 and the U.S. Supreme Court's ruling in *Board of Curators of the University of Missouri v. Horowitz* (1978) are especially relevant to incidents involving impaired students in the university setting.

Problem Identification

Health professionals are resistant to expressing impairment concerns to or about their peers. Similarly, many faculty are reluctant, in their view, to

---

*This association has recently changed its name to the American Association for Counseling and Development (AACD).

place the career of a student on the line over a problem that is bound to correct itself over time. In the terms of addiction theory, faculty are unfortunately often "enablers" for impaired students because of their misplaced efforts to help through silence.

Certainly, faculty have an ethical responsibility to act positively on knowledge that (1) a student is not meeting the standards set for adequate performance, (2) a student is a danger to himself/herself, and/or (3) a student poses a danger to others (APGA, 1981). On the other hand, faculty must not take liberties to broaden the concept of impairment beyond these three criteria. For example, to identify a student as "impaired" because of negative views expressed about the profession or similar expression of controversial beliefs would violate the student's right of inquiry and expression (AAUP, 1968).

Confidentiality

Knowledge of student impairment should be kept confidential to the extent that confidentiality can be maintained and still protect the well-being of the student and/or others. The faculty member always has the option of seeking consultation from experts to better define a particular student problem.

Although some students will report their problems to faculty, most impairment problems come to the attention of faculty through reports of other students, others in the community, or most frequently, in the process of clinical performance evaluation. Some examples are: (1) a student reports that a classmate is stealing drugs from the hospital, (2) the campus police report to the dean's office that a student has been found overdosed in the dormitory, or (3) in observing a student's clinical practice, a faculty member notes poor performance and depressed affect. Regardless of the means of learning about student impairment, there is an ethical obligation to begin positive action and respect confidentiality.

Educational institutions should keep academic and disciplinary records separate to minimize the risk of improper disclosure of disciplinary action. Noncurrent disciplinary records should be destroyed (AAUP, 1968).

Confronting Poor Clinical Performance

Many faculty are reluctant to document the poor clinical performance of students who score high on written examinations. To do so is viewed as risk taking in academia. Written examinations are thought to be a source of "hard" data on performance whereas clinical evaluations are considered "soft" and sensitive to subjectivity. Some faculty are concerned that negative clinical evaluations in the presence of high grades may lead to student grievance and legal liability for the institution. But the Supreme Court's *Horowitz* decision supports and has the effect of encouraging faculty to be honest in their evaluation of students in the clinical setting (Kapp, 1981).

Charlotte Horowitz, a medical student with excellent grades, was dismissed in 1971 from the University of Missouri–Kansas City because of poor clinical performance. She filed in federal court against the university claiming that the dismissal infringed her civil rights. In addition, the university had not granted her a formal hearing to challenge the dismissal. In a 9–0 decision, the court approved the decision of the university and further stated that a formal adversary hearing should not be required after a negative academic evaluation that results in dismissal. A more recent court decision set forth the elements required for due process in academic affairs. These elements included: (1) the student must be allowed to explain reasons for poor performance, and (2) the student must be allowed to provide information to show that future performance would be acceptable (Stoller v. College of Medicine, 1983).

Although it is not suggested here that Horowitz was an impaired student, the court decision is a precedent upholding faculty and university responsibilities to honestly evaluate students. If this is done, impairment problems will surface along with other student problems such as inadequate cognitive, affective, or psychomotor abilities.

Performance evaluations must be based on written criteria that are made available to students before beginning a practicum. Students must be evaluated without regard to race, sex, or religion. Students have the right under the Family Educational Rights and Privacy Act of 1974 to examine and copy any records pertaining to them that are maintained by an educational institution. This includes clinical evaluations. Finally, students should be informed of a performance problem as soon as possible (Kapp, 1981).

Problem Evaluation and Response

Although faculty are in a favorable position to identify the impaired student, particularly in the process of performance evaluation, in general they should not engage in a detailed mental health evaluation of these problems. Furthermore, faculty should not counsel or otherwise provide therapy for their students (APGA, 1981). Since faculty have a primary relationship with their students that is supervisory and evaluative, it is unethical to encourage self-disclosure that might pose a conflict of interest or place the student in academic jeopardy (Callis et al., 1982). The only exception to this ethical principle is if another competent professional is not available for referral. In such a situation, as in short-term crisis intervention, the faculty member should avoid discussing aspects of the problem that might create a conflict of interest.

The following case illustrates an ethical approach to faculty knowledge that a student is impaired.

> A college student approaches his psychology teacher after class and indicates that he has been extremely depressed lately and even thinking about suicide. He asks the teacher for help since she is also on the staff of the college counseling center. The teacher expresses her concern but explains that she believes it would be inadvisable to work with him as a client since they already have a teacher-student relationship. She recommends another counselor and walks with him over to the center to assist him in arranging for an interview with this counselor. (Callis et al., 1982, p. 46)

Faculty responsibility to provide rapid and appropriate referral to impaired students will be discussed in more detail in the next section.

FACULTY INTERVENTIONS

Faculty roles in effective intervention for impaired students include advising, mentoring, and referral for counseling or treatment. Faculty with counseling expertise may serve as counselors for impaired students from other schools or for programs within their schools for which they do not have teaching responsibilities.

Advising

Advising is the faculty role of providing information, recommendations, approvals, disapprovals, or warnings to students on matters directly related to the curriculum. Many schools assign each student a faculty advisor to provide guidance and academic supervision throughout the program. In addition, for each course or practicum, faculty meet with most students individually at one time or another in an advisory role. Impairment issues come up routinely in advising students on work loads, adding or dropping courses, integrating part-time work with part-time or full-time study, improving study habits, meeting deadlines, granting or rejecting requests for time extensions, etc.

Faculty have many opportunities to help impaired students in the advising role. The ongoing advisor is able to chart the progress of the student through the program and note downward trends in grades or clinical performance. Discussion about these trends can be effective in assisting the student to recognize impairment risks.

Advisement is the best means of intervening with high achievers who are attempting unrealistic work loads. Examples are the graduate nursing student who wishes to pursue full-time study and a full-time head nurse position, the M.D.-Ph.D. student asking permission to take an elective in addition to an already overloaded schedule, or the clinical psychology student who requests independent study hours the first semester in order to get an early start on a dissertation proposal. The advisor who is sensitive to impairment risk will routinely encourage and often require students to maintain reasonable work loads. Reinforcing unrealistic self-expectations and needs for constant high achievement among students is a mistake commonly made by faculty advisors in the health sciences. A *laissez faire* approach to advising is also discouraged. The student moving through the curriculum of one of the health professions is certainly at risk for loneliness, isolation, and early burnout without the active and concerned advice of faculty. This appeal for advising with the student's personal life considered is not an endorsement of mediocrity. Again, the central impairment concern is performance. Advisors should help students plan goals and schedules that will support consistent quality performance in the long run.

As advisors, faculty have the obligation to observe the personal demands of the curriculum on advisees, individually and collectively. These observations should be reported, maintaining confidentiality regarding individual student concerns, to the curriculum committee and other decision-making groups or individuals in the educational setting. A common problem of students is the competing expectations of the various courses in which they are enrolled. The faculty advisor should report these concerns to those in a position to evaluate the curriculum as a whole and therefore institute changes where needed.

Mentoring

Mentoring is gaining increasing recognition as a faculty-student relationship that can "help healthy students grow into well rounded professionals" (Flach et al., 1982). A mentor serves as a senior colleague, role model, and friend, not as a professional counselor or therapist. Mentoring need not include formal academic advisement, although some students select their advisors as mentors.

Although mentoring is usually not thought of in terms of intervention for impaired students, the relationship has potential to help troubled students in ways that advising and counseling cannot. Mentoring can be a viable adjunct to helping an impaired student, as long as needs for counseling or treatment are being met by another professional outside the mentoring relationship. In situations where a student is in an early stage of impairment, or has corrected impairment through counseling or treatment, mentoring may be quite successful without concurrent professional counseling. If a faculty member chooses to make mentoring dependent on concurrent counseling, this should be stated clearly to the student as part of the mentoring agreement.

How does mentoring begin with an impaired student? Students with performance problems either seek out faculty help, or faculty must contact these students to discuss the problems. During these discussions, faculty should not volunteer or agree to be the student's counselor. However, faculty may offer office time to the student to discuss career development, problem solving within the context of the curriculum, and other school-related concerns. Faculty should make the differences between counseling and mentoring clear enough that a student can discuss them.

Because counseling one's students poses ethical problems, the only viable ongoing relationship with students, beyond teaching, advising, and clinical supervision, is mentoring. A consistent theme in mentoring theory and research is the reciprocal nature of the relationship (Flach et al., 1982; Vance, 1982). Mentor and student experience decreased isolation in their organization. The mentor is able to relate his/her experiences, knowledge, and philosophy to a protégé following the same professional path. The student receives coaching and acceptance from one who has reached the status that he/she seeks. Simply put, mentoring in teaching is getting to know students and allowing students to know you within the context of a genuine and caring relationship.

Faculty-student mentor relationships are best not assigned, as advisors would be assigned to each student upon entering school. Rather, mentoring best develops on the basis of faculty-student attraction, similar specialty interests, or other factors that enhance the mutuality of the relationship. For the impaired student, or one with a history of impairment, faculty with special knowledge of impairment or faculty who have recovered from impairment are probably the best mentors. For example, the student recovering from alcoholism is more likely to find an understanding mentor among faculty acquainted with alcoholism through personal experience, study, or clinical practice. Similarly, women students may prefer women faculty for mentors (Flach et al., 1982; Hall & Sandler, 1983; Vance, 1982), and men students may prefer men faculty. However, the benefits of specificity in matching mentors and students can be overstated. One of the remarkable qualities of the mentoring relationship is its capacity for broadening the interests and increasing the sensitivity of mentor and student.

There are a number of variations on traditional one-to-one mentoring that are effective in early intervention or long-term coping for impaired students. Support groups for students are in many ways a group mentoring activity. These groups tend to emphasize helpful interaction with older students and faculty without supervisory or therapeutic overtones (Dickstein, 1982; Plaut et al., 1982). Students experiencing worry and anxiety about success in the educational program may be attracted to these groups. In addition, these groups are an excellent forum to encourage new students to seek one-to-one mentoring from upper classmen and faculty.

Other variations on the mentoring process that have the effect of reaching out to all students, including those in distress, are: (1) develop a course that deals with "how to make it" concerns and assists students in balancing personal goals with those of the school and profession; (2) hold open forums where professionals who are recovering from impairment speak candidly to students—include time for informal one-to-one and small group discussions; and (3) conceptualize and plan orientation for new students as mentoring, rather than initiation.

Counseling

The faculty role in counseling or other treatment is referral. Depending on the degree of impairment and other circumstances, the referral may be presented to the student as optional or mandatory for continuing in the program. By far, most referrals are suggestions to students and are indeed optional. An optional referral involves meeting with the student, pointing out your reason for concern in performance terms, and suggesting professionals or agencies in the community for counseling. Of course, referrals for those students who must have counseling or treatment in order to continue, or have hope of continuing, are the most difficult to manage.

An effective mandatory referral is based on student cooperation, clinical consultation, administrative support, and adequate follow-up. A "blind" mandatory referral, without feedback or follow-up, is not ethical or workable in the health professions, where students are involved in patient care. There must be assurances in the referral process that students are indeed involved in appropriate counseling or treatment, and that they are not impaired in the clinical setting. Phases of managing an effective mandatory referral are (1) confrontation, (2) clinical evaluation, (3) counseling or treatment, and (4) follow-up.

Educational institutions in the health professions should have a written policy regarding counseling or treatment for students. Informal support from program directors and deans is also crucial. Before making a mandatory referral, be sure the action is consistent with written policies and has the support of the program director. In the confrontation phase, ask a faculty colleague to validate your conclusion that the student's impairment is such that professional intervention is required. This should be a faculty member with current knowledge of the student's performance. If there is agreement, a meeting is called, with the two faculty members and student present. Avoid involving more than one other faculty member in the confrontation. More than two faculty members are sure to intimidate the student. On the other hand, a single faculty member will not have the impact that two are able to achieve. The performance problems are presented, personal and professional concern is expressed, and the need for professional evaluation and possible treatment is emphasized.

The paramount goal in the clinical evaluation phase of referral is to assure an effective match between the student's problem and the counseling or treatment he receives. Therefore, second only to protecting the safety of the student and others, an in-depth, objective, and eclectic professional evaluation of the impairment problem is a top priority. The student health or counseling service may be the best resource for evaluation, but not necessarily. There is no substitute for knowing the strengths and limitations of the resources for referral in your community. Find out if the programs for recovering health professionals in your state are open to students. Perhaps you are fortunate enough to have a special program for health sciences students such as the Mental Health Program for Physicians in Training at UCLA (Borenstein & Cook, 1982). Take special care in referring students with what appears to be an early burnout syndrome or a drug-related impairment. These problems are not yet widely understood among mental health professionals. If you must use one referral agency, such as the student health or counseling service, be sure they are up-to-date on the types of problems students in the health professions might present. Any drug-related impairment should be evaluated by an addiction specialist.

It is only after the evaluation that decisions should be made regarding status in the educational program, specifically, whether student status will continue during treatment or whether the student must withdraw during treatment. Every impaired student should have the benefit of appropriate counseling or treatment before a decision is made to dismiss the student for academic reasons. Impaired students who are uncooperative in seeking treatment are subject to academic dismissal. Those impaired students who have violated university rules, or state or federal laws, may or may not be provided an opportunity to seek treatment and continue in the program. This depends on the seriousness of the violation. For example, for the addicted student, possessing drugs for one's own use is viewed very differently than selling drugs to others.

Once the impaired student has been matched with an appropriate counselor, therapist, or treatment program, the follow-up phase of referral begins. The purpose of follow-up is to determine whether performance is being or can be restored to acceptable levels. If the student remains in the course or practicum, the faculty member continues to evaluate performance much as before. If the student must withdraw for treatment, the burden is on him/her to contact the school with a desire to return to school with evidence of potential for acceptable performance.

GAINING INSTITUTIONAL SUPPORT

Faculty cannot work in isolation to identify and assist impaired students and hope to be successful. Whether through long-standing committees on student health or new committees on "the well-being of students" (Weinstein, 1983), policies can be developed to support prevention and early intervention. To implement these policies, attempts must be made to spread interest through forums, seminars, or guest speakers. Administration must support the policies, both formally and informally. It is helpful for faculty to become involved with other health professionals within the university and the community who are involved in similar activities within their schools or programs. In addition, faculty can attend state and national conferences on impairment to learn innovative institutional strategies, or meet some of their requirements for research and publication by investigating the well-being of their student body. These findings can be used to reinforce the need for prevention and early intervention policies and resources.

SUMMARY

There is much the individual faculty member can do to assist the impaired student. Honest evaluation of performance is the first step. Willingness to use advising and mentoring as opportunities to provide practical help to troubled students is also very important. Faculty can prepare themselves to effectively intervene when a student's performance indicates a need for counseling or treatment. These interventions are greatly facilitated by progressive institutional policies and availability of referral resources suited to the special needs of students in the health professions. No doubt, there is an element of risk taking in helping an impaired student. Initially, other faculty, administration, or the student may protest. In the end, the student may be dismissed despite all efforts. However, the satisfaction of assisting recovery, once experienced, is more than enough to make intervention worthwhile.

REFERENCES

American Association of University Professors, U.S. National Student Association, Association of American Colleges, National Association of Student Personnel Administrators, & National Association of Women Deans and Counselors (1968). Joint statement on rights and freedoms of students. *AAUP Bulletin, 54,* 258–261.

American Personnel and Guidance Association (March 19, 1981). *Guidepost,* Suppl. A-D.

Bjorksten, O., Sutherland, S., Miller, C., & Stewart, T. (1983). Identification of medical student problems and comparison with those of other students. *Journal of Medical Education, 58,* 759–766.

Board of Curators of the University of Missouri v. Horowitz, 435 U.S. 78 (1978).

Bojar, S. A. (1971). Psychiatric problems in medical students. In G. B. Blaine & C. C. McArthur (Eds.), *Emotional problems of the student* (pp. 350–363). New York: Appleton-Century-Crofts.

Borenstein, D. B., & Cook, K. (1982). Impairment prevention in the training years. *Journal of the American Medical Association, 247,* 2700–2703.

Brill, P. L. (1984). The need for an operational definition of burnout. *Family & Community Health, 6*(4), 12–24.

Callis, R., Pope, S., & Depauw, M. (1982). *APGA Ethical Standards Casebook* (3rd ed.). Falls Church, VA: American Personnel and Guidance Association.

Dickstein, L. (1982). The student hour: A support system for freshmen medical students. *Journal of American College Health, 31,* 131–132.

Edwards, M. T., & Zimet, C. N. (1976). Problems and concerns among medical students—1975. *Journal of Medical Education, 51,* 619–625.

Flach, D. H., Smith, M. F., Smith, W. G., & Glasser, M. L. (1982). Faculty mentors for medical students. *Journal of Medical Education, 57,* 514–520.

Hall, R. M., & Sandler, B. R. (1983). *Academic mentoring for women students and faculty: A new look at an old way to get ahead.* Washington, D.C.: Association of American Colleges.

Harris, P. L. (1984). Assessing burnout: The organizational and individual perspective. *Family & Community Health, 6*(4), 32–43.

Kapp, M. B. (1981). Legal issues in faculty evaluation of student clinical performance. *Journal of Medical Education, 56,* 559–564.

Kay, J., Howard, T., & Welch, G. (1980). Health habits of medical students: Some perils of the profession. *Journal of the American College Health Association, 28,* 238–239.

Kramer, M. (1974). *Reality shock.* St. Louis: Mosby.

Lenhart, R. C. (1980). Faculty burnout-and some reasons why. *Nursing Outlook, 28,* 424–425.

Pepitone-Arreola-Rockwell, F., Rockwell, D., & Core, N. (1981). Fifty-two medical student suicides. *American Journal of Psychiatry, 138*(2), 198–201.

Pfifferling, J. H. (1984). Viewpoint: The role of the educational setting in preventing burnout. *Family & Community Health, 6*(4), 68–75.

Plaut, S. M., Hunt, G. J., Johnson, F. P., Brown, R. M., & Hobbins, T. E. (1982). Intensive medical student support groups: Format, outcome and leadership guidelines. *Journal of Medical Education, 57,* 778–786.

Ray, G. J. (1984). Burnout: Potential problem for nursing faculty. *Nursing and Health Care, 5,* 218–221.

Reidbord, S. P. (1983). Psychological perspectives on iatrogenic physician impairment. *Pharos, 46*(3), 2–8.

Schwartz, A. H., Swartzburg, J. L., & Slaby, A. E. (1978). Medical school and the process of disillusionment. *Medical Education, 12,* 182–185.

Stoller v. College of Medicine, 562 F. Supp. 403. U.S. District Court, M.D. Pennsylvania (1983).

Tweed, S. (1979). Alcohol isn't the answer. *Imprint, 26*(1), 48–49.

Vance, C. N. (1982). The mentor connection. *Journal of Nursing Administration, 12*(4), 7–13.

Weinstein, H. M. (1983). A commitee on well-being of medical students and house staff. *Journal of Medical Education, 58*, 373–381.

Welch, R. L. (1980). The battered student syndrome. *Radiologic Technology, 51*, 613–616.

Chapter 10

Clinical Behavioral Scientists: Consultants and Teachers in Family Practice Residencies

Sylvia Shellenberger, Ph.D.,
and Gary Wellborn, M.D.

Behavioral scientists are becoming permanent members of many health care teams. The clinical behavioral scientist can provide a variety of services including teaching, patient care, and consultation within the medical community. These types of services, the advantages of having clinical behavioral scientists as permanent members of health care teams, and recommendations for training professionals in this role are described. The chapter deals with the behavioral scientist's role as consultant to and teacher of students, residents, fellows, and administrators, and as personal confidant and researcher. These roles are observed collaboratively from the two perspectives of the behavioral scientist and the physician. In addition, methods for clinical behavioral scientists to establish a professional support network and maintain their own intrapersonal balance are discussed.

ESTABLISHING CREDIBILITY

Establishing and maintaining openness, credibility, and acceptance by physicians are essential to the behavioral scientist if he/she is to be effective. One way of developing this credibility is to demonstrate interest in the physicians' work. By attending hospital rounds with the physicians, spending time in the ambulatory care center, attending medical conferences, and accompanying residents/faculty to the emergency or delivery room, the behavioral scientist communicates a willingness to participate in activities for the purpose of gaining a better understanding of the physicians' responsibilities and perspectives. In addition, presence in the milieu establishes the behavioral scientist as a true team member rather than as someone to be called only when there is a major psychosocial problem.

Another way of gaining credibility in the medical setting is by becoming attuned to the cognitive style, language, and goals of physicians. Accommodating to the medical model facilitates acceptance by those who use that particular problem-solving and decision-making approach.

There are a number of appropriate and often neglected areas of the students' and residents' training where the behavioral scientist can gain the respect and confidence of those he/she serves, and make a positive contribution to the educational process. After establishing a personal relationship with the residents, the behavioral scientist can participate with them in their struggles with hospital administration and faculty. Likewise, consulting with the residents regarding their patients and teaching them relevant techniques for managing the psychosocial components of patients' problems enhances the behavioral scientist's value as a team member.

DEVELOPING PERSONAL RELATIONSHIPS IN THE MEDICAL SETTING

In most residency programs the person who is likely to (overtly) demonstrate interest in feelings is the behavioral scientist. Both by personal interest and professional training, he/she is seen as the individual of choice to act as confidant, counselor, and informational source for the personal problems of students, residents, staff, and faculty. For example, residents frequently consider it improper to express strong emotions in the presence of a departmental chief who is their primary evaluator. They may fear that the chief will reject the demonstration as inappropriate, a sign of weakness, or worse. The expectations of residents when seeking the counsel of the behavioral scientist are that he/she will be accepting, understanding, less critical, and possibly even helpful in resolution of their problems.

Struggles between residents and the various forms of administration are ubiquitous. The behavioral scientist can act as mediator, advocate, or facilitator as dictated by the situation. Clear communication of grievances and motives can ameliorate the majority of these conflicts and help maintain stability in the face of time restraints, patient care requirements, and other stresses. The addition of logical analysis and effective problem-solving techniques is seen as a constructive contribution by those most closely engaged in such confrontations, and the behavioral scientist is in a prime position to apply both those skills between the residents and the administrators.

Further consolidation of the relationship comes in helping residents cope with the stresses around them. Pfifferling (1983) lists numerous methods of helping the residents cope with the stresses of training and practice. The literature which deals with the stresses and stressors of medical professions often mentions the loss of social contacts and interests as one of the major aspects of dysfunction (Coombs & Fawzy, 1982; Davis, 1981; Leichner & Kalin, 1980; Loes & Scheiber, 1981; Nelson & Henry, 1978; Pasnau & Russell, 1975). In rap sessions where they meet to discuss patient or personal problems, residents often suggest meeting as a group for social activities. Although these spontaneous suggestions would often be dropped because of the time involved in coordinating such an activity, the behavioral scientist can maintain the momentum with reminders, proposals, or organizing efforts.

Dealing with expectations of self and others is a source of constant irritation for a great number of physicians. The ideals and goals most physicians set for themselves early in training tend to be unrealistic and, more often than not, unattainable. The resulting frustration (when internalized) or anger (when externalized) interferes with patient care and personal growth and development. The behavioral scientist, through modeling, reframing, and giving permission for limits, makes acceptance of human frailty a palatable process in resolution of these dilemmas. The acceptant, yet structured approach to human difficulties generalizes to the physician's experiences with the unrealizable expectations of his/her patients, families, and faculty. This also aids him/her in helping those people develop expectations that are more realistic and compatible with the physician's own goals and limits.

CONSULTING WITH RESIDENTS AS A MEMBER OF THE PATIENT CARE TEAM

Clinical social sciences are viewed by many physicians as vague, imprecise, inefficient, ineffective disciplines best left to those who have the time to pursue them. Family practice residents work 80 to 100 hours a week learning the wide range of technological skills needed to provide comprehensive primary medical care. Thus, they view the prospects of open-ended, long-term counseling of an individual as a less cost-effective investment of time when compared to the number of organic illnesses they could manage in the same time period. To address these problems effectively, the behavioral scientist must devise concise, specific approaches to particular problems that can be administered in brief counseling sessions (e.g., 30 to 45 minutes), with specific goals (e.g., relief of psychosomatic pain), with a specific predetermined duration (e.g., weekly sessions for six weeks), and usually with a predetermined contractual consequence if the counseling is ineffective (e.g., referral for more intensive treatment).

Although some psychosocial problems require more time than is generally available to the family physician–behavioral scientist team, a surprisingly wide range of psychopathology can be effectively treated in this system. Identification of more extensive problems that are not amenable to this therapeutic model (and should be referred or have consultation), such as complex family issues or frank psychosis, is a valuable aspect of this approach for both members of the team, thus helping to define the boundaries of counseling appropriate for family physicians.

The role of the clinical behavioral scientist as consultant can be a powerful force in the education of a new physician in dealing with many common complaints of patients and their families. Some of the most difficult problems encountered by generalists are those arising from interpersonal relationships, such as patients' and their families' responses to chronic diseases or terminal illnesses. Physicians spend nearly 20 years in preparation for the job of dealing with organic disease and usually less than six months preparing to deal with the myriad of individual personalities. The therapy for organic disease is a comparatively direct, though frequently complex, task when compared to the treatment of people, which is often a wide-ranging endeavor requiring cognitive information, flexibility, and empathy. The behavioral science consultant and physician acting together constitute a formidable team, and through this association, the consultant becomes a potent role model from which the physician profits in all his/her encounters with patients.

The behavioral scientist becomes proficient in administering behavior modification plans and suggesting relevant reading material and other specific activities designed to reinforce the points of previous counseling sessions and to prepare the patient for subsequent sessions. For example, the patient with a psychosomatic pain disorder may be given brief instruction in relaxation techniques and then presented with a programmed cassette tape with which he/she is to practice the procedure at specific intervals until the next counseling session. Similarly, a patient with anxiety attacks may be asked to keep a log of the conditions under which he/she feels an attack beginning. With the aid of this log, a desensitization program can be devised that the patient can follow between meetings.

The psychologist gains new perspectives working directly with physicians and their patients. The time restraints of the situation are better comprehended, and techniques that incorporate greater speed and effectiveness are developed. Manipulation of the doctor-patient relationship can greatly improve patient compliance. Observation of the resident and patient often reveals problems in that relationship which can be addressed to improve the resident physician's effectiveness. The consultant becomes expert in streamlining his/her counseling to the particular problem at hand and at minimizing side issues in order to keep the sessions brief enough to be practical for the residents.

If the psychologist can maintain a noncritical, helper orientation, the bond between the behavioral scientist and physician will help to shape their efforts to become more effective clinicians both as a team and as individuals. If the physician can state his/her impressions and beliefs about the patient's psychological functioning in an open, supportive environment, he/she will build more self-confidence in approaching these nonorganic aspects of medical practice. In addition, the physician gains the benefits of greater expertise, efficiency, and competence in handling psychosocial problems.

The real beneficiary of this approach is the patient. The presence of the physician at the counseling sessions fosters trust in the psychologist as the peer and cotherapist of the physician with whom the patient has a previously established relationship and helps to legitimize the problem. It is the team approach that allows the rapid progress often observed in this setting.

TEACHING THE CONTENT OF BEHAVIORAL SCIENCE

Behavioral science is woven into all aspects of teaching programs in family medicine. The faculty physicians, along with the behavioral scientists, raise behavioral issues as a problem-solving consideration in the same context as issues related to the differential diagnosis, medication, and other aspects of medical problem solving.

A principal method the clinical behavioral scientist uses for teaching the content of behavioral science is consultation or cotherapy with the residents and students. Conferences cover the core content of the material residents need to master in order to assist in evaluation or cotherapy. Then psychosocial assessment and therapeutic techniques that are appropriate for utilization by family physicians are practiced in joint sessions with patients. For example, a model for marriage counseling is presented as a conference. Then residents practice the model with their patients in conjoint sessions with the psychologist.

The conference series is a major component of the behavioral science teaching program. Topics covered include family dynamics, the impact and meaning of illness to the patient and family, psychological assessment techniques for use in medical practice, behavioral analysis and management, development of contracts with patients, psychiatric classification of illness, and pharmacological treatments of mental illness. In addition to coordinating conferences on these topics, the psychologist works with residents as they prepare presentations on problems seen with high frequency in practice. Examples of these topics include management of children who are school phobic, hyperactive, or failing in school; counseling parents whose children have temper tantrums; dealing with adolescents who have anorexia nervosa or are suicidal; and working with adults who have psychosomatic problems, anxiety reactions, or situational depression. The conference series supplies residents with core content for understanding the psychosocial aspects of their patients' problems and introduces management methods appropriate to these factors.

Another aspect of the behavioral scientist's teaching role, as for other faculty, is giving feedback to residents regarding their performance with patients. After observing the residents with patients in the hospital, in the examining room, or in the psychologist's office, the psychologist gives constructive feedback regarding their communication, therapeutic, and patient education skills.

The use of objective psychological testing has been proven to be an effective diagnostic tool which has helped to establish credibility of the psychologist both with residents and with the patients. The physicians are exposed to various testing instruments for specific (e.g., anxiety scales) or general (MMPI) applications. They become familiar with the applications as well as the reliability of the various tests and have used the tests to confirm suspected diagnoses or as investigative procedures to determine the nature of a patient's problem when the interviews have been ambiguous or confusing. In addition, the patients seem to be more willing to accept the interpretations of such tests rather than the conclusion of the clinicians after a less structured interview process. Similarly, the resident physicians, who have been trained to approach problems objectively, accept the results of objective testing with little more skepticism than when they receive serum chemistry determinations from the laboratory.

The behavioral scientist facilitates professional contacts with organizations and nonphysician professionals from the community who provide support and services of value for both psychological and/or paramedical patient care. These nonphysician professionals can expand the resources of the behavioral science program. This provides residents with an opportunity to distribute some of their patients' problems to organizations that were established specifically to meet those needs, thus allowing the residents to concentrate on the remaining difficulties.

Finally, the behavioral scientist's teaching role carries with it the responsibility to assist residents in integrating the social problems with the organic ones. In an analytical sense, the behavioral scientist needs to be able to help residents determine the psychosocial aspects of an illness in as logical a fashion as they diagnose physical ailments. The development of protocols for management of these concurrent problems has been an effective means of defining as well as treating these aspects of illness. If viewed as an integral part of the process of assessing disease, the psychological aberrations can be anticipated and addressed before they become clinically manifest in doctor-patient relationships, thus allowing the residents and their patients to enjoy mutually rewarding, effective, and supportive interactions.

APPLYING EVALUATION SKILLS IN TEACHING

Since many behavioral scientists have expertise in the area of evaluation, they are often called upon to assist in developing evaluation mechanisms, interpreting the data, and applying the results. For example, the psychologist interprets standardized test scores of residents in training and assists in developing remediation plans for residents who are having difficulty with certain aspects of their clinical decision making or acquisition of knowledge. From an analysis of the department's group data, the psychologist identifies strong and weak areas in the training program and suggests curricular changes.

RESEARCHING EDUCATIONAL AND PSYCHOLOGICAL QUESTIONS

Engaging in research is another role the clinical behavioral scientist assumes. Through his/her own study, the behavioral scientist contributes to the body of knowledge and practice of psychology, family medicine, and related disciplines. In addition, the behavioral scientist models effective research skills and consults on the research projects of others including students, residents, staff, and faculty. This systematic inquiry occurs in a wide range of settings in the medical and educational environment. These investigations are for the purpose of exploring issues related to education, administration, communication, and patient care, recommending changes that enhance health care delivery, and strengthening the education of students and residents. Staff attitudes, alcohol intervention approaches, effects of certain drugs, and educational techniques are examples of the types of variables explored.

PROBLEM SOLVING IN THE CLINICAL ENVIRONMENT

The clinical behavioral scientist is an observer of and consultant for change of human behavior in the health care setting. The consultant observes all aspects of the clinical environment including the physical surroundings, the patients, the hospital and clinic staff, students, residents, and faculty. From these observations of the clinical milieu, the behavioral scientist finds areas where a closer look is desirable. Diagnosis may be undertaken in a formal (e.g., using sociometric techniques) or informal (e.g., conversation with various individuals) manner in order to determine the aspects or areas that warrant attention and intervention. For example, there may be staff members or faculty who need problem-solving skills or who want to learn more effective communication skills. In addition to the behavioral scientist's skills in these areas, a mutually respectful relationship with administration, staff, students, and residents is essential to success in this setting. The behavioral scientist's level of acceptance in the clinical environment will determine the depth to which he/she can go in problem identification and resolution. Prevention of problems can be the focus of the behavioral scientist as experience in the setting is obtained and as all parties come to feel comfortable with this role of the observer/consultant.

The training of the behavioral scientist includes a background in creative thinking, motivational techniques, problem solving, group dynamics, and evaluation of group and individual performance. Physicians need these skills and intuitively learn many of them. Psychologists have specific training in these areas and can offer the physicians a conceptual framework and a more systematic approach as a result of their formal training. Residents, staff, or administration, for example, may be nudged out of their usual problem-solving styles by the behavioral scientist's encouragement to combine the obvious in unusual or different ways, to brainstorm, or to hitchhike ideas. To illustrate, a resident was frustrated at his inability to find the ideal case to illustrate the points he wanted to make in his grand rounds lecture on children's school problems. The behavioral scientist's simple suggestion that he look at his own life as a possible example led him to recall some of his past experiences. His self-exploration afforded him not only an increased understanding of his childhood perplexities, but also led to the construction of a powerful autobiographical example for his lecture.

Department chairpersons, business managers, directors of medical education, and others within the medical arena confront complex administrative dilemmas that can become clearer when under the scrutiny of an outside observer/consultant such as the clinical behavioral scientist. A psychological and systemic perspective can elucidate underlying reasons for maladaptive behavior, such as overreaction to a minor problem. Complaints about the call room's malfunctioning refrigerator may symbolize a larger concern to residents. In reality, the residents may be feeling isolated, vulnerable, or frustrated because of a lack of privacy or a lack of control over how they organize their time. Residents seem to progress through a series of cycles, able to tolerate the pressures of residency at times and less well able to tolerate them at others. The clinical behavioral scientist who is sensitive to the cycles and to the underlying causes of residents' reactions to minor distresses can provide administration with insight and direction for identifying the roots of the problem and developing methods for resolving the issue. It is predictable that if the larger concern is not addressed, another complaint would soon surface. By contrast, dealing with both the immediate difficulty and the underlying issue can move residents to a clearer understanding of the origin of their grievances.

In this example, the anger and frustration the group felt over the broken refrigerator probably represented the struggle the residents were facing as designs were being finalized for new call rooms for the three residencies in the hospital. Residents felt excluded from the design process and feared their call rooms would be inadequate.

When these vulnerabilities were voiced and a committee with representatives from each residency department was formed to review the architect's plans, the anger and frustration quickly dissipated.

Another role the clinical behavioral scientist assumes is to encourage administration to be tolerant of individual resident's differences. Allowing flexibility in programming is an example. For instance, a resident whose husband worked a 3:00-to-11:00-P.M. shift in a corporation was frustrated because she was unable to find any time to spend with her husband. In discussing her dilemma, it was proposed that she schedule her office patients from 5:00 P.M. backward to 1:00 P.M. instead of the usual chronological fashion. This would at times provide extended time over the lunch hour to spend with her husband rather than leaving the office earlier in the afternoon when her husband would have already left for work. In this dilemma, the clinical behavioral scientist acted as facilitator and mediator with administration.

Because administrators are frequently barraged with complaints and problems by everyone—staff, residents, students, and faculty—they often find it difficult to maintain an air of optimism. The clinical behavioral scientist can be supportive and empathetic and can also help to identify positive, productive approaches to resolution of complaints and problems.

To illustrate, the department's business manager complained that her staff never listened when she told them there was no need to feel what they were expressing to her. Since this was observed to be a common pattern for her, the behavioral scientist mentioned that she might instead try empathizing with the staff's feelings so that they would perceive an attitude of acceptance and understanding from their supervisor, thus facilitating their acceptance of her suggestions.

In group settings, whether participants are nurses, faculty, or residents, the behavioral scientist models effective interpersonal skills. He/she encourages quiet participants to share their ideas with the group and summarizes or harmonizes as needed. The unproductive behavior of participants who are overly aggressive or domineering is noted and addressed at appropriate times.

MAINTAINING PERSONAL JOB SATISFACTION

In order to ensure that behavioral scientists will continue to be available to serve others, they need to be able to turn to friends and colleagues who will be supportive and healing. Setting aside time for informal case discussions or attending conferences with colleagues of the same discipline will enable behavioral scientists to discuss important professional and personal matters with individuals who have similar backgrounds. Likewise, steps can be taken to bring in interns, consultants, or fellows of the discipline to provide objectivity, support, and understanding.

Faculty retreats provide opportunities for strengthening relationships, identifying problems, and setting priorities for individuals within the department. In this manner, the faculty group is brought together in a way that can facilitate their mutual supportiveness.

Just as behavioral scientists assist others in setting realistic and attainable goals, we must do the same for ourselves. Acknowledging personal limits and establishing priorities are key steps in caring for ourselves so that we are physically and emotionally able to care for others.

TRAINING CLINICAL BEHAVIORAL SCIENTISTS

The training of the clinical behavioral scientist to work in this broad role includes core content in personality theory, psychopathology, developmental psychology, and family dynamics, as well as clinical skills in diagnosis and treatment of individual and family disturbances. Thus, the bases for application of psychological principles are similar to the bases needed to work in other applied settings. Beyond this, experience in family medicine is important for developing an understanding of how to apply the skills learned.

In addition, competence in evaluation and curriculum development will allow flexibility and breadth of the job role. Training and experience in teaching methods is important since the behavioral scientist's primary responsibility is teaching residents the psychosocial perspectives they need to practice family medicine in a comprehensive manner.

National guidelines for training health psychologists are currently under development (Stone, 1983). They suggest that a generic doctorate in clinical, counseling, or school psychology be obtained with health psychology specialization at the postdoctorate level. Until this type of extended training is available, it is important for trainees to spend at least a year or more in the family medicine setting before taking on the extensive responsibilities described in this chapter. A limited number of pre- and postdoctoral internships are available to meet this need (Treadwell, 1983).

In the physician's view, the personal characteristics of the clinical behavioral scientist need to be compatible with the medical community. The consultant must realize the priorities and pressures experienced by physicians in training and practice. For example, the psychosocial difficulties will often be a lower priority than a life-threatening physical problem, and there may be insufficient time to address both simultaneously in many situations. The behavioral scientist needs to be flexible and realistic in setting the goals that can be accomplished during the residents' limited time in the program and the practitioners' limited time during the work week.

In order for the behavioral scientist to build credibility with the residents and physician faculty, it is essential that they see patients along with them. Videotaping resident-patient encounters and providing feedback is highly desirable; however, it is with face-to-face contact with patients alongside the residents that the clinician's value increases as perceived by the residents.

SUMMARY

Learners in a graduate education program have many needs for which they look to their faculty, including advocate, counselor, confidant, educator, researcher, therapist, consultant, and role model. No individual faculty member, physician, or behavioral scientist can meet all these needs. Because of the differences in training and priorities of physicians and behavioral scientists, in some settings the behavioral scientist will have the opportunity to contribute some dimensions that may not otherwise be represented. Each residency program is different and has different needs. We have discussed the basic areas of involvement to illustrate the scope of such an undertaking. Familiarity with the issues presented in this chapter should make it easier to determine the specific needs of a particular residency program.

The roles of advocate and advisor are fostered by the behavioral scientists' credibility. Being perceived as a valued team member tends to generalize from the residents to their faculty. Demonstrating clear communication, basic managerial skills, and an academic orientation, the behavioral scientist can improve the efficiency and satisfaction of the personnel at all levels of the training program as well as among the administrators with whom the program deals. This results in greater stability within the residency, thus diminishing anxiety and stress and allowing that unproductive energy to be applied more constructively. As an advisor or advocate, the behavioral scientist has the natural advantage of being a nonphysician and often can offer a different perspective, which in a conflict merits consideration.

In conclusion, the behavioral scientist can reinforce and augment the presence of humanity in family practice training programs. It is difficult because of time constraints for the physician educator to focus a primary interest on a patient's psychological status when trying to instruct the residents in the appropriate use of increasingly complex medical technology. Although it is often ignored in medical training programs, it is the humanity that separates the technicians from the physicians. By allowing the residents to express feelings, the behavioral scientist legitimizes the feelings of the residents and thus allows the residents to legitimize the emotions of their patients. Practicing good nuturing skills, he/she fosters personal growth and provides for the benefits of constructive criticism to those he serves. Exhibiting effective communication and counseling skills, he/she extends the benefits of those skills to all the people with whom the program is involved. By actively becoming involved with consultation, instruction, and research, the behavioral scientist can engender interest and respect, as opposed to frustration, for the wide variety of people served by family physicians. It is the goal of family practice to allow all of us, as patients or professionals, access to this type of care and caring.

REFERENCES

Coombs, R. H., & Fawzy, F. I. (1982). The effect of marital status on stress in medical school. *American Journal of Psychiatry, 139*, 1490-1493.

Davis, R. M. (1981). Sleep deprivation in graduate medical education. *Illinois Medical Journal, 16*(3), 146-149.

Leichner, P., & Kalin, R. (1980). Results of the first Canadian psychiatric knowledge self-assessment for residents. *Canadian Journal of Psychiatry, 25*(4), 281-289.

Loes, M. W., & Scheiber, S. C. (1981). The impaired resident. *Arizona Medicine, 38*(10), 777-779.

Nelson, E. G., & Henry, W. F. (1978). Psychosocial factors seen as problems by family practice residents and their spouses. *The Journal of Family Practice, 6*(3), 581-589.

Pasnau, R. O., & Russell, A. T. (1975). Psychiatric resident suicide: An analysis of five cases. *American Journal of Psychiatry, 132*(4), 402-406.

Pfifferling, J. H. (1983, October). Coping with residency distress. *Resident and Staff Physician, 105*, 111.

Stone, G. (Ed.). (1983). National working conference on training in health psychology, Arden House, Harriman, New York, May 23-27, 1983 [Special issue]. *Health Psychology, 2*(5).

Treadwell, T. W., Jr. (1983, May). Rationale for a training program for non-medical professionals. In T. W. Treadwell, Jr., S. Shellenberger, K. Watkins Couch, J. Day, & D. Ransom (Presenters), *Extending the concept of faculty development in family medicine: Internships for behavioral scientists and educators*. Symposium conducted at the meeting of the Society of Teachers of Family Medicine, Boston.

Chapter 11

Coping with Stress During Internship

John L. Ziegler, M.D., and Nick Kanas, M.D.

The Fourth Medical Division regarded itself as the top service at the Boston City Hospital, the elite in the sharpest and brightest of all the teaching hospitals in town. We were the iron men, we told ourselves. The lights in the laboratory on the top floor of the Peabody Building were never turned off at night; the house staff never slept.—Lewis Thomas, *The Youngest Science*, 1983, pp. 49–50

The days of the "iron men," recalled by Lewis Thomas, refers to the time-honored tradition of medical internship. The rigors of internship—long hours, sleep deprivation, high standards of competency and comportment, time pressures, life-and-death decisions, and endless "scut" work—are widely regarded as necessary rites of passage to physicianhood. Survival of this incredibly stressful period results in such virtues as "commitment" and "responsibility," according to seasoned educators. But what are the costs, psychologically, emotionally, and professionally, of this prevailing attitude toward postgraduate medical training?

This chapter will examine the issues of stress and coping in medical internship. The experience of the first postgraduate year provides an instructive window to view patterns of individual and group behavior under severe stress. Our observations derive from a four-year experience of a weekly stress discussion group for medical interns during which participants shared stressful issues, feelings, and coping methods (Ziegler & Kanas, 1984). We shall describe the major issues causing stress that were raised by the interns, speculate on the inner sources of stressful feelings that appear to be common to interns, and comment on the adaptive and maladaptive coping mechanisms we have observed.

THE INTERN STRESS DISCUSSION GROUP

Participants were medical interns from the School of Medicine, University of California San Francisco, who were on an eight-week rotation to the Veterans Administration Medical Center. The group leaders were the authors (an internist and psychiatrist) and the medical chief resident. Attendance was voluntary, and interns were asked to discuss issues or events that caused stress (defined as a perceived threat) in their lives. The interns turned over their beepers to their residents for the discussion hour. Group leaders kept track of the discussion topics, and a questionnaire evaluating internship stress and coping behavior was sent out to the interns at the end of the first year (Ziegler & Kanas, 1984). Twenty-one returned the questionnaire.

Attendance averaged five (three men, two women) out of a possible eight interns on each rotation. On the questionnaire, the interns reported attending an average of five sessions and missing two sessions. Reasons for missing sessions included schedule conflicts and lack of time; no interns checked "not interested" or "group not helpful."

Although this was not a psychotherapy group, we monitored group climate for the first year to determine the discussion atmosphere (Kanas & Ziegler, 1984). The results of this analysis disclosed that the interns were involved and open, yet respectful of each other's privacy. Much of the group process was shaped by the leaders, who were supportive and empathetic.

The members found the group to be useful. On the questionnaire, 55% of the participants said it was "moderately" or "very" helpful in dealing with stress, and none rated it as "not at all" helpful.

ISSUES CAUSING STRESS

. . . the absolute asceticism of the residency recreates, for the young physician, the sacrificial ethic of monastic medicine. That ethic is severe: immediate response to the needs of the patient, to the call of the emergency room, to the demands for reports; unmitigated responsibility for correct decisions made promptly and communicated clearly; flagellating denial of sleep, self-indulgence, and frivolity, even to the point of depression and deterioration of personal life, of friendship and love. This practice, which is intense in the year of noviceship and less so in succeeding years, must instill into many medical minds the monastic principle of altruism. Guilt should always be felt in the future when a call is to be answered, a patient seen, or a consultation completed. The physician's conscience will ever after cry out when self-interest intrudes on patient care. At least this seems to be the hidden rationale of this training. (Jonsen, 1983, p. 1534)

A major complaint of the interns in the group was related to the lack of time available to do all that was asked of them. This contributed to an ongoing sense of not being in control of their lives. Time pressure was symbolized by the incessant "beeper" calls, often for trivial tasks or questions. An intuitive need to visit and chat with their patients was frustrated by the demand for completing paperwork, tracking down X rays and laboratory reports, attending conferences and rounds, and learning medicine. The interns also voiced a need to complete all work on their patients before leaving for the day, thus sparing the on-call intern additional calls or procedures during the night. Caring for difficult or dying patients added to the sense of inefficiency. A very ill patient in the intensive-care unit was not only emotionally draining but would usurp valuable time from other duties.

Coping patterns varied. Predictably, there was universal anger against the "system," blaming the outdated internship tradition, excessive bureaucracy, emphasis on technology, uncaring staff, and economic constraints. Anger at the system tended to unite the interns against a common enemy. The system appeared immutable; anger and complaining yielded little change and often labeled the intern as a troublemaker. A second coping mechanism was resignation, conservation of energy, and sheer "survival." Most interns chose to contain angry feelings, get the job done, and go home at a reasonable hour. Others viewed the maze of daily "scut" work as a challenge—a "game" to be played to subvert or circumvent the harassment of the system.

The interns could discern that their stress was often the result of high self-expectations. They acknowledged that they had altruistic ideals, fantasies of healing the sick, and heroic images of themselves when they entered medicine. To achieve these goals, many interns had developed compulsive, type A behavior patterns oriented toward achievement and approval. As the internship year progressed, these ideals were seriously threatened. They could not accomplish all that needed to be done, they could not cure illness or even make much difference in their patients' lives, they could not learn or know everything: a "larger-than-life" performance was impossible. In reality, the demeaning, endless "scut" work, the patronizing attitude of senior faculty, and bottom rank in the medical hierarchy served to lower self-esteem. In coping with this gap between their fantasized roles and the reality of internship, some interns developed an attitude of cynicism and bitterness. In others, there was gradual erosion of their "ideals" and reluctant acceptance of the pragmatic realities of medical practice. Still others denied that the internship was stressful at all, preferring to wall off their feelings.

Another generic issue that caused stress for interns was the doctor-patient relationship. There were four related aspects to this issue: dealing with seriously ill or dying patients, coping with the "hateful" patient (Groves, 1978), finding time to practice humanistic medicine, and moral stress.

Seriously ill and dying patients cause considerable anxiety and frustration in medical staff (Artiss & Levine, 1973). Physicians are trained to diagnose and treat, with improvement or cure as the expected outcome. When patients worsen and die despite their doctors' best efforts, the outcome is viewed as a failure. Interns went through a painful realization that cure is sometimes not a realistic goal. This disillusionment was further compounded by the threat of a dying patient to the interns' own view of mortality. Denial of death is a common human trait, and the fantasy of immortality is strongly held by doctors (Konior & Levine, 1975). The interns' experiences with dying patients awakened anxieties over death and resulted in considerable tension or confusion in their relationship with patients.

Coping with individuals who are irascible, rejecting, demanding, angry, excessively dependent, or denying is a challenge under ordinary circumstances (Artiss & Levine, 1973). When interns, relatively inexperienced in interactive techniques, must care for such individuals who are also stressed by illness, they react in a predictable manner: hostility, avoidance, rejection, denial (Gorlin & Zucker, 1983; Groves, 1978). Interns confessed to angry feelings about difficult patients and then felt guilty over the awareness that they were angry—an unacceptable emotion for a physician to display.

Finding time for "humanistic medicine" was a major frustration for interns. The system rewards industry, efficiency, memorization, diagnostic acumen, and "therapeutic distance." Therefore, time spent talking and listening to patients was time lost in accomplishing the tasks of the day. On arrival at the hospital, the choice of a bedside visit or completing the medical record was easy for the intern: the chart came first. The consequence of an incomplete record would raise eyebrows on rounds, and the fear that undiscovered laboratory data would have serious clinical consequences inevitably drove the intern to paperwork. This attitude was intuitively disturbing and frustrating to interns. They felt isolated and abandoned in an environment that left little room for emotions, compassion, and empathy for the patient.

The doctor-patient relationships also produced moral stress in the form of management decisions. The ethics of the "do not resuscitate" order, judgments about potentially morbid diagnostic and therapeutic procedures, economic considerations, and conflicts between personal values and institutional policies created considerable anxiety. Interns, because of their novitiate status, were often at odds with senior staff or consultants regarding clinical decisions with ethical consequences. Their desire to be autonomous and independent, particularly since they were ultimately responsible for their patients, was frustrated by the mandates of their seniors.

We infer that much of the anxiety, guilt, and anger that underlie doctor-patient issues derive from dependency conflicts. George Vaillant (1982), a Harvard psychiatrist, aptly describes the situation: ". . . we like taking care of other people because we are dependent, yet we tend to keep our dependency needs secret from ourselves" (p. 20). Thus, patients will view their physicians with the expectation of fulfillment of their need for nurturance, love, happiness, and security. Physicians likewise have unconscious needs from their patients, such as approval, gratitude, respect, admiration, and getting well (Jensen, 1981). These mutual dependency needs cannot realistically be met, and severe "role strain" develops in the doctor-patient relationship (Tokarz et al., 1979). Although a more in-depth analysis of dependency in physicians is beyond our scope, the literature on the subject supports the hypothesis that unfulfilled childhood needs are strong determinants in physicians' behavior (Artiss & Levine, 1973; Jensen, 1981; Tokarz et al., 1979; Vaillant et al., 1972).

Stressors varied during the course of the year. Table 1 ranks important contributors to perceived stress as judged by all interns returning the questionnaire. At the beginning of the year, issues involving multiple simultaneous demands, lack of knowledge, lack of sleep, and high self-expectations were perceived as most stressful. After at least six months of internship, these issues became less problematic. Some items became more stressful as the year progressed, especially high expectations and demands from others, and the amount of work. Interactions with friends, relatives, and fellow physicians produced little stress.

COPING WITH STRESS

The preceding discussion highlights the key issues, coping patterns, and sources of stress in medical interns. Although the discussion group did not attempt to teach stress management, the interns reported that sharing common experiences and feelings offered some relief. They were also pleased to encounter empathetic and supportive faculty members. Since the group was

Table 1

Contributors to Perceived Stress in Medical Interns

Issue	Responses indicating moderately/very much/extremely (%)	
	Beginning of year	After 6+ months
Multiple simultaneous demands	95	80
Lack of knowledge of medicine	90	48
Lack of sleep	86	76
High expectations from self	81	62
The amount of work	71	76
Demanding patients	60	65
Care of chronically ill or dying patients	52	48
Interactions with non-M.D.s (esp. R.N.s)	50	44
High expectations from others	43	57
Personal relations outside of the medical center	38	43
Interactions with attendings	30	35
Interactions with residents	20	10
Interactions with other interns	5	5

discussion-oriented, issues were allowed to be raised and developed over the course of each session. Coping mechanisms were freely discussed, with the goals of providing mastery and attempting realistic problem solving. Table 2 shows some of our accumulated wisdom concerning house staff coping methods.

In coping with stress, one should not underestimate the value of talking with friends and peers. Table 3 illustrates that much support was derived from friends and relatives outside the medical center, and from fellow interns and residents. Two thirds of the questionnaire respondents derived help from appreciative patients. Surprisingly, little support was given by attendings and non-M.D. staff, such as nurses. Perhaps the latter groups were perceived as stressors in their own right. Alternatively, intergenerational and inter-professional factors may have created emotional barriers between the interns and these groups.

Owing to the short rotations of interns in the VA program, we viewed a more structured seminar on stress management as too overwhelming and impersonal. Other training programs have made such attempts with varying success (Kelly et al., 1982; Siegel & Donnelly, 1978; Wise, 1977). When time and program structure permit, we recommend that time management, self-awareness and sensitizing techniques, assertiveness training, and relaxation methods be introduced to interns.

Table 2
Suggested Ways for House Staff to Reduce Job-Related Stress

Goal	Suggested methods
Recognize stressors	• Make a commitment to identify and reduce stress in your life • Be sensitive to emotional responses to stressors (feelings of guilt, frustration and anger, depression and hopelessness, tension and anxiety) • Try to identify major stressors using systematic self-monitoring • Take *early* action to reduce stressor and initiate coping before emotional response "takes over"
Time management	• Negotiate tasks with colleagues • Delegate responsibilities to others • Reduce beeper interruptions (e.g., be available on ward for questions at set times; instruct callers to leave messages and indicate "stat" or "at your convenience" for return calls) • Set aside an hour as "inviolate" and relax, walk, run, meditate, or otherwise get it together • Be selective in choosing what you read and learn— you remember best what interests you and what applies to your patients
Behavior modification	• Learn to be appropriately assertive (as opposed to aggressive) • Learn techniques of active listening, imagery, and constructive criticism
Social support	• Establish as a priority spending quality time with friends and family; structure the time so that you are not called away and are rested and relaxed; seek out peer relationships; join support groups, community organizations, or team sports
Environment	• Take steps to establish as relaxing and aesthetic an environment as possible (e.g., radio or tape recorder in your office, pleasant art work, carpeted floor) • Inform colleagues or co-workers of your favored work habits so that you will not be interrupted needlessly
Relaxation techniques	• Explore various techniques such as yoga, meditation, biofeedback. • Ensure adequate diet and exercise regularly • Engage in self-awareness techniques to discover "highly prized beliefs" (myths) that may not work for you • Cultivate relaxation habits with the same energy and commitment that you apply to your work

Table 3
Support in Coping with Stress

Support	Responses indicating moderately/very much/extremely (%)
Personal relations outside of medical center	95
Other interns	90
Residents	88
Appreciative patients	67
Attendings	33
Non-M.D. staff (esp. R.N.s)	22

We have examined the genesis of stress in internship and commented on the value of a support group. Having listened for the last three years to these issues, we are convinced that the training environment for house officers should be changed. The days of the "iron men" have long since passed, and today's interns are sensitive barometers of the excessive pressures of modern medicine. Maladaptive coping and the "impaired physician" are perhaps at the tip of the iceberg.

CONCLUSION

It is paradoxical that physicians should be called upon to counsel patients to lead less stressful life-styles when they themselves engage in appallingly stressful practices. It is further curious that physicians receive virtually no formal training in stress management, either for themselves or for educating their patients.

One way of examining this paradox is to look at the "mythology" of medical practice. Omnipotence, omniscience, and invulnerability are heroic qualities ascribed to physicians by patients. Altruism, sacrifice, and commitment are the expected behaviors. The grandfather of modern medicine, William Osler, advised his trainees:

> You cannot hope, of course, to escape from the cares and anxieties incident to professional life. Stand up bravely, even against the worst. Your very hopes may have passed on out of sight, as did all that was near and dear to the Patriarch at the Jabbok ford, and like him, you may be left to struggle in the night alone. Well for you, if you wrestle on, for in persistency lies victory, and with the morning may come the wished for blessing. But not always; there is a struggle with defeat which some of you will have to bear, and it will be well for you in that day to have cultivated a cheerful equanimity. Remember too that some-

times "from our desolation only does the better life begin." Even with
disaster ahead and ruin imminent, it is better to face them with a smile,
and with the head erect, than to crouch at their approach. (Osler, 1947,
pp. 7–8)

Yet, as we have observed in our intern group and as described eloquently
by others (Mawardi, 1979; McCue, 1982), medical practice has changed
drastically. The old myths do not stand the test of reality: omnipotence gives
way to the power of the "system," not the individual; omniscience yields to
the overwhelming information explosion; and invulnerability succumbs to
the mere humanness of physicians (Hilfiker, 1984).

Derek Bok has described incisively the dilemmas of medical training in
the modern era:

> Professor Donald Selden aptly summarized the traditional view in his
> 1981 presidential address to the Association of American Physicians:
>   Medicine is a very narrow discipline. Its goals may be defined as
>   the relief of pain, the prevention of disability, and the postpone-
>   ment of death by the application of the theoretical knowledge
>   incorporated in medical science to individual patients.
> This conception of the doctor's role has had a marked effect on the
> nature of medical education. In a profession that emphasizes scientif-
> ically determined findings, rather than the rough judgments charac-
> teristic of lawyers and business executives, professors are inclined to
> impart knowledge didactically, as truths to be described rather than
> problems to be discussed. Matters outside the domain of science com-
> mand little attention. Although everyone knows that psychological and
> behavioral factors can influence health, doctors have tended to regard
> these matters as unscientific and have left them largely to
> others—psychologists, social workers, public health officials, and the
> like. It is only natural, then, for medical schools to push such subjects
> to the margins of the curriculum. Similarly, since ethical issues and
> patient values have little effect on the scientific determination of disease,
> they have not loomed large in the thinking of physicians or faculty
> committees, at least until recently, when the law courts and the media
> began to make such problems too prominent to ignore. Much the same
> has been true of other subjects relevant to health, such as the prevention
> of disease, the cost and equitable distribution of medical services, and
> the development of health policies and regulations. Because these topics
> are peripheral to the scientific analysis of illness, they have either been
> relegated to secondary status in the curriculum or left to other faculties
> such as public administration and public health. (Bok, 1984, p. 36)

The implications of this "narrowness," he goes on to say, are to foster precisely the most undesirable qualities in the medical trainee. Enlarging on the issue, J. Michael Bishop (1984) bemoans: ". . . the average medical student I encounter from year to year displays a literal and unsupple state of mind whose quality prefigures a dreary performance at the bedside" (p. 96). What is needed, clearly, is a new point of view. The "system" *can* be altered given enlightened leadership. More time *can* be made available to trainees through more creative use of ancillary personnel, computers, and other hospital economies. Most important, the process skills of communication, self-awareness, problem solving, and humane bedside behavior *can* be taught *pari passu* with other medical knowledge and skills. Psychiatrists and educators have long wondered whether the goals of rigorous house staff training are really met. A consensus is developing that it is time to reexamine premedical requirements to provide more breadth in medical training, to attend more carefully to teaching noncognitive skills, to create a learning environment that rewards humane behavior over technical competence, and to foster adaptive and curious habits of mind over rote learning (Bishop, 1984). Within this new framework should be a prominent curricular emphasis on self-awareness and stress management, skills that will help ensure personal well-being and professional satisfaction.

REFERENCES

Artiss, K. L., & Levine, A. S. (1973). Doctor-patient relation in severe illness. *New England Journal of Medicine, 288,* 1210–1214.

Bishop, J. M. (1984). Infuriating tensions: Science and the medical student. *Journal of Medical Education, 59,* 91–102.

Bok, D. (1984, May). Needed: A new way to train doctors. *Harvard Magazine,* p. 36.

Gorlin, R., & Zucker, H. D. (1983). Physicians' reactions to patients. A key to teaching humanistic medicine. *New England Journal of Medicine, 308,* 1059–1064.

Groves, J. E. (1978). Taking care of the hateful patient. *New England Journal of Medicine, 298,* 883–887.

Hilfiker, D. (1984). Facing our mistakes. *New England Journal of Medicine, 310,* 118–122.

Jensen, P. S. (1981). The doctor-patient relationship: Headed for impasse or improvement. *Annals of Internal Medicine, 95,* 769–771.

Jonsen, A. (1983). Watching the doctor. *New England Journal of Medicine, 25,* 1533–1535.

Kanas, N., & Ziegler, J. L. (1984). Group climate in a stress discussion group for medical interns. *Group, 8,* 35–38.

Kelly, J. A., Bradlyn, A. S., Dubbert, P. M., & St. Lawrence, J. S. (1982). Stress management training in medical school. *Journal of Medical Education, 57,* 91–99.

Konior, G. S., & Levine, A. S. (1975). The fear of dying: How patients and their doctors behave. *Seminars in Oncology, 2,* 311–315.

Mawardi, B. H. (1979). Satisfactions, dissatisfactions, and causes of stress in medical practice. *Journal of the American Medical Association, 241,* 1483–1486.

McCue, J. D. (1982). The effects of stress on physicians and their medical practice. *New England Journal of Medicine, 306,* 458–463.

Osler, W. (1947). *Aequanimitas.* Philadelphia: Blakiston.

184   Heal Thyself

Siegel, B., & Donnelly, J. C. (1978). Enriching personal and professional development: The experience of a support group for interns. *Journal of Medical Education, 53*, 908–914.

Thomas, L. (1983). *The Youngest Science*. New York: Viking.

Tokarz, J. P., Bremer, W., & Peters, K. (1979). *Beyond survival* (p. 11). Chicago: American Medical Association.

Vaillant, G. E. (1982). When doctors fail to care for themselves. *Harvard Magazine*, p. 20.

Vaillant, G. E., Sobowale, N. C., & McArthur, C. (1972). Some psychologic vulnerabilities of physicians. *New England Journal of Medicine, 287*, 372–375.

Wise, T. N. (1977). Utilization of group process in training oncology fellows. *International Journal of Group Psychotherapy, 27*, 105–111.

Ziegler, J. L., & Kanas, N. (1984). A stress discussion group for medical interns. *Journal of Medical Education, 59*, 205–207.

Chapter 12

The Health Professional in Treatment: Symptoms, Dynamics, and Treatment Issues

Herbert J. Freudenberger, Ph.D.

During the past 5 to 10 years there has been an ever-increasing concern with impaired professionals. What specifically constitutes impairment? Freudenberger (1984b) states that "physical and mental disability, alcoholism, substance abuse, debilitation through aging, loss of motor skills, and sexual involvement with patients would constitute impairment" (p. 2).

As had been previously conjectured, the health professional is not immune to these illnesses and, as a group, may be considered at essentially a higher risk than the general population. Nagy (1981) wrote, "In part this is a function of easy 'accessibility,' as well the continued stresses and pressures with which the professional is functioning" (p. 36). According to a recent article (Steyer, 1981), perhaps as many as 10% of the country's doctors are considered unable to perform properly due to alcoholism, drug abuse, senility, emotional problems or mental illness."

FACTORS CONTRIBUTING TO IMPAIRMENT

According to Dennis Jaffe (1984), "new regulations are undermining the kinds of certainty that physicians felt they once had—total autonomy without outside interference, freedom to set fees and the assurance of a livelihood" (p. 43) all contribute to impairment. The pressures of maintaining one's daily practice are heightened by "inflation, rising office expenses, keeping accurate records, peer review, geographic population shifts, increased competition, and a glut of specific professionals in dense urban areas" (Freudenberger, 1983). All these environmental concerns add to the pressures felt by professionals.

An additional contribution to impairment is the need for high achievement (Freudenberger & Richelson, 1980), which often constitutes a major internal pressure for many impaired professionals. Often from an early age, these people have set up significant and highly demanding goals for themselves. Their values and desire for performance, accomplishment, perfect grades, and scores are always present in their lives. They often find that they have little time for fun, and even less time for living. Their major emphasis is on "accomplishing," sometimes at significant cost to themselves.

Other professionals have their own contextual matrix for burnout. The nursing profession is plagued with "nurse administrators who relentlessly overextend themselves by working extra long hours" (Clark, 1980, p. 41). Farber and Heifez (1982) speak at length about the impact of psychotherapeutic practice on psychotherapists. Sheridan and Sheridan (1980) speak of the inherent pressure that the legal professional experiences. He comments on the fact that law is a "public contact occupation" and as such has been shown to be more stressful than other professions" (p. 47).

Perusing the literature, one soon recognizes that librarians, dentists, social workers, nurses, attorneys, judges, physicians, psychologists, rehabilitation counselors—all who work in the service arena find that a percentage of their colleagues sooner or later are impaired in their functioning. This impairment makes its impact on their lives, their families, as well as on their job functioning.

WHO ARE IMPAIRED PROFESSIONALS? WHAT ARE THEY LIKE?

During the past few years, this therapist has treated at least 75 psychologists, social workers, attorneys, physicians, nurses, clergy (ministers, priests, nuns, rabbis) (Freudenberger, 1982c), pharmacists, police officers (Freudenberger & Robbins, 1982), judges, and alcohol-drug counselors in his private practice.

The mean age of most of the individuals who seek treatment is 38 years.

The general age range is between 35 and 45. This is essentially in agreement with Bouhoutsos and co-workers (1983), who found that 42 years of age was the mean for 96% of the therapists she treated; approximately 40% were married, 25% single, and the rest recently divorced, widowed, or separated. Eighty percent were male. However, during the past few years, there has been a noted increase of impaired women seeking treatment (Freudenberger & North, 1985). The group is largely composed of physicians, librarians, social workers, attorneys, and psychotherapists. The mean age of this group is approximately 32. The increase of women becoming impaired is a function of what Pines (1981) refers to as professional women who "felt they had less freedom, autonomy, and influence in their work as well as less variety, less challenge, and a less positive work environment" (p. 87). These are major factors leading to impairment of professional women. The men reported in this paper have been practicing their profession for approximately 15 to 25 years. The women, on the average, have been working in their career approximately 10 years.

PRESENTING SYMPTOMS AND REASONS FOR SEEKING TREATMENT

Presenting symptoms range from depression, exhaustion, anxiety about their lives and work, feeling a sense of cynicism or boredom creeping into their demeanor, and questioning what made them initially enter their chosen profession. Some seek assistance because they are experiencing problems with their family, friends, or patients. Some lose a number of patients and do not know the cause of this downturn in their practice.

Others are facing ethics charges with their state certification boards for a variety of reasons. The rather typical one is sexual involvement with patients, facing narcotics charges, or threat of disbarment because of pending financial embezzlement. Charges such as these may promote entrance into treatment. But some professionals may need to be threatened by colleagues or staff that if they do not seek treatment they will be turned in, reported, or asked to leave their facility or practice. This has sometimes been referred to as invoking "the snitcher's law," but it appears it is more sensible to "snitch" than to allow an impaired colleague to continue to jeapordize others. Another group is "threatened" into treatment by a spouse, lover, or partner who has found them frequently drunk, drugged, emotionally impaired, or acting "strange."

A typical story is that of an internist who was referred by his practitioner partners. He is 40 years old, married, with three children. In the past few years he has begun screaming at the staff, both in the office and the nurses in the hospital. His behavior is erratic; for instance, he may spend excessive office time with one patient and give another a cursory examination. He is given to crying, mood swings, and frequent bouts of depression. He was found to be an abuser of cocaine and Valium for the past five years.

Another instance is that of a 43-year-old recently separated dentist who was arrested while intoxicated in a neighboring state. Further perusal revealed that he has been stopped repeatedly by the police in his local community and was often escorted home and told "not to drink so much." It is not unusual to find that a "community as a whole" often covers up for the impaired professional. This cover-up is certainly to the detriment of the person as well as his clients.

Additional factors include overwork, trying to get ahead, and equating volume with quality; dissolving a professional relationship, bankruptcy; serious illness of spouse; illness of a child, death of a child, or the ending of a long love or marital relationship. Others feel the demands not only of the family, "but also society which seems to have overwhelmed them. They often feel they must be all things to all people" (Vincent, 1969).

Women frequently experience role conflicts, ambiguity about their multiple role functions. In time, difficulty emerges with the decision-making process, conflicts of assertion and aggression, and planning successfully on a day-by-day basis. They often speak of working extremely long and tedious hours, having little or no time for social life, and finding their marriages falling apart. One young woman, a 30-year-old attorney, knew she was close to a breaking point when she found herself collecting scissors and spending hours in her apartment getting drunk and staring at them. In the process she always wondered what it would be like to stab herself. She was close to a psychotic break when she was brought to the office. She was accompanied by a former patient of mine, who was a close friend of the woman and became concerned about her frequent drinking bouts and serious mood changes in the office. She revealed that, in order to become a partner in the law firm, she had had no vacation in two years and worked 80 to 100 hours per week, with little if any life left for herself.

Still other men and women are referred by their physician—usually an internist, cardiologist, or dermatologist. Initially they sought assistance because of physical symptoms, e.g., rashes, hives, heart palpitations, migraine headaches, hypertension. In time the symptoms were viewed as nonphysical in origin and a psychological-therapeutic intervention approach was suggested as the course of treatment.

TREATMENT ISSUES AND APPROACHES TO TREATMENT

Usually, the healer-helper has a difficult time viewing himself/herself in the role of patient. He fears a loss of dignity, loss of sense of self, or loss of power; he feels impotent and rather early on voices a loss of self-esteem. He may present himself as masochistic, guilt ridden, feeling ashamed concerning his behavior and deeds, and may believe that he cannot ever again feel comfortable in facing family, friends, or colleagues, once the truth is known.

Further exploration revealed that part of the dynamic is that these physicians have allowed their power or narcissism to get in the way of their functioning. In time, both will serve as serious deterrents to treatment. Their potential power and its abuse by the professional is enormous, especially if it is in the hands of a person who initially feels inadequate and insecure and is easily threatened by the world around him.

In the initial psychotherapeutic treatment phases the helper's dynamics of narcissism is not readily accessible to the therapist. Any intrusion into the narcissistic defense system is viewed as an attack that must be repelled at all costs. The initial approach to this narcissism is not to attack, but rather to discuss with the person his general demeanor, issues, and behavior that he himself believes have changed over the years, and to ask him to discuss what he believes may be troublesome areas. An attack or confrontation will only lead to rejection of the comments, and probably will serve to discontinue treatment. Since we are dealing with a bright person, asking to speak to observable problems leads to a more significant interaction since both patient and therapist are working on a problem together. This often serves to diminish a potential power struggle, and the need to maintain control. The narcissism may also be accompanied by a subtle or not so subtle delusion that the physician can help all and do everything to perfection. Certainly the drive to perfection, and the need to "help all" are fertile grounds for burnout.

Treatment is further complicated by counterphobic mechanisms in which initially there is continuous denial that anything is wrong. Physicians may deny that they are tired, ill, work too hard, or are having serious difficulty at home (Freudenberger, 1984a). A typical story of denial is that of a 39-year-old social worker, who was becoming increasingly abusive to his wife and children, was given to arguments, frequently threatened to leave, and suffered from long periods of silence when "no one was allowed to talk to Daddy"; all comments were dismissed by him as "just working a little too hard, and needing a vacation."

The denial mechanism further manifests itself in subtle shifts to an inflexibility of thinking, a rigid orthodoxy of treatment approaches, wherein to question the approach is to leave one open to receiving verbal abuse of being stupid or professionally ignorant. This rigidity is heightened when the professional is confronted with having committed an error or errors. The dentist, for example who, in seeking to work with more and more patients and longer hours, has become sloppy in his work quality and finds himself involved in a number of malpractice suits.

Other examples of this confrontation are: the psychiatrist who lost one of his patients to suicide; the oncologist who really began to like the 24-year-old physician patient (a son of his medical school colleague), who died of carcinoma; the attorney who, after extensive preparation in proving a client's innocence, and believing it, had the client confess in court to the murder and sexual assault of an 80-year-old woman. All these situations served to undermine the capacity of the professional to be objective and hold onto distancing feelings. They often found themselves caring too much and in time collapsed with a whole range of burnout-stress symptoms.

It is imperative that, once treatment has begun, the client is assured of confidentiality (Burgess, 1980). This is important if treatment is to occur within a safe environment. It is further necessary for the therapist to be professionally appropriate with the impaired person, not to regress the treatment into a "buddy" situation. One helpful approach is to immediately establish that he now is the helper and that the person is the patient and the one who is in need of assistance. Do not "Red Cross nurse" the colleague. Also do not undermine your therapy in a subtle underground fashion (giving the impression that you are a friend and colleague, yet still doing therapy simultaneously). This approach will most assuredly lead to the malfunctioning of the need for assistance and the continuation of treatment.

Initially the clinician must separate out the crisis and acute features of the treatment from long-term goals for treatment. Ascertain how much time the professional is willing to give to therapy—short term or longer term. If it is short term, then promote as soon as possible a therapeutic alliance—where the therapist seeks to establish a "cooperative framework, wherein the patient will give meaningful information, be discouraged from the use of vague generalizations. Throughout emphasize that only specific and tangible examples will help the work" (Sifneos, 1979, p. 69).

As soon as possible, work on breaking down resistances to treatment by eliciting, from the patient, the real reasons for being in treatment, e.g., excessive gambling, drinking, drugs, exhaustion, family arguments, diminished functioning at work, or loss of objectivity (Freudenberger, 1982b). Help the patient evaluate the life-style value system he functions within. For example, has he functioned predominantly in a framework of dedication, competence, or high achievement? It may be necessary to help him perceive that these values have placed him in a high-risk category for burnout, especially if they are accompanied by a rigidity of perception and functioning.

Others may find that they arrived at this point of burnout because of "personal unresolved issues" (Meyer, 1982)—issues that in early or middle adulthood manifest themselves because of the cumulated years of stress (Freudenberger, 1982b).

Part of the treatment also needs to focus on the reasons for the occupational choice and on lifetime goals. Here it is significant to point out that self-worth is intimately associated with educational, personal, and occupational achievements. If, during the course of work and life, the values of prestige, self-worth, power, and the acquisition of material goods are accompanied by the desire for caring, giving service, and doing for others, the physician may find himself in a serious conflicted situation. On the one hand, he may want to be selfish, and on the other hand, to "do for others." As one young Hispanic woman physician said, "I did not know that my pushing so hard and proving so much would end in my becoming ill." She was referred because of serious periodic depressions.

The therapist also needs to be aware of his/her countertransference feelings. One needs to be alert to the fact that as one works with a healing-helper colleague one may have a tendency to be caught in the trap of overidentifying with the patient. This process of overidentification may prevent the therapist from looking at the colleague objectively. One needs to recognize that because the impaired person may be a therapist, it does not automatically mean that he has overcome long-unresolved, personal issues.

Help the colleague to look at what he wants out of life and at how his behavior and life-style attitudes may have served to immobilize him. Work on short-range goals that will permit change. Suggest, for example, that to begin to pay attention to rest, relaxation, fun, nutrition, exercise, and appropriate distancing from clients.

We often do not appreciate the degree to which burnout may have intruded on cognitive functioning. Impaired sense of time, difficulty in keeping appointments, and overbooking are all part of the burnout process. The therapist needs to work on the reclarification of values, as well as identifying characteristics that may be inherent within the organizations within which the professional is functioning, which may have furthered the burnout process.

The therapist needs to assist the professional to reestablish communication and contact with family and friends. With this end in mind, couple or family therapy is appropriate. It is often through the family, friends, or colleagues (all of whom may appropriately be called on during this crisis) that one gains further information as to what is occurring in this individual's life.

SUMMARY

On the whole, recovery from impairment is relatively high. Treatment calls for assisting the individual to look at his values and assumptions and to observe how learned helplessness has impacted on his life. Teach him to be more supportive of himself, more caring, less critical and help him to achieve and enhance self-esteem as well as consolidating and nurturing familial, friendship, and colleague resources.

For the addicted alcoholic or drug abuser, a 28-day detoxification program may be called for, with subsequent ongoing therapy, as well as attendance at Alcoholics Anonymous or Narcotics Anonymous meetings.

The impaired professional will need to learn how to cope with infirmities and aging and how to plan for his physical, psychic, and financial survival. He will need to relearn how to relax, have fun, laugh, enjoy, take vacations—often a very difficult thought for the impaired professional to accept.

REFERENCES

Bouhoutsos, J., Holroyd, J., Lerman, H., Forer, B. R., & Greenberg, M. (1983). Sexual intimacy between psychotherapists and patients. *Professional Psychology, Research and Practice, 14*(2), 185–196.

Burgess, A. W. (1980). Stress and burnout. *Career Foundation Letter*, No. 64. Belle Mead, N.J.: Carrier Foundation.

Clark, C. C. (1980). Burnout: Assessment and intervention. *Journal of Nursing Administration, 10*(9), 39–44.

Farber, B. A., & Heifez, L. J. (1982). The process and dimension in psychotherapists. *Professional Psychology, 13*(2), 293–301.

Freudenberger, H. J. (1981). *Burnout: How to beat the high cost of success.* New York: Anchor Press/Doubleday. (Reprinted in paperback, New York: Bantam.)

Freudenberger, H. J. (1982a). Coping with job burnout. *Law and Order, 30*(5), 3–6.

Freudenberger, H. J. (1982b). Counseling and dynamics—Treating the end-stage burnout person. In W. S. Paine (Ed.). *Job stress and burnout: Research, theory and intervention perspective.* Beverly Hills, CA: Sage Publications.

Freudenberger, H. J. (1982c). Rabbinic burnout: Symptoms and prevention. *Central Conference of American Rabbis, Yearbook*, Vol. 92. Columbus, Ohio, pp. 44–52.

Freudenberger, H. J. (1983). Hazards of psychotherapeutic practice. *Psychotherapy in Private Practice, 1*(1), 83–89.

Freudenberger, H. J. (1984a). Burnout and job dissatisfaction: Impact on the family. In J. C. Hansen (Ed.), *Perspectives on work and the family*, Rockville, MD: Aspen Publications.

Freudenberger, H. J. (1984b). Impaired clinicians: Coping with burnout. *Innovations in clincial practice: A source book*, Vol. 3. Sarasota, FL: Professional Resource Exchange.

Freudenberger, H. J., & North, G. (1985). *Women's burnout. How to spot it, how to reverse it, and how to prevent it.* New York: Anchor Press/Doubleday.

Freudenberger, H. J., & Richelson, G. (1980). Burnout: How to beat the high cost of success. New York: Anchor Press/Doubleday.

Freudenberger, H. J., & Robbins, A. (1982). The hazards of being a psychoanalyst. *Psychoanalytic Review, 66*(2), 275–296.

Jaffe, D. T., & Trubo, R. (Eds.) (1984). Burnout: When the doctor's bag gets heavy. *Medical World News*, March 26, pp. 41–50.

Meyer, J. H. (1982). Burnout: Developmental influences. *Canadian Counselor*, p. 16.

Nagy, B. R. (1981). Help for impaired physicians. *New York State Journal of Medicine*, September, 1531–1534.

Pfifferling, J. H. (1980). The problem of physician impairment. *Connecticut Medicine, 44*(3) 587–591.

Pines, A. M., Aronson, E., & Kafry, D. (1981). *Burnout—From tedium to personal growth.* New York: Free Press.

Sheridan, E. P., & Sheridan, K. (1980). The troubled attorney. *Barrister, 7*(3), 42–56.

Sifneos, P. E. (1979). *Short-term dynamics psychotherapy*. New York: Plenum.

Steyer, R. (1981). Thy brother's keeper: The impaired physician, *MD, 25*(12), 33–42.

Vincent, M. O. (1969). Doctor and Mrs.—Their mental health. *Canadian Psychiatric Association Journal, 14*, 509–515.

Chapter 13

The Inner Strains of Healing Work: Therapy and Self-Renewal for Health Professionals

Dennis T. Jaffe, Ph.D.

Working as a health professional—physician, nurse, dentist, or psycho-therapist—creates a unique set of inner pressures and demands. These demands often set apart the health professional, especially the physician, into a special category of social status, prestige, respect, and mystery. People go to health professionals when they are experiencing pain and suffering, for help, relief, and healing. The health professional in turn spends his/her day seeing people whose suffering tends to make them dependent, and who often expect the health professional to know how to bring them relief. Although health professionals share many occupational stressors with other service professions—such as difficult work conditions, frustrating demands of client/patients—there are a few environmental factors that set them apart: their proximity to suffering and death and the great emotional and physical needs of their patients. The question explored in this paper is "What are the negative effects of being close to all this pain on the health professional?"

The practice of healing deeply affects the personal experience, and the

194

personal life, of the health professional, yet that effect is rarely explored. How does a healer cope with the continual demands and his/her frequent incapacity to deliver true healing? How does this special pressure affect the healer's capacity to live fully and to find peace and satisfaction?

I shall discuss these questions from the personal perspective of being a psychologist and family therapist, with a large part of my practice focused on health professionals and their families who are in personal crisis, facing serious personal illness, and in family conflict. As an outgrowth of my clinical work, I have for many years led workshops and taught seminars in coping with the stress of being a health professional. These seminars are based on the inner exploration by participants of the effects of being a healer on their inner selves, as well as on their external practice. Finally, as a researcher I have been interviewing physicians in transition, particularly physicians who have had a major personal crisis, and have made important changes not only in their lives, but in their values and approach to medicine.

NUMBING, DENIAL, AND BURNOUT

The psyche's first response to painful and traumatic emotional material is numbing and denial. Other people's pain makes us anxious—we tend to try to make others feel better, most often by covering up their pain. Seeing another in pain activates a sense of helplessness in the observer as well. People who are in attendance in disasters, for example, experience a variety of physical and emotional stress symptoms. Seeing another's pain sets up a resonance within the self, where personal memories of pain are activated. Empathy is a natural process, but the health professional must learn to temper that with a professional demeanor that has been termed "detached concern."

It is difficult to sustain emotional openness to other people in pain over time. The dentist, in addition to working in close quarters under pressure, must face the fear and avoidance of patients who see him as creating pain. Even family members and friends in pain become difficult to be with over time. In many ways, we have learned ways to avoid experiencing pain. The life of the health professional is spent in contact with pain, and no matter what the training, the personal strain of this experience takes a toll.

When a young health professional in training first enters a hospital, the experience is overwhelming. Added to the proximity to pain and suffering is the obligation and expectations to do something about it. The student is confused, often helpless, and overwhelmed with facts and procedures to learn.

People enter medicine, nursing, and psychotherapy with a desire to care for others, to do social good, and often to achieve social status and avoid competitive, aggressive, and commercial settings. When they think about being with people in pain, the usual fantasy is that they will be able to release them from their suffering, earning respect and deep gratitude. The ability to handle intense pain is not a criterion for entering the profession. Rational intelligence and school performance are demanded. The student must make the choice for a health career early and, therefore, has little opportunity to develop other areas of the self—social, personal, or creative—in the quest to enter a select profession. The young health professional often lacks social and emotional maturity. Yet, the healer-to-be must cope with a world of pain and life and death, with only minimal skills and even less emotional maturity and social support.

In training, and in professional interaction, the emotional effect of doing health work is rarely spoken about. There are several myths about professional conduct that support such behavior. First, the health professional is taught that his/her needs have no place in health work and that a competent health professional has learned to submerge all needs except an abstract desire to be helpful. Second, the professional's feelings are also considered not relevant and, when they erupt, are considered to get in the way of effective treatment. A health professional is not supposed to feel, or to share, sadness about death or to respond emotionally to the pain of patients and their families. Even among colleagues, the sharing of feelings or the presence of personal needs is taboo. Cynical detachment is the expectation. This can often lead to serious consequences for the inner life of the health professional and his/her ability to have deep emotional relationships with family and friends.

The result is a response of numbing, deadening, and turning away from feelings. Ford (1983) notes, "The applicant to medical school who professed an altruistic interest in helping patients has by the end of his internship become a hardened cynical house officer whose relationship to patients has become adversarial rather than nurturing" (p. 209). The effect on his inner life is no less drastic. Although the young physician often marries during this period, the marriages of physicians (whether or not they are perceived as satisfying by the participants) are often characterized by emotional withdrawal and detachment. The experience of pain and demands from patients and the continual pressure to respond lead to emotional deadening. Eventually, this has important consequences for the health professional's life.

Another familiar inner process focuses on the gap between what the student expected from the healing profession and what he actually does. The inner image of the benevolent healer, who gives life to patients and is appreciated, is confronted with the reality of the overworked technocrat, who does not have the time or skills to get to know patients and cannot give them what they so deeply desire. The added frustrations of mounting debts, difficulty starting a practice, diminished opportunities, uncertainties of the future of the profession, and a spouse who has waited patiently for added companionship and an end to overwork, all come together to create further pressure that the young health professional often copes with by continued withdrawal.

The final nail on the coffin of the healer's feelings is the disinterest of colleagues and institutions in these processes and the lack of social support and validation for looking at these pressures. Common modes of response to this situation range from drug use to alcoholism, professional burnout, dissatisfaction, and depression. Very few health professionals are able to maintain the façade of personal availability and achieve satisfaction in their work.

A common response to the pressure of continual demands from patients has been professional burnout. Maslach and Jackson (1981) note that "helpers are often forced to spend considerable time in intense involvement with [troubled people, and these exchanges commonly become] charged with feelings of anger, embarrassment, frustration, fear and despair" (p. 99). Cherniss (1980) traces the cycle of loss of idealism, detachment from the problems of patients, frustration with professional bureaucracy, and lack of peer support, which occurs in the first year of professional practice. The stresses and depersonalization of health work lower the self-esteem and the personal accomplishment of the practitioner, which leads in turn to increasing isolation, in a cycle that gets continually worse.

FAMILY EMOTIONAL SUPPORT

One of the most pressing needs of health professionals is emotional support. Yet, paradoxically, they often arrange their lives so that they do not get it, or they remain unaware of their need. The marriages of health professionals, especially physicians, cannot resolve or contain many of these feelings. The physician or healer comes home emotionally drained and has little to offer his spouse and children. His family is often experienced by the health professional as not very different from patients—as a source of pressure to perform and give. Emotional relationships are seen as draining; so the healer often comes home and pulls back from yet another demand. The family and the spouse feel deserted again, after the desertion of the long days and frequent evening and weekend absences. Traditionally, the family of the physician was expected to "make sacrifices" because of the specialness of the physician's work. It has been observed that family members often gain a physician/husband's attention by getting sick. Many health professionals also respond to the pressure of their work by becoming helpless and dependent and expecting emotional nurture and no demands from their families. They become resentful when the nurture they not quite consciously expect does not come to them.

Another constellation of family dynamics can be found in women health professionals. Although women find the nurturing, emotionally giving role of health professionals closer to the traditional feminine role, they try to continue that role at home. A woman physician I knew, with a full practice, would run home and prepare dinner and take care of her three children, while her husband, also a physician, would relax and watch television. Women in healing professions often have to continue their role at home, often without having a source of nurturing for themselves, or even seeing their need for it. Thus, both male and female health professionals have difficulty in mobilizing their families or personal worlds as settings for self-renewal, from the pressures of being a healer.

SELF-AWARENESS OF THE WOUNDED HEALER

At the risk of oversimplifying, my thesis is that there is a significant problem in overlooking the effects of being a health professional and the way that doing this work changes one. The healer has needs, feelings, and deep reactions to what he/she experiences, and at some time in a career, these effects and inner experiences need to be acknowledged and taken into account. The professional myths that the healer has no needs, that these needs detract from the provision of adequate service if acknowledged, that feelings are not relevant, and that we can simply turn off our responses to human pain are untenable and contribute to the distress that helping professionals experience in their work and lives. What is needed is for the health professional to learn how to renew himself each day from the strain of health work.

Recently, there has been a new focus and conception of healing work, which has been labeled "holistic" (see Jaffe, 1981; Gordon et al., 1981). This emerging perspective has led many health professionals to look at themselves, and their work, differently. The new focus is characterized by an enlarged focus of concern, where the physician explores emotional, social, and spiritual dimensions of the patient and therefore has more avenues for intervention; a healing relationship based on shared responsibility between health professional and patient, which takes some of the pressure off the helper; and a recognition that self-care of the health professional is important, that the health professional needs to respect his/her needs in order to be effective. Many health professionals accept the major tenets of this model and thus have begun to modify their style of work and their relationship to themselves.

At some point in time, the cumulative effects of numbing, burnout, or emotional withdrawal no longer provide psychic protection. A personal crisis often triggers the shift from numbing to a more self-renewing response to the demands of the healer's life. The crisis takes many forms. Some experience a personal illness, emotional breakdown, or depression. For others, a spouse generates a marital crisis, reacting to deficiencies in the relationship that were not addressed by the health professional/spouse. The precipitating crisis can also take the form of a change at work, such as a clinic closing, or a financial setback that opens up other questions about motivation, meaning, and satisfaction of health work. Sometimes, a shift occurs when the personal psychotherapy process leads to important questions about inner meaning of healing work or the needs it serves.

These crises shift the focus from the external work of the healer to the inner process of the healer. The individual, who is used to being the helper, in control, and dispensing wisdom now experiences pain and suffering within himself. A single crisis often focuses attention on many submerged effects of healing work, precipitating rapid change, as if the dam had burst.

For example, a woman physician experienced a life-threatening illness. She was the only child of a physician and a nurse. She entered medicine and found it intellectually challenging but draining. She felt that if she looked at her feelings about patients dying around her, she would lose her effectiveness and ability to function. Her physical illness led her into psychotherapy, where she explored her decision to enter medicine in relation to her family. Therapy facilitated an examination of her own reaction to healing work and a redefinition of her work style to take her neglected personal needs into account. As a consequence, she decided to have a child and consciously rearranged her work to have more time with her family, producing a more balanced approach to her personal and family life.

CLINICAL IMPLICATIONS

When the physician becomes a patient, the role shift is difficult. The very factors that make a person a good health professional make one a bad patient. In situations where the spouse initiates therapy, usually because she is not able to gain the health professional's emotional involvement or attention, the initial response is confusion. One physician, responding to the sense of abandonment felt by his family because he had not been home on time for supper for many years, was assuming that his whole family just shared the sense that these things had to be sacrificed. He did not feel he had to accord his family even the emotional involvement he reserved for patients, because he felt they were extensions of himself. When he realized that his family needed him, he began to increase his involvement and find ways to spend less time at work.

Many times the crisis helps the health professional to accomplish some personal growth that had been neglected or delayed in the long haul through professional school and career development. Much of my therapy with young health professionals can be seen as emotional teaching. What it means to be emotionally available is not known, and the role of feelings in their lives has been neglected. This inattention to feelings is often supported by staff in hospitals and clinics. Feelings are to be avoided, certainly in staff, and in patients as well.

The crisis also illuminates another difficulty in the healer's life. He/she finds it easier to feel adequate in a situation where the patient needs him but where he is in control. Many physicians find it easy to be intimate with patients, because they are in control of the relationship, and they are looked up to as authorities. That may be why there are so many situations of sexual relationships between physicians and patients, when these same physicians have difficulty in other intimate settings. The physician or therapist loses a sense of control when he/she comes home, where others may seek a more mutual or peer relationship. The traditional medical marriage is structured like the traditional doctor/patient relationship. New sex and family roles toward mutuality and shared work, shifts in expectations of emotional support in marriage, and demands for more intimate sharing make the traditional arrangement less common, and less workable, for both parties.

The need for the health professional to confront his/her own vulnerability, pain, and personal response to the work of healing has always been recognized. Ancient Greek mythology assigned the power of healing to a "wounded healer." In the myth, the healer obtains the wisdom and knowledge of life and death, but cannot use it to heal his own incurable wound. The healer then participates in the sickness he/she seeks to heal. Today, "medical student's disease" (experiencing symptoms after reading textbook accounts) is one way in which young healers participate emotionally in the sicknesses they seek to master, and the curious phenomenon of physicians tending to die or struggle with the diseases they specialize in suggests that there is some inner wisdom in this formulation. For our purposes, we can assume that, as the cumulative effects of working with sick and suffering people build up, the health professional will have to become aware of his own inner response, and do something about it, or else face serious disability, burnout, impairment, or serious limitation as a human being.

Jess Groesbeck (1981), a Jungian analyst who has written on the wounded healer, writes of a dream he had during his own training and its import:

> In the dream I was alone and suddenly viewed my hands as both being cut off. I said to myself, "I am just like Mrs. W, who teaches

my two daughters." I suddenly began to cry and sense a real loss. Upon awakening I was tearful and associated to old memories of my early life when the middle finger on my right hand was traumatically severed. At the time of my dream I was living separated from my family during a transitional move. My daughters were going to a small country school where they were being taught by a teacher whose hands were crippled. I had met the teacher once. Apparently in the few years previous to this time this woman had been burdened with a very difficult family life, many personal tragedies and no way even to support herself. She was not pleasing to look at and became involved at school and later as a teacher all by being "a pest to others." Finally, through the encouragement of my mother-in-law, she went back to school and became a certified teacher. Her popularity with children was unusual and her ability to teach was the finest. Even with her crippled hands she was able to deal with this handicap effectively and teach the children in a special way. My daughters described her as a beautiful person.

The meaning of the dream came clear to me as an answer to the needs of my psychology. Hitherto I had believed that, as taught in medical school and psychiatric residency, one must always show forth strength and hide all weaknesses in order to be the best kind of physician. Through many of the experiences, dreams, and work with patients, it became apparent that in analytical work one cannot hide wounds or weaknesses; one in fact must confront and make them conscious if he is ever to have the hope of becoming a genuine wounded healer. As noted above, attempts to hide or disavow one's weaknesses may result in disaster and failure. (p. 143)

HELPING THE HEALTH PROFESSIONAL

The wounded-healer myth suggests that the health professional has to look at and explore his/her personal feelings. One of the most important ways that I have helped health professionals to do that is to explore the inner meanings and needs of healing work to them. Several interesting patterns were found.

First, I have found that a decision to become a helping person is usually one that is made, if not consciously, very early in life. Often, when I ask people in my training groups about their early family life, they picture a family role where they were a helper. As a child, they felt they had to help their parents deal with their problems or conflicts, such as alcoholism, or be the good child who was always expected to help with the others and not be a bother. This early childhood role is one that they try to repeat as a health professional. For example, they want to keep things going well and be seen as helpful and therefore good. Or their family may have been so stressful that they kept themselves under control by taking care of things. Thus, they already found it hard to achieve mutuality in relationships and coped by arranging for a lot of control. Or they based their self-image on being helpful and taking care of others, and that is the only role they feel comfortable in. They are not attuned to their inner needs and are not used to asking for help from others—a common story told by health professionals.

People often enter a profession in part carrying out some hidden agenda or acting out some personal need from childhood. In healing work, it is particularly important to explore this inner constellation because the work itself is so demanding, that they can in effect smother themselves by working in this way. Exploring this role usually makes a helper aware of factors that lie behind their burnout, such as, for example, an expectation of deep appreciation from patients, which is not often found. They also can explore their difficulty in creating a helping relationship that does not mirror precisely their early family role. Thus, after self-exploration, they may be able to adopt a more flexible role in their health work, whereas previously they were inhibited by one way of working.

Psychological work with health professionals must also focus on their original sense of purpose, the almost spiritual sense of mission that brings many people to health work. Recalling the original intention and commitment to health work, and exploring why that has dimmed, often initiates an interesting set of reflections. For example, the professional may look at the unintended costs of various compromises, how a particular work setting has kept him from doing the kind of work he would like to, or how emotional exhaustion or overwork has limited his ability to really respond to human problems.

Another issue that emerges in working with wounded healers is separating their personal needs from their work. This means asking the healer what his/her deepest personal needs are. Health professionals are notorious for having little outside life, for having their primary lives and deepest, most meaningful involvements within their healing world. Often, for example, their family or community life cannot compete in intensity with their healing work. Therapists may find that their families cannot offer them the intimate connection, the attention, and the respect that they feel from their patients. They may try to be therapeutic or helpful with their families and feel hurt when their interventions are neither respected nor appreciated. That is why therapists or physicians are asked not to treat themselves or their families.

The health professional usually needs to develop a life outside of health work or else runs the risk of becoming overly dependent on certain responses from patients and his work family. For many healers, this means taking the risk of becoming close to other people and opening up to new areas of themselves in relation to emotions and intimacy. This means shifting their sense of the healer's role and allowing more openness, mutuality, and flexibility in professional relationships. It also means redefining priorities, boundaries, and commitments between family and work.

For example, much of my family therapy with physicians revolves around the assumption that the physician cannot make dependable commitments to family, and that they therefore feel unimportant and abandoned. Afer a while they cannot continue to subordinate themselves to work demands, and they withdraw or conflict. Physicians, at first feeling that they cannot compromise or make changes, find that medical work can be limited and support systems can be created to offer complete time off and shorter hours. Many health professionals, after exploring their needs and seeing the effects of health work on them, find ways to limit their practices and make changes. This often renews and strengthens their ability to deliver high-quality service.

The process of becoming aware of inner needs and feelings is not enough to resolve the issues of the pressure of health work. Although much can be done by personal work, there is also a need for burnout interventions to focus on the aspects of healing work and environment that are counterproductive for both the health professional and the patient. There is some evidence that the distant and uninvolved stance may have negative effects on the healing process itself.

An intervention by psychiatrist Samuel Klagsbrun (1979), who was asked by the nursing staff to help with the staff burnout problem on an oncology ward, illustrates how this self-examination can affect an entire healing philosophy. The nursing staff were quitting and getting sick because of the pressure of dealing with the mainly terminal patients, who faced frightening and painful treatment. The nurses were not allowed to share their feelings, and they felt that their work consisted mainly of being servants to the patients. Everyone together was depressed.

At first, Klagsbrun ran a group for staff to share feelings. The group soon proposed an experiment in the structure of the service. A self-care experiment was devised, where patients all shared the work, if possible, and were encouraged to help each other. Everyone ate together and began to talk about feelings more openly. The nursing staff, since patients were helping more, were freer to talk about their own feelings and to be involved with the patients. Surprisingly, these changes made everyone, even the physicians who were initially resistant, feel better about their work. Curiously, patients on this service began to do better in treatment as well. The primary learning of this intervention was that when staff feel burned out, it may be remedied by a structural change in the nature of the way that people engage in their healing work, which allows the sharing of the inner experience of staff. The nurses reported that they were able to cry with patients, ask for help, and get close to patients, whereas previously they had been stuck in their detachment.

As a health professional learns that his/her inner awareness is related to effective work, several types of support systems must be strengthened. Support systems can be defined as places where open communication and sharing can take place, and emotional support is exchanged. The first type of support system a health professional needs is an inner one to his/her self. A channel of information and respect must be opened so that the health professional is aware of his emotional responses to work and the meaning of work to his life and takes them into account in daily life. The second support system is personal support through intimate relationships with spouse, friends, family, and lovers. These are the people who can listen to feelings and meet one's needs in ways that patients cannot. Finally, as in the above intervention, there need to be support groups at health care settings that allow healers to air feelings and share experiences. A professor of internal medicine I know has made great shifts in the work of his teaching hospital by initiating meetings where his staff can share feelings about patients and about their work. This simple step has profoundly affected their work.

What has been suggested in this chapter is that the current concern with health professional burnout, and the stress of health work, is in large part due to the emotional response to continual proximity to human pain and suffering. The health professional must see that he cannot simply give and remain detached from these feelings, but must begin at some time a process of looking inward at personal needs, responses, and roles. Often, this leads to major personal changes and changes in the way of doing health work. This new view is a more human and balanced view of self than that of the detached, omnipotent healer. The personal pressures and health problems of health professionals seem to stem from the impossibility of taking care of oneself and hiding or ignoring the emotional effects of health care work. At some point, some sort of personal exploration process needs to take place. This can be done in individual or family therapy, or as part of a seminar/workshop where the person of the health professional is the focus, not the work he/she does. Such retreats for self-renewal are increasingly being adopted in many types of service work.

REFERENCES

Cherniss, C. (1980). *Professional burnout in human service organizations*. New York: Praeger.
Ford, C. V. (1983). *The somatizing disorders*. New York: Elsevier.
Gordon, J., Hastings, A., & Fadiman, J. (1981). *Health for the whole person*. New York: Bantam.

Groesbeck, C. (1981). The archetypal image of the wounded healer. Unpublished manuscript.
Jaffe, D. (1981). *Healing from within*. New York: Knopf.
Klagsbrun, S. (1979). Cancer, emotions and nurses. In C. Garfield (Ed.), *Stress and survival*. St. Louis: Mosby.
Maslach, C., & Jackson, S. (1981). The measurement of experienced burnout. *Journal of Occupational Behavior, 2*(2), 99.

III

Emergent Strategies:
Designs for the Future

Chapter 14

Health Promotion—
A Challenging Approach
to Health Care

Cynthia D. Scott, Ph.D., M.P.H.

Looking forward, the entire health care system is going through some important changes that will affect the format and composition of work and professional life dramatically. The kinds of health care services, the personnel who perform these services, and the method of financing these services are all undergoing substantial restructuring at this time and need to be taken into consideration when discussing the well-being of professionals. Some of this change is occurring because the burden of illness is shifting from infectious and acute toward chronic, life-style, and environmentally induced diseases. Another change in emphasis is occurring in response to the expanded base of research and policy analysis that supports the development and use of health promotion, disease prevention, and self-care in clinical medicine.

Health care practice in the coming decade will be influenced by advances in these areas:

1. *Computer technology* will provide major assistance in scheduling, billing, record keeping, and diagnostic and treatment procedures.
2. *Composition of illness.* "New illnesses" will emerge, and old syndromes may be redefined with an advanced biomedical understanding of preventive and diagnostic approaches.

209

3. *Behaviorial science* will have increased experience in addressing and managing the emotional and behaviorial aspects of health care, with the expanded use of health psychologists involved in the provision of health care.

4. *Integrative approaches* will include integration of modern and ancient traditional therapeutic modalities into current health practices.

5. *Prevention/health promotion* will lead to increased emphasis on lifestyle, health enhancement programs in business and industry, and wellness insurance.

Many of these changes will have direct impact on how professionals are trained and how they practice. To put these changes into perspective this chapter will provide an overview of the following areas: the basic assumptions upon which health professional education is based and how health promotion, health education, and self-care programs challenge and enhance these assumptions; and the practical aspects of establishing and maintaining health promotion and self-care practices in educational and practice settings.

THE ASSUMPTIONS OF THE BIOMEDICAL MODEL AND NEW RESPONSES

Every system of education is based on a set of philosophical values that form the basic assumptions and underlying framework upon which a curriculum is structured. These assumptions can be explicitly stated or, more often, are implicitly understood. In the field of medicine, the primary assumptions of training have developed from the biomedical model, which holds that the world is rational, scientific, or mechanistic. The practice of health care that has evolved from this model has emphasized analysis, action, and a highly developed technology. Biomedical scientists believed that once the offending pathogen was discovered, they would be able to develop a treatment that would repair the damaged organ or replace the missing chemical in an individual patient.

Most recently, this model and the treatment approaches developed from it have been criticized from a wide variety of perspectives (i.e., the spiritual, political, ecological, consumer, and cross-cultural). These critiques have produced their own sets of assumptions from which other models and treatment approaches have developed. A few of these assumptions will be reviewed here and the newly developing responses explored.

Assumption 1

Good health is a service that is "delivered" by health care professionals and "consumed" by patients. Health is a temporary absence of medically defined illness and not a reflection of social and personal responsibility and life-style. The health care professional is responsible for making the patient healthy.

Response

Health is increasingly being seen as the result of a partnership between a lay person and a professional. Both share the responsibility for maintaining an individual's health. The healing process consists of mobilizing self-help and self-care practices in tandem with other approaches. The role of the health professional is to elicit from the patient the inherent ability, inner knowledge, and physical, mental, and spiritual resources to participate in the healing process. The health professional's role is to shift this sense of responsibility for health maintenance to the individual and assist him in becoming active in his own health maintenance and self-care practices. Health is created and recreated, that is, maintained—not delivered.

> It is supposed to be a professional secret, but I'll tell you anyway. We doctors do nothing. We only help and encourage the doctor within. (Albert Schweitzer)

Assumption 2

Health care is basically a function of trained health professionals with lay persons and families undertaking only minor and supplementary responsibilities.

Response

If anything, almost the reverse is true. Illness and disorders are a common, almost ongoing, feature of family life in the United States. Levin (1977b) cited a study of 273 households in Ohio and found an average of 12.4 acute illnesses or injuries per family in a 30-week period, averaging 57.4 total illness days per household. These illnesses are by and large taken care of at home. The United States hospitalization rate is roughly 96 to 97 hospitalizations per 1,000 persons per year, yet acute illness or injury requiring reduced activity is experienced at the rate of 2,068 serious illness or injuries per 1,000 persons per year. This represents about 20 acute illnesses or injuries handled outside the hospital for every one that is handled inside the hospital. These conditions require large amounts of nonprofessional or lay care. In addition, some illnesses are cared for exclusively by families with no professional intervention whatsoever. Alpert and co-workers (1967) found that low-income families are at especially high risk for health problems of all kinds. Ninety-three percent of families reported one or more symptoms over a 30-day period, and the ratio of medically nonattended symptoms to medically attended symptoms was 7:1. Since nonprescription drugs are more commonly used than prescription drugs, a significant amount of self-medication is carried out as an alternative to professional care.

Many health problems are regarded by families as requiring attention, but professional care is either not sought or often not perceived as completely effective or palliative at best. The following problems often fall into this category: osteoarthritis, chronic pain syndromes (e.g., low-back pain, headache), certain types of cancer, problems peculiar to the elderly and to females, etc. In addition, psychophysiological dysfunctions, so-called psychosomatic illnesses (e.g., irritable-bowel syndrome, some ulcers, neurodermatitis, and possibly labile hypertension), are areas that modern medicine is just beginning to investigate and address in practice and in the training of health professionals.

Families also do a significant amount of symptom monitoring; 84% of homes have clinical thermometers. Richardson (1969) found that 50% of persons with illness episodes consult one or more family members before seeking any kind of outside advice or help.

Assumption 3

Disease originates externally to the individual and is, therefore, treated as an entity external to the person and is more often than not explained as an accident. The disease is the focus of care—not the person who "has" the disease.

Response

As Sir William Osler, the most famous physician of the nineteenth century, noted: "You need to know what kind of person has the disease, not what kind of disease a person has." Predisposition to disease may originate from environmental and hereditary factors, and before the clinical manifestations present, an individual's immunological defense/balancing mechanisms are called into action. Many factors contribute to the individual's being able to maintain his internal balance (e.g., previous and current health status, level of physical fitness, including quality of nutrition, and psychological states such as level of self-esteem, ability to be flexible in new situations, and feeling fulfilled by work). The healing process, centered in the patient, is encouraged by many activities individuals may incorporate into their day-to-day activities. Disease may be viewed as a metaphor for a concern in an individual's life (i.e., you might ask a person with neck spasms who or what is a "pain in the neck" to him, or you might ask someone with stomach pains who or what situation is making him "sick to his stomach"). Can we, as health professionals, completely separate the physical pain of angina from the emotional pain and suffering that an individual feels when he is hospitalized and separated from his loved ones?

The failure to understand the human condition has caused medicine to come to emphasize the importance of seeking cures rather than the relief of suffering. Health professionals are often trained in a dichotomous Cartesian framework, where concerns of the mind are separate from the functioning of the body. This mind set has led to a formulation of medical treatment that circumscribes a whole array of emotional concerns of the patient, ignoring the main task of medicine—the relief of suffering, both physical and psychological. Disease has been viewed and treated outside the context of the person, his family, community, and spiritual relationship. What is currently being developed is a multidimensional understanding of suffering that is leading to new models of professional training and treatment approaches and settings (Cassel, 1982).

Assumption 4

Disease and death are negative and to be avoided at all costs. They must be fought and overcome by health professionals.

Response

"Dis-ease" may represent a lack of "ease," an imbalance either within the individual or between the individual and his environment. Granger and Westberg have observed that "the most important factor that facilitates the onset of illness is an inadequate philosophy of life: no goals, no beliefs about the nature of existence, no sense of purpose in life" (Kotz & Fielding, 1980, p. 18). Imbalances in an individual can be the result of experiencing many potentially stressful life changes. Gunderson and Rahe (1974) found that clusters of life changes preceded the onset of reported illness, and that increased life changes in the years preceeding the study period repeatedly showed a positve, significant correlation with illness during the study period. The Schedule of Recent Experiences developed by Holmes and Rahe (1967) and modified by Sarason and co-workers (1979) provides a way for individuals to assess the recent changes in their lives and their evaluation of their situation. Many instruments like these have been developed and are being used in clinical practice.

Assumption 5

The health of the health care professional is secondary to his intellectual ability in measuring effectiveness as a healer. Assessment of proficiency is primarily related to one's academic achievements and one's adherence to certain personality characteristics (e.g., excessive thoroughness, attention to small details). These abilities are only circumstantially related to the health of the health professional.

Response

Recently, there has been increased emphasis on the connection between the health and well-being of health professionals and their ability to be effective in their professional role.

Before this recent examination of the health of health professionals, the self-care needs of this group had been denied or largely unsupported. Many students have felt like they signed "a delayed gratification contract" when they entered training in the health field. Their own needs go unmet, while they attempt to learn to meet the health needs of others. This contract often becomes a lifelong pattern of self-denial that leads to both physical and emotional exhaustion. To complicate this situation further, this attitude about not taking care of yourself often leads to a tendency to deny the need for emotional support and help when problems do arise, making interventions difficult.

The health, both emotional and physical, of the health professional can have a direct influence on patient care. Physical exhaustion taxes decision-making capacity, and emotional upset precludes the complete observation of patients' emotional states. At the core of this interaction is the philosophical understanding that one of the functions of a healer is to lend strength to another until he recovers (Cassel, 1982). How can a professional who is exhausted and emotionally depleted himself participate fully in the healing interaction with a patient? And yet the entire health training system supports, both explicitly and implicitly, the physical and emotional incongruity between the prescriptions that health professionals give their patients and the lack of a prescription for self-care. It is no wonder that the statistics on impairment and ill health among health professionals are staggering.

The health professional is now being seen as an important "instrument" in the health care process, deserving support in maintaining his/her own well-being. "Physician heal thyself" is becoming the focus of new curriculums and programs in health care.

THE EMERGENCE OF HEALTH PROMOTION, HEALTH EDUCATION, AND SELF-CARE

Historically, the major forces operating to lower mortality and morbidity from infectious diseases in the last 100 years have been economic and social changes, environmental control measures, immunization, health education, and other public health activities. Treatment services have played a secondary role. The contribution of medical care in lowering mortality and morbidity from noninfectious diseases has been useful but limited—once pathological changes reach the stage where they produce symptoms requiring treatment, it may no longer be possible to reverse the disease process. Treatment, therefore, is only a secondary line of defense, with prevention solidly the first choice (Terris, 1980, pp. 180–188). The recent Surgeon General's Report on Health Promotion and Disease Prevention, *Healthy People* (1979), cites that further improvements will be achieved through a renewed national commitment to efforts designed to prevent disease and promote health (Kotz & Fielding, 1980). Before going any further, we offer the following definitions of the major elements of disease prevention discussed in this chapter.

Health promotion emphasizes the development of programs and approaches that enhance the physical and mental well-being of individuals who do not feel well but have no obvious organic diseases. These programs often consist of risk appraisal (evaluating sources of individual stress and coping styles, nutrition, fitness, environmental and ecological factors, life-style behaviors), physical and emotional assessment, counseling, behavior change, etc. (Gordon, in Hastings et al., 1980, p. 19).

Health education provides information and education about evaluating and improving health behavior, coping with illness, making appropriate use of health care facilities and other resources, and taking increased responsibility for one's own health and well-being.

Self-care is a process whereby a lay person can function effectively on his/her own behalf in health promotion and decision making and in disease prevention, detection, and treatment at the level of the primary health resource in the health care system (Levin, 1977a). This represents a change in the basic patterns of responsibility and decision making in individuals regarding their health.

BUILT-IN RISKS

These developments in the public sector and the rapid growth in scientific knowledge and technology have resulted in some major risk factors being built into our present health care system.

- Today 100,000 patients will be discharged from hospitals and 5,000 of these patients will have had hospital acquired infections, many preventable.
- In one day, about 2,300 Americans will die of cardiovascular disease—half before their 75th birthday, and largely due to factors over which they have some control—smoking, diet, exercise, and blood pressure. (Kotz & Fielding, 1980, pp. 32–33)

These iatrogenic (physician-generated) problems are of great concern to health professionals. Levin (1977a) adds that "every time you add a care giver, you are adding an unknown risk of iatrogenesis." He sees the main job of public health as protecting the public not only from the insult of disease but also from the assault of the health care system. Besides the direct risk of contracting additional physical health problems, there is also the risk of encountering additional emotional and physical suffering in the name of "treatment." Cassel (1982) explores the paradox of how even "successful treatment" may cause undue bodily and mental suffering. Often these factors are not weighed into the equation of developing treatment plans.

Looking again at the broad picture, this balance of prevention and treatment is accurately reflected in the definition of health by the World Health Organization, "health is a state of complete physical, mental and social well-being and not merely the absence of disease." Therefore, health cannot solely be a product of the medical care system, but is a multifaceted result of services, environment, life-style, and attitude. To attain this state requires a combination of both social and *individual* responsibility. It is this combined responsibility that most accurately reflects the overall direction of health promotion, health education, and self-care programs.

CURRENT DEVELOPMENTS

Programs in health promotion, health education, and self-care are woefully underdeveloped and undersupported in the health policies of the United States. Currently, 95% of the national health budget is allocated to disease care, whereas 5% goes to prevention and promotion. This situation exists despite ample studies which show that health status is not primarily attributed to the quality or quantity of medical care but rather to the effects of life-style, health habits, and the quality of the ecological and social environment (Cooper & Rice, 1979; Terris, 1980, 1981).

Behind the current economic crisis in health care is a growing awareness among the public and professionals that the present approach to health and illness are out of balance and inadequate for meeting the needs of our complex society. Costs seem beyond containment, and third-party payers (insurance companies) are raising their premium prices and lowering their coverage. Hospital costs have increased by almost $3 billion each year as a result of workers' illnesses. This has led to increased interest in health promotion, health education, and self-care. The shift comes from many directions: preventive medicine, public health, family practice, business and industry, government, and the general public. For example, business and industry are attempting to keep their health care budgets in line by supporting new programs on health education and health promotion in the workplace. Currently it is the business and hospital industries which, for mainly economic and productivity reasons, are taking the lead in designing and marketing health promotion and health education programs (Jones, 1982; Keenan, 1982).

Health Promotion in the Workplace

For example, numerous businesses and professional groups are supporting health promotion in the workplace (The Chamber of Commerce of the United States, The Health Insurance Association, The President's Council on Physical Fitness and Sports, The American Hospital Association, and The American Association of Fitness Directors in Business and Industry). More than 1,000 national organizations have started health promotion programs (e.g., Chase Manhattan Bank, General Foods, Ford Motor Company, Prudential Life Insurance Company, NASA, and Exxon). A healthy workforce is becoming an investment in productivity and lowered health care costs.

Some of the key concepts that are being incorporated into these health promotion programs are the following:

—risk identification often using computerized health risk appraisals
—health risk reduction—engaging in behavior change
—focusing on high risk employees
—redesigning the work place to support healthful practices. (Jennings & Tager, 1981)

Hospital Environments

The development of health programs in the work setting has specific significance for workers in hospitals. Hospitals have been shown to be particularly stressful employers. In a recent study by the National Institute for Occupational Health and Safety, Colligan and co-workers (1977) studied the relative incidence of mental health disorders in 130 major occupational categories. When these data were ranked, seven of the top 27 occupations were related to health care operations (health technologists, licensed practical nurses, laboratory technicians, nursing aides, health aides, registered nurses, dental assistants). Both the complexity of the organization (multiple levels of authority, heterogeneity of personnel, work interdependence, and specialization) and the responsibility for people causes more stress (Calhoun, 1980). This situation makes hospitals a likely starting point for sponsoring health promotion programs, both for their employees and for the surrounding community. Several hospitals are offering fitness counseling services and fitness facilities and undertaking fitness research (Ardell, 1981; Carpenter, 1980). The American Hospital Association has established the Center for Health Promotion to help hospitals become involved in patient education, community health education, and employee health education. For example, a number of hospitals (e.g., Smaritan Health Services, Phoenix, Arizona; Swedish Medical Center, Englewood, Colorado; Union Hospital, Lynn, Massachusetts have developed innovative wellness/health promotion programs.

Education in Prevention

Within medical education the development of training opportunities in prevention has lacked political and economic clout. Only 4% of every general health care dollar is spent for preventive activities, and only 1.5% of the nation's 350,000 practicing physicians are engaged in full-time preventive medicine practice (i.e., aerospace medicine, public health, general preventive medicine, and occupational health) (Barish, 1979).

The development of family practice as a recognized specialty in 1969 with their mandate to train physicians to provide general personal health services, including prevention, added new life to the field of preventive medicine. A survey of the 1979–1980 American Association of Medical Colleges *Curriculum Directory* showed that 99 of 130 accredited medical schools had some required teaching in preventive and community medicine, although this was often in the form of epidemiology or biostatistics and not about actual clinical practice. A recent study by Barker (1981) found that the teaching of preventive medicine has achieved only limited development of its potential role in medical education. Although several curriculum development projects are underway, the major shifts will need to occur in the basic assumptions of medical training and demand more than just an additional class or lecture.

In addition to prevention in its more traditional focus, a few medical schools have redesigned their curriculums to emphasize more than applied biology and include an understanding of human behavior and social process.

For example, the College of Medicine at Pennsylvania State University includes courses in health ecology, religious science, literature, and philosophy.

One notable exception is the major revision in curriculum undertaken at the Texas College of Osteopathic Medicine. They are designing a program that shifts emphasis from the diagnosis and treatment of established and advanced disease toward the promotion of health and prevention of disease. In this program, increased emphasis is placed on the patient's responsibility for his/her own health and on the physician's role as a teacher of healthful living, especially by example. A major emphasis is on developing health oriented physician education. This curriculum is based on the assumption that a major factor producing disease orientation in the health professions is the educational process itself. The chief elements of this program are prevention orientation, problem-based instruction, computer assistance, healthy living for the participants, and professionally trained medical educators (Jonas, 1981). In addition to the above components, students continue to be trained to practice on both sides of the prevention-treatment equation (Korr & Ogilvie, 1981).

In addition, the profession of nursing must be credited with maintaining a "whole-person perspective" in much of their training and practice. Nurses, as professionals, are playing an active part in this health care revolution. The Nurse Practitioner/Physician's Assistant Program at the University of California, Davis, has developed a self-care curriculum that focuses on the health of the nurse practitioner/physician's assistant and on developing skills in education and self-care approaches to use with patients (O'Hara-Devereaux, personal communication, 1967).

SELF-CARE FOR THE HEALTH PROFESSIONAL

An important focus of this newly developing interest in health care is on the health professional. How can professionals promote their own health, educate themselves to be good health educators, and maintain their best level of wellness in a demanding environment? These questions have become a challenge to the health profession's training programs, health centers, continuing professional education, and professional organizations.

Examples of training and educational approaches, organizational innovations, new practice options, and professional interventions will be fully described in the following chapters. These programs represent attempts to address the structural and individual difficulties inherent in the design and implementation of health care services and the career trajectory of its professionals. It is hoped that these examples will plant the seed of vision and innovation for others who are interested in humanizing health care for the patient and professional.

REFERENCES

Alpert, J. J., Kosa, J., & Haggerty, R. J. (1967). A month of illness and healthcare among low income families. *Public Health Reports, 82,* 705–13.

Ardell, P. B. (1981). Hospitals join the wellness movement. *Medical Self-Care, 13,* 30–31.

Barish, A. M. (1979). The influence of primary preceptorships and other factors on physician's career objectives. *Public Health Reports, 94,* 36–47.

Barker, W. H. (1981). The teaching of preventive medicine in American medical schools, 1940–1980. *Preventive Medicine, 10,* 674–688.

Calhoun, G. L. (1980). Hospitals are high stress employers. *Hospitals, 54*(12), 171.

Carpenter, D. C. (1980, Summer). Promoting health and fitness—A new role for hospitals. *Hospital and Health Services Administration,* pp. 16–30.

Cassel, E. J. (1982). The nature of suffering and the goals of medicine. *New England Journal of Medicine, 306*(11), 639–645.

Colligan, M. J., et al. (1977). Occupational incidence rates of mental health disorders. *Journal of Human Stress, 34*(3).

Cooper, B. S., & Rice, D. D. (1979). The economic costs of illness revisited. *Social Security Bulletin, 39,* 21–36.

Gunderson, E. K., & Rahe, R. H. (Eds.) (1974). *Life stress and illness.* Springfield, IL: Thomas.

Hastings, A. C., Fadiman, J., & Gordon, J. S., (1980). *Health for the whole person.* New York: Bantam.

Healthy People, The Surgeon General's Report on Health Promotion and Disease Prevention, 1979, DHEW Publication No. (PHS) 79-55071. U.S. Department of Health, Education and Welfare, 1979.

Holmes, T. H., & Rahe, R. H. (1967). The social readjustment rating scale. *Journal of Psychosomatic Research, 11,* 213–218.

Jennings, C., & Tager, M. J. (1981, summer). Good health is good business. *Medical Self Care.*

Jonas, S. (1981). Health-oriented physician education. *Preventive Medicine, 10,* 700–709.

Jones, L. (1982). Health promotion. *Hospitals, 56*(11), 88–90.

Keenan, C. (1982). Health promotion. *Hospitals, 56*(11), 92–96.

Korr, I., & Ogilvie, C. (1981). Health orientation in medical education, United States: The Texas College of Osteopathic Medicine. *Preventive Medicine, 10,* 710–718.

Kotz, H. J., & Fielding, J. E. (Eds.) (1980). *Health Education and Promotion: Agenda for the 1980's.* Health Insurance Association of America.

Levin, L. S. (1977a). Forces and issues in the revival of interest in self-care. *Health Education Monographs, 5*(2), 115–120.

Levin, L. S. (1977b). Gaining a realistic perspective on health intervention: Implications for health education, Conference on Consumer Health Education and the Health Care Delivery System, School of Public Health, University of Michigan, Ann Arbor.

Richardson, W. C. (1969). Poverty, illness and use of health services in the United States. *Hospitals, 43,* 34–40.

Sarason, I. G., Johnson, J. H., & Siegel, J. M. (1979). Assessing the impact of life changes, in I. G. Sarason & C. D. Spielberger (Eds.), *Stress and anxiety.* Washington, D.C.: Hemisphere Pub. Co.

Terris, M. (1980). Preventive services and medical care: The costs and benefits of basic change. *Bulletin of the New York Academy of Medicine, 56,* 180–188.

Terris, M. (1981). The primacy of prevention. *Preventive Medicine, 10,* 689–699.

Chapter 15

The Role of Professional Organizations in Developing Support

Emanuel M. Steindler, M.S.

The role of medicine in responding to physician impairment can be characterized as active intervention in a highly sensitive area with few preexisting guideposts to direct and channel that activity. It can be seen as an expansion of professional concern for the health and well-being of both the members of that profession and the patients they serve.

It has been undertaken at one time or another, and with varying degrees of intensity, by all segments of the profession, including medical schools, hospitals, and specialty societies, but most notably and consistently by one national association of physicians and its constituent societies in states throughout the country.

This chapter is a retrospective overview of the strategies that have evolved in the performance of that role by that national association—the American Medical Association. It is a prospective look, as well, at some of the trends that have begun to emerge to give new direction and shape to this performance in the future.

STRATEGIES OF ORGANIZED MEDICINE

The major strategies we will be looking at can be grouped under the following headings:

1. Articulating and propagating a professional and ethical responsibility to take appropriate action.
2. Recognizing and encouraging alternative ways of exercising this responsibility.
3. Exploring and explicating viable relationships between the public and private sectors.
4. Providing mechanisms for constructive interchange of ideas and experience.

Those strategies were not devised by a small cabal and sprung full-blown from the confines of a remote, smoke-filled conference room. Indeed only rudimentary and embryonic forms could be discerned with the first stirrings of action in the early 1970s. Rather, these strategies developed and took on substance and meaning as thoughtful and concerned men and women throughout the country responded in diverse ways to a panoply of events and circumstances.

The Ethical Imperative: The Blueprint Is Created

The time was mid-1971. The occasion was a meeting of the Council on Mental Health of the American Medical Association. The order of business reached the principal item on the agenda: a draft statement concerning medicine's obligations to cope with the problems of "disabled doctors."

Medical societies in two states—Oregon and Connecticut—had asked the AMA to propose ways to deal with problems created by physicians whose practices were being adversely affected by alcoholism, drug dependence, or mental illness.

In response, the Council on Mental Health conducted two surveys. One was directed to state medical societies. "What," the Council asked in effect, "are you doing about this situation?" The other was directed to three state medical boards to find out if actions against licenses involved these conditions in a significant way.

Answers from the boards—in Connecticut, Oregon, and Arizona—indicated that disciplinary action was being taken fairly frequently. Over an 11-year period in Arizona, for example, 3.2% of the physicians in that state had been disciplined because of alcohol problems, 1.7% because of drug problems, and 1.3% because of mental illness.

Answers from the medical societies revealed that seven had committees active in this area. Most, however, had no committees and were not even thinking of starting them. Three even expressed indignation at the implication that they had alcoholics, drug addicts, or mentally ill persons in their membership.

The Council decided then that a significant problem did exist, but that little was being done to deal with it.

At the meeting, the Council reviewed what the drafting committee of two of its members had presented. Some minor modifications were made, and the draft report was approved for forwarding to the Board of Trustees and House of Delegates.

When the House adopted the report in 1972, it became official AMA policy. It contained these key elements:

- A declaration that it is a physician's ethical responsibility to recognize impairment in a colleague and take constructive action.
- A call to all state medical societies to form a specific committee to deal with the problem—to identify and help the impaired physician.
- A commitment to develop model legislation for states to modify their medical practice acts so that a range of disciplinary and monitoring choices could be available to the boards and to medical societies.
- A recommendation that medical schools and residency programs offer meaningful instruction on alcoholism and drug abuse, so as to reduce the incidence of impairment in practitioners of the future.

These were to become the guideposts for AMA involvement in the ensuing years.

Options for Medical Societies: The Continuum of Concern

State medical associations—and, within a few states, county medical societies as well—have undertaken a variety of approaches to physician impairment and well-being. So have some medical specialty societies, hospitals, and medical schools.

A menu of options—most of them identified in the 1972 AMA report and others developed through field experience—runs the gamut from primary prevention through detection, intervention, and monitoring.

Primary prevention means shoring up personal and family strengths, learning how to cope with stresses, and improving the environment in which medical training and practice take place. Increasingly, medical students and residents have become involved in these activities, both in their own groups and in organized medicine and medical society settings.

Detection consists of providing a viable mechanism for colleagues and other concerned persons to report a physician they believe may be impaired—a mechanism that promises support and advocacy for the physician rather than punishment and retribution.

Most state medical societies now have such a mechanism in place. In a few states, it is simply there to be accessed; there is a minimum of publicity about it. In the others, however, there are varying degrees of outreach, including sustained educational campaigns through the county medical societies, auxiliaries, and other professional societies whose members come in contact with physicians. The typical message is "Bring the troubled physician to us now, before his ability to practice is affected, before the state medical examiners have to restrict or revoke his license. The sooner he enters treatment, the better chance he has for recovery."

After detection, or identification, comes intervention—confronting the physician, overcoming the denial that is usually made, and persuading him to enter treatment. Again, this has been an integral part of most medical society impairment programs.

Treatment itself takes place not under direct medical society auspices but through referral to treatment facilities or individual therapists. Many medical societies, however, monitor treatment, in the sense that they determine at the outset that a therapeutic relationship has been established, and go on to evaluate the progress of treatment. In the more comprehensive programs, monitoring will continue when treatment is over, when the physician needs encouragement and support to resume his professional life or, if necessary, to embark on another career.

Public and Voluntary Approaches: Building Bridges

Because medical practice acts and regulations differ from state to state, just as medical society programs differ, each state has had to work out its own pattern of relationships between the public and private sectors with regard to physician impairment.

The licensing or examining board in most states today can refer a physician to treatment and monitor that treatment, much as a medical society does. It is not "all or nothing" when it comes to license revocation. That this is so is in large measure a result of adoption in more than 35 states of major features of the AMA's model legislation.

Still, the state board is perceived as an adversary by many physicians, and this perception often inhibits case finding and reporting. The boards in some states have for this reason referred cases to medical societies where there is little or no threat or danger to patient health, and most have agreements, tacit or otherwise, with their medical societies that they (the societies) should take the lead in detection and intervention, referring to the board only those cases that constitute a hazard to the public.

Opportunities for Interaction: Doing by Learning

A conscious and consistent strategy pursued by the AMA over the years has been to facilitate the exchange of information and ideas among those working in programs throughout the country. Principally this has been accomplished by sponsorship of a series of six national conferences, through 1984, and the publication of a quarterly newsletter on physician impairment with a circulation that has grown to more than 3,000 copies.

From the first conference in San Francisco attended by 125 persons to the sixth in Secaucus, New Jersey, attended by nearly 400, there has developed a network of impaired-physician professionals, consisting of members of state medical society impairment and well-being committees, medical society executives who staff the committees, auxiliary members, concerned medical students and residents, directors of treatment programs, members of licensing and medical examining boards, medical educators—and a few physicians who are themselves impaired and seeking help. Leaders and leadership have thus not arisen and operated in isolation.

Through the national meetings, through the newsletter, through ongoing informal consultations that cross state lines and discipline boundaries, practical learning has taken place, learning that has been applied to specific problem areas. As a consequence, there has been a growing cohesiveness, not so much one of uniformity, because state and regional differences demand diversity, but rather one of building consensus on what works and what does not work all along the continuum of concern.

EMERGING ISSUES

Substantial advances in the impaired-physician issue have been made on several fronts during the past 12 years. They will become the foundation for even greater advances in the years ahead.

Unresolved issues remain, however, and the following are among those that may grow in importance.

Defining Impairment

The AMA has defined the "impaired physician" as one whose ability to practice medicine is affected adversely by mental illness, alcoholism, or drug dependence.

Operationally, the term has been narrowed or broadened depending on time, place, and circumstance. Thus, several state medical societies have, for purposes of their own programs, excluded mental illness as a parameter of impairment unless it is associated with chemical dependence. A few, on the other hand, have extended their programs to include cases of senility, sexual deviance, and incompetence. Some licensing boards have merged impairment with incompetence and even unlawful practice.

Nevertheless, on the whole, there has been reluctance on the part of programs to spread themselves thin by responding to every problem of physician disability, incompetence, poor judgment, moral turpitude, or ignorance. Occasions do arise, of course, when the boundary lines are not clear-cut, when to be rigid would mean to ignore some individuals and situations that could benefit from intervention.

The issue of detecting and dealing with psychiatric illness more effectively will continue to demand attention. If more psychiatrists become active in state programs, it might cause outreach efforts to encompass, not exclude, physicians who do not have primary problems of alcoholism or other substance abuse.

It may be that we are tending, in fact, toward a more inclusive definition of impairment comprising both illness and distress, a definition that would characterize an impaired physician as one whose behavior is consistently detrimental to self or dangerous to patients.

Refining Research

Counting the number of impaired physicians depends a great deal on how impairment is defined. But even when there is agreement on definition, reported prevalence rates have varied widely, from as low as 1% to as high as 20%. None of these estimates has been based on well-designed studies —almost all involve relatively few cases or extrapolations from other populations.

The epidemiology of impairment, including confrontation and treatment efficacy and relative significance of various etiological factors, requires precise formulation so that more realistic and workable methods of prevention and therapy can be devised and pursued.

Overcoming Stigma

We need to be assertive and forthright in our determination to combat the stigma that still too often attaches to anyone who has had problems with alcoholism, drug dependence, or mental illness.

This becomes especially crucial when physicians attempt to pick up the pieces of their lives, after successfully undergoing treatment and rehabilitation, or when medical students who have had these problems and are not in school try to resume their training.

Providing the Funds

We need to address in a more concerted and comprehensive fashion the matter of adequate funding for impaired physician activities, including both medical society programs and government agency programs.

And we need to address the financial problems of impaired physicians themselves as they enter and continue in treatment and begin to reestablish themselves in their communities.

Involving Other Professions

Medicine needs to extend its hand to other health professions and offer them what it has learned, and will yet learn, about this problem in physicians; in turn it may gain valuable insights from the perspectives of others.

Nurses, dentists, psychologists, pharmacists, veterinarians, all have begun to look at their own problems of impairment and well-being and to take steps to deal with them, often in concert with organized medicine.

CONCLUSION

It is clear that national professional organizations are taking an active role in the definition and response to a broad spectrum of problems of impairment. Organized medicine, medical societies, and public licensing boards are becoming increasingly concerned and mobile in the development and implementation of a wide range of intervention programs and research projects. These organizations are thus demonstrating that they can, in fact, guide policy and program development, both to assist individuals with problems and to make organizational changes that can prevent the development of these problems in the future.

Chapter 16

State Medical Societies: Their Perceptions and Handling of Impairment

Robert C. Larsen, M.D., M.P.H.

In the last decade state medical societies have developed committees and programs to address the problem of impairment in the profession (Rubin, 1983). The purpose of this study has been to describe the efforts directed toward this group of doctors by the state medical organizations. Furthermore, the data were collected with the intention of allowing for a description of the population of physicians designated as impaired.

A questionnaire was developed with the assistance of the AMA, the California Medical Association, and five state medical society committees known to be active in the arena of the impaired physician. Surveys were then sent to chairpersons of the committees in the 50 states and the District of Columbia beginning in the fall of 1983. Forty-eight surveys were returned.

This chapter reports the findings that pertain to the composition of these committees, the characteristics of the impaired physician population, the nature of the problems presented, and the feedback from committees regarding their function to date. Interpretation of the results is consistent with

This report is the result of research conducted while the author was a Robert Wood Johnson Clinical Scholar at the University of California, San Francisco Medical Center, 1982–84.

an evolving field in need of standardization and increased collaboration. Recommendations include the concept of an integrative model with the state medical society's role dependent on interchange with organized medicine at both local and national levels.

COMMITTEE COMPOSITION AND SERVICES

The committees were officially formed from 1973 through 1983 with most states forming a committee in the last four years. Seventy-three percent of committees meet quarterly or less frequently. Only two committees meet more than once per month. The mean number of members per committee was 13.5, with 12.9 physicians per committee. Experts in chemical dependency are well represented with 36% of the membership, or 4.5 members per committee. Thirty-one percent of committee members are physicians with personal histories of impairment, and 27% are psychiatrists. Six of 44 committees that responded to questions regarding committee composition had no members with prior histories of impairment. Interestingly, committees with a greater-than-average proportion of physicians with histories of impairment (>31%) tended to have a lower-than-average number of psychiatrists (<27%). Likewise, committees overrepresented with psychiatrists (>27%) were underrepresented with "recovering" M.D.s (<31%).

Data regarding services provided indicate that almost all committees provide identification (93%), intervention (100%), treatment referral (100%), follow-up (91%), and preventive or educational services (89%). Assistance with practice reentry (72%) and financial assistance (39%) are provided by some committees. Medical reeducation (24%) and direct treatment (15%) are made available by a smaller number of committees.

Nineteen of 48 states have an organized program of treatment for impaired physicians. In 14 of these the medical society conducts the program, though it may not be under the committee's control. In 12 states participation in the program allows for avoidance or diversion from disciplinary or legal action. In 29 states there is no organized program per se for treatment of impaired physicians. However, referral mechanisms are in place in 21 of these states, leaving eight states with no established referral protocol.

As the charge of these committees is to deal with the problem of impaired colleagues, each respondent was asked to give the committee's definition of physician impairment. Twenty-six responses noted a condition that included chemical dependency, psychiatric illness, or a physical disorder. Four definitions related solely to chemical dependency. An additional parameter of the definition involved the impact on the individual's ability to function. Twenty-three respondents noted that the impaired physician functioned poorly in caring for patients or in other realms of medical practice. Only 11 responses mentioned that poor functioning might be present in personal or social roles in addition to professional roles. Seven committees have no specific definition of impairment. One respondent replied with "We know it when we see it."

DATA ON IMPAIRED M.D.s

Forty-five committees had 1,087 referrals in the past year for an average of 25.8 referrals/committee (range = 1–200) or 2.75 referrals/1,000 licensed M.D.s (range = 0.84—24.8). Two hundred physicians had been referred in the prior two months to 43 state committees (range = 0–15/committee). These referral rates give an estimate of approximately 100 physicians per month referred to state medical societies across the nation.

Committees were queried as to the means by which referrals were made to their committees. Though much has been written about colleagues in medicine protecting or denying impairment in physicians, 63% of respondents stated that colleagues were often the source of referral (Chappel, 1981). The physician's family (20%), legal authorities (17%), and local medical societies (13%) were noted as referral routes with lesser frequency. Self-referral (7%) and a physician's own doctor (2%) are infrequent routes. Other routes, such as nonphysician hospital staff and pharmacists, were identified by a small number of committees. After having presented to the committee, the impaired physician typically remains under the committee's attention for approximately two years.

A profile of the impaired physician can be gleaned from the committees' cumulative experience. As a means of approximating the histories of impairment for physicians referred to committees, questions were asked about the "average impaired physician." Eighty-nine percent of respondents typically have had no prior committee contact with the doctor referred. Thirty-two percent of committees describe the impaired colleague as having been in treatment before coming to the medical society's attention. Fifty-seven percent of committees noted that the referred physician tends to have had contact with other official bodies such as licensing boards, hospital staff committees, or professional conduct committees. Committees were asked to estimate the mean age of the physician population they see. Cumulative results place the average age at 46.3 years, which is consistent with data reported elsewhere (Herrington et al., 1982; Johnson & Conelly, 1981; Larsen, 1983). The youngest and oldest impaired physicians were 29.2 years and 73.3 years, respectively, on average.

The literature on physician impairment notes that denial and delay are common phenomena in the sick or troubled physician (Little, 1971). These characteristics have been supported by case reports and relatively small samples of physicians (Vaillant et al., 1970). In this study 66% of respondents estimated that physicians delay presenting to their committees in the majority of cases. Ninety percent of respondents feel that the potential stigma associated with being identified as impaired is a major reason for delay.

As in any area of medicine, evaluation of the presenting problem is a critical step in developing an individualized approach to each referral. Thus the evaluation process was examined. Emotional stability was identified as the variable given most attention or emphasis in evaluating the impaired physician. Ninety-two percent of committees noted this to be "very important" as compared to physical condition (67%), the doctor's home life (67%), contact with other physicians (31%), the quality of friendships (28%), or involvement in community affairs (8%).

All committees are presented with problems of alcoholism, drug abuse, and mixed-substance abuse. Eighty-eight percent of committees are presented with psychiatric disorders at least sometime. Problems of aging (37%), behavioral problems (33%), physical disorders (31%), and educational deficiency (14%) are categories that present less frequently.

The issue of causation is controversial and difficult to establish as it applies to impairment in physicians. Rather than look for cause-effect relationships, associated concerns were examined via questions regarding "the nature of the problem" of physician impairment. The physician's psychological disturbance and the implications for patient care were designated as requiring much, if not the most, attention by committees in 97% and 95% of responses, respectively. The physician's medical condition (87%), his social functioning (74%), the legal aspects (50%), and the implications for the "image of medicine as a profession" (48%) are of less concern.

COMMITTEE SUGGESTIONS

The final section of the survey used open-ended questioning to collect data on the committees' experiences in working with impaired doctors. Twenty-three respondents noted that denial, concealment, and noncompliance by impaired physicians and colleagues was the most difficult aspect of the work. Problems with physician attitudes and raising awareness regarding impairment were mentioned by nine committees. Eight responses focused on early identification and intervention as difficulties. Four committees noted a lack of appropriate treatment and rehabilitation planning or resources. A similar number felt confidentiality was a problem area.

In response to questioning regarding successes experienced, 16 committees noted cooperation, commitment, and concern of committee members and physician networks in helping impaired colleagues. Eight respondents attributed successful function to support from the medical society. Effective identification and intervention, improved awareness and educational efforts, cooperation with the licensing board, and involvement by recovered physicians in the committee's operation were also frequently mentioned factors contributing to the committees' successes.

Given that these committees represent the frontline in organized medicine's dealing with impaired physicians, the committees were asked for suggestions for local, state, and national societies. Thirteen responses recommended increasing educational efforts to the medical community about impairment and its treatment. Other frequently mentioned suggestions included the need for a program director at the state level, an increase in funding, heightened involvement of local societies and hospital staffs, a need to alter attitudes and awareness in the medical community, and the desire for more staff support for the state committees.

The state medical societies potentially represent a link between the local society and the national association levels in the development of a comprehensive approach to caring for disabled doctors. In addition to resources such as the AMA Impaired Physician Newsletter, committees desire statistics on incidence and outcome data, reporting of successful intervention and treatment models, funding suggestions, and model legislation, especially in regard to reporting. Local societies and hospital staffs were identified as having a key role as the primary contact with the impaired M.D. State committees value the liaison with the medical community for identification and treatment referral purposes. However, many respondents noted infrequent use of the local medical societies. A model emerges that utilizes the local medical professional as the point of interaction with the impaired colleague. The state society's purpose might best be seen as providing a coordinating function and resources to the local level. The national society would function as a clearinghouse for data, models, and methods for addressing the problem.

INTERPRETATION OF DATA

In looking at the data collected, it becomes apparent that there is variability in the approach taken by state medical society committees. Some committees have no members with personal histories of impairment, yet this has been noted as important to the success in other states. A core of basic services is made available by virtually all committees with a degree of uniqueness provided by certain special services.

Though the AMA has provided a definition of physician impairment, there are committees with a less comprehensive operating definition (Report of the AMA Council on Mental Health, 1973). A number of states restrict the medical cause for impairment to substance abuse alone. An even larger group make no mention of the impact on personal and social functioning aside from the physician's professional role. Finally, a noteworthy number of committees have no specific definition for impairment at all.

The data allow for an estimate of the frequency of presentations to such committees. These referral rates represent one approximation of the incidence of impairment in medicine. In one year's time more than 1,000, or three tenths of 1 percent of all physicians, were referred to state committees. Geller and Bissell (1979) have estimated a prevalence rate of 23,000 for alcoholic physicians alone. A commonly used approximation is that the lifetime risk for impairment in M.D.s is about 10%. If current epidemiological estimates are correct, then state medical societies are dealing with only a fraction of the total problem in medicine.

The wide variation in referral rates is accounted for, at least in part, by some committees being newly formed and others associated with active re-gionalized treatment programs. Yet one cannot help but wonder how many physicians in need exist in locations with markedly lower referral rates to their state committee.

The majority of physicians referred have no prior treatment, yet contact with official bodies is a common occurrence. The physicians evaluated by committees typically represent the age spectrum of physicians. Chemical dependency is the type of problem most frequently seen by committees. This finding is consistent with reports from state programs published elsewhere (Gualtieri et al., 1983; Shore, 1982; Talbott et al., 1977). Psychiatric illness is evaluated to a lesser frequency. Yet the emotional stability of the physician is the evaluation parameter that is most important. Furthermore, though concern was noted by respondents for the potential effect on the doctor's patients and for the physician's physical health, the psychological disturbance of impaired M.D.s is given the most attention by the committees. The "psychological vulnerabilities of physicians" described by Vaillant and col-leagues (1972) appear to be of importance to the committees' evaluation process. Smith and Steindler (1982) have argued that the use of psychiatry early in the physician's professional career may promote well-being and ameliorate potential emotional dysfunction.

These data support the premise that delay in seeking assistance is a common phenomenon in sick doctors. The stigma of impairment is perceived by committees as the primary reason for this reticence. Denial, as a frequently used defense, noted by other authors, is commonplace in these committees' experience.

A possible bright spot in the data is that colleagues are the most frequent source of referral. At what point colleagues make such referrals is unknown, but the referral for assessment comes from other doctors more than any other source including family or authorities.

This study has taken a cross-sectional view of a field in transition. Gone are the days of organized medicine's implicit disregard for troubled physicians. However, a unified approach is not present as yet. Delineating and testing of models for evaluation, treatment, follow-up, reentry, and education is now possible. The experience of the state medical society committees reveals much about the characteristics of the impaired physician population, certain favorable programmatic avenues, and the degree of unmet need for further support of the committees' necessary operation. State medical societies are caring for disabled doctors, yet this study raises questions about physicians who may be dysfunctional and not coming to any committee's attention.

REFERENCES

Chappel, J.N. (1981). Physician attitudes toward distressed colleagues. *Western Journal of Medicine, 134,* 175-180.

Geller, A., & Bissell, L. (1979). *The impaired physician: Advances in primary care.* Baltimore: Williams & Wilkins.

Gualtieri, A.C., Cosentino, J.P., & Becker, J.S. (1983). The California exerience with a diversion program for impaired physicians. *Journal of the American Medical Association, 249,* 226-229.

Herrington, R.E., Benzer, D.G., Jacobsen, G.R., et al. (1982). Treating substance-use disorders among physicians. *Journal of the American Medical Association, 247,* 2253-2257.

Johnson, R.P., & Conelly, J.C. (1981). Addicted physicians: A closer look. *Journal of the American Medical Association, 245,* 253-257.

Larsen, R.C. (1983). *The California diversion program for impaired physicians.* Presentation to the meeting of the American Psychiatric Association, New York.

Little, R. (1971). Hazards of drug dependency among physicians. *Journal of the American Medical Association, 218,* 1533-1535.

Report of the AMA Council on Mental Health (1973). The sick physician. *Journal of the American Medical Association, 233,* 684-687.

Rubin, H.L. (1983). Substance abuse and the professional. In J.P. Callan (Ed.), *The physician: A profession under stress.* Norwalk, CT: Appleton-Century-Crofts.

Shore, J.H. (1982). The impaired physician: Four years after probation. *Journal of the American Medical Association, 248,* 3127-3130.

Smith, R.J., & Steindler, E.M. (1982). The psychiatrist's role with the impaired physician. *Psychiatric Journal of Ottawa, 7,* 3-7.

Talbott, G.D., Richardson, A.C., Jr., & Atkins, E.C. The MAG disabled doctors program: A two-year review. *Journal of the Medical Association of Georgia, 66,* 777-781.

Vaillant, G.E., Brighton, J.R., & McArthur, C. (1970). Physicians' use of mood-altering drugs: A 20-year follow-up report. *New England Journal of Medicine, 282,* 370-386.

Vaillant, G.E., Sobowale, N.C., & McArthur, C. (1972). Some psychological vulnerabilities of physicians. *New England Journal of Medicine, 287,* 372-375.

Chapter 17

Implementing a
Self-Care Curriculum

Janet Mentink, R.N., M.H.S., and
Cynthia D. Scott, Ph.D., M.P.H.

During the late 1970s, health care became increasingly oriented toward family-based care, resulting in the establishment of family practice residencies and programs to train nurse practitioners and physician assistants. This rekindled interest in primary care was targeted toward a perceived maldistribution of health care services (both inner city and rural), a lack of providers for certain cultural groups, and a perceived imbalance between technological and humanistic individually focused interventions (Davidson, 1981).

Family practice, as defined by the American Academy of Family Practice and the American Board of Family Physicians, emphasizes first-contact care and assumes ongoing responsibilities for the patient in both health maintenance and therapy of illness. This personalized care acknowledges the interaction between the patient and physician and the use of consultants and community resources (Rakel, 1977). This comprehensive focus necessitated the development of a curriculum that matched the task set out for family practitioners (physicians, nurse practitioners, and physician assistants).

This curriculum is of interest because it emphasizes the development of skills enabling the nurse practitioner to make "contact" with the patient and to learn to take care of himself or herself in the context of providing health care assistance for others.

This chapter will outline the development of a behavioral science curriculum in the Family Practice Department, Family Nurse Practitioner and Physician Assistant Program, at the University of California, Davis. This process took two years, 1979–1980, and resulted in a four-quarter sequence that is taught in conjunction with the physical medicine courses. The major steps in the development of the curriculum will be described along with examples of the course format.

THE PROCESS OF CLARIFYING VALUES

The essence of education . . . is the transmission of values, but values do not help us pick our way through life unless they have become our own. The task of education would be, first and foremost, the transmission of value, of what to do with our lives. There is no doubt also the need to transmit know-how, but this must take second place. . . .More education can help us only if it produces more wisdom. Science and engineering produce "know-how," but "know-how" is nothing by itself; it is a means without an end, a mere potentiality, an unfinished sentence. (Schumacher, 1973, p. 82)

In designing a new curriculum it was important as a faculty to clarify and understand our own philosophical approach to the newer values emerging in health care, such as the shift from infectious disease to chronic disease, increasing emphasis on life-style and environmental intervention, and introduction of health promotion, health education, and self-care practices in order to develop a new behavioral science curriculum. The exploration was based on the premise that the means to developing a new curriculum were not separated from the ends and therefore careful monitoring of our own behavior and responses throughout became key to this process.

This portion of the program was undertaken with strong leadership from the program directors and with the assistance of professional consultant resources. A series of seven off-site, two-day workshops were held over a two-year period to articulate values, translate them into curricular structures, and train ourselves to teach/model the new curriculum.

This process of clarification of both personal and professional values was exciting and confrontive and provided a forum for extensive self-examination. As educators, we wanted to practice the process of self-education as defined in the original Latin *enducere*, which means "to lead out that which is within." This clarification process resulted in renewed commitment and, for some, surfaced conflicts.

As discussions progressed, seven major themes emerged:

- The means are not separate from the ends in the practice of health care.
- Self-care, self-awareness, and self-referenced behavior are essential practices for educators in order to "teach" these skills to our students.
- Relationships with our patients are focused on assisting them to return to a state of physical, mental, and emotional well-being.
- The real art of health care is based on the humanistic application of scientific knowledge.
- The patient must be seen within the context of his culture, family, and environment.
- A desire to reemphasize the importance of attitudinal, interpersonal, and self-care issues is necessary in the education of health professionals.
- The task of educators is to provide the best possible technical training along with the transmission and articulation cf ideas and values.

From these themes the faculty crafted a mission statement elucidating our values and objectives in an educational program. What follows is a condensed version of the statement that was circulated to prospective students and faculty.

MISSION STATEMENT

Caring for ourselves is an essential part of being a health care professional. This entails acquiring information and self-care practice for maintaining health, wholeness, and integrity. Such factors as diet, exercise, self-awareness, awareness of others, and ecological awareness are basic aspects of real health consciousness (for ourselves and for others with whom we come into professional contact).

Health consciousness necessitates an appreciation of the interrelationships between personal, social, cultural, economical, and environmental factors. The key difference in this approach to health care is the conscious emphasis on health balance and integrity; the primary-care emphasis is *not on disease*. This may seem incongruent; despite the fact that you will be learning a great deal about disease, its identification (diagnosis) and treatment, it will only be a "part" of your professional responsibility. The diagnosis and treatment of disease will be addressed within a professional framework that teaches values and skills to promote a broader spectrum of health, balance, and integrity.

It is an intrinsic part of each health care professional's job to be an educator and a promoter of health, to express health via personal example and information exchange, as well as expertise in carrying out the other technical aspects of primary care.

Reflecting the goals above will necessitate that student and faculty develop the capability of doing the following:

- Exercising expertise in traditional areas of health care practice: to be a scholar of disease patterns and to be efficient in carrying out basic health care tasks.
- Understanding and explaining alternative conceptions of health and illness, being teachers and educators in the fullest sense of the word.
- Being aware of the integral relationship between body and mind: emphasizing the vital connection between physical wellness and positive thinking, disease, and negative thinking.
- Exercising self-care, self-referenced, and affirming/supporting this in others. Support for nourishing ourselves and facilitating that in others, being able to be composed and centered, especially during times of work pressure.
- Establishing wholesome, easy contact and communication with others: being in touch, being available physically and psychologically to patients during working hours. This will be reflected in the constructive use of your senses as basic tools in your everyday work, i.e., sensory awareness, touching, seeing, listening easily and competently.
- Cooperating with patients, other health care colleagues, intimate associates; listening to different points of view; taking time to formulate and articulate goals that become the basis for working together; much of our opposition is the result of not being interested in "harmonizing" different viewpoints around agreed-upon goals.

FACULTY DEVELOPMENT

An integral part of the process of clarifying our values was the development of a functioning team among faculty members. This process was facilitated by outside organizational development consultants and consisted of structured exercies, discussions, and conflict management. Woven throughout this ongoing development was a program to develop (1) self-awareness, (2) communication skills, and (3) group process skills. As a consequence of this exposure to new ideas and approaches, individual faculty members developed special interests in geriatrics, health promotion, patient education, ethical issues, and behavioral medicine, which they incorporated into their teaching.

CURRICULUM COMMITTEE

A curriculum committee of the entire faculty was developed to address designing both the technical-medical-diagnostic and treatment areas as well as the behavioral science curriculum. The intent was to present the behavioral science material in concert with the medical information to provide an integrated hierarchy of skill development. Following are excerpts from the introduction to the behavioral science course and a brief outline of each quarter's goals, format, and content.

To implement this curriculum, it was necessary to develop specifically targeted reading packets and experiential techniques in addition to available textbooks. (Specific information may be obtained directly from the first author.) Following is the student information for the behavioral science curriculum.

INTRODUCTION TO BEHAVIORAL SCIENCE SERIES

Your coming year will be a very exciting, stimulating, and challenging one. This year is one of growth and change, and with change often comes stress. As this will be a year of many changes, we encourage you to be aware of this, to deal with these changes positively, and to know that the faculty is available to assist and support you through this year.

It is imperative that you assess valuable relationships and protect them as they will be extremely important to you during this year. "Self-care" is essential for you to be there for yourself, your family, your friends, and your patients. We strongly encourage you to take time for yourself and to be self-nurturing. This will greatly facilitate your participating fully in this exciting and important year and will promote your sense of well-being.

We welcome you to our program and are looking forward to a great year of working and growing together!

We, as a faculty, believe behavioral science, with an emphasis on "self-care," is the discipline that differentiates family practice, Family Nurse Practitioners (F.N.P.s), and Physician Assistants (P.A.s) from other medical specialties. It is the ability of these clinicians to provide personal continuity of care and to oversee all aspects of his/her care that distinguishes us as a "new" and distinct discipline. Central to this new discipline is the clinician/patient relationship. Our role as clinicians is to assist the patient to maintain and/or return to a state of health—physical, mental, emotional. The real art of care is based on the skillful and humanistic application of scientific knowledge. The goal is the understanding of the person in his/her entirety, in the whole course of his/her life, and in the context of his/her culture and environment.

As we are all aware, there is clinical evidence reinforced by research that indicates a correlation between the physical state of disease and mental and emotional states of disease. Inherent in this belief is the necessity to view the person as a "whole," disregarding the traditional mind/body split.

The current behavioral science curriculum has been designed to reflect our belief that the "art" of delivering humanistic care embraces inherent and learned skills. This conviction has evolved over time and resulted in a curriculum that embraces student self-care, growth, self-awareness, and the prospect for developing skills that promote growth in clients as reflected in more awareness, healing, behavioral changes, prevention, a high level of wellness, as well as medically curative interventions.

As health professionals, we routinely contact individuals with disease, we daily have numerous opportunities to be in relation to toxicity, negativity, sadness, and unhappiness. To imagine that this continual exposure has no significant effect on our own well-being would be a serious misunderstanding of how human beings affect each other. Since we already know that health care people have a higher rate of certain "disease" (i.e., suicide, drug and alcohol abuse, to mention a few), we are interested in educating clinicians who are self-aware, self-referenced, and sensitive.

The intent of the behavioral science curriculum represents a focus on both content areas and process format for students that enhances self-awareness and sensitivity to imbalances, as well as sensitivity to the needs of themselves and others. The focus is on promoting learning of techniques for dealing with negativity which are "healthier" than drugs, alcohol, or getting sick oneself. The intent is to teach skills that allow the clinician to assist patients to realize the outcome they desire.

OVERALL COURSE FORMAT

The series will be taught over four quarters and in the internship. Classroom methods of presentation will be group interaction, role playing, formal lectures, and review of patient encounters. Knowledge and skills gained will be directly applicable to patient care and daily life; students will gain mastery there.

The curriculum represents two types of activities: One is process, tending to be oriented toward personal growth, and the other, more focused on didactic material, is oriented toward content. Video and audio tapes of the student interviewing will be used in nonthreatening dyads or triads.

The grading is on a letter basis, A to F. The grade will be determined by the communication portion on site visits and practical examinations and, when relevant, on a paper-and-pencil evaluation on content areas. Each of the site visits contains a communication skills checklist. This is used to assess the development of the student's patient interaction skills at all site visits. An example is given in the appendix of this chapter (pp. 253-256).

Each quarter will contain the following elements:

- Attendance and participation in all sessions.
- Evaluation on communication portion of the site visit.
- Written paper-and-pencil quarterly examinations. Written examination may be combination short answer, multiple choice, true/false, with a take-home essay portion.
- Participation in one or two audio recordings of patient encounters for learning.
- Videotaped practicum:

  Twice during the program, and at the end of the fourth quarter, the students are given an oral examination that incorporates the entire behavioral science curriculum and medical curriculum. This consists of a programmed patient presentation which is video recorded. The presenting problem has both a medical and psychosocial/emotional component. The criteria for evaluation are based on the site visit protocol with a special component for this particular problem. The student/actor introduction is observed and videotaped. The student is expected to demonstrate good communication skills, gather data on all problems, and explore any relevant psychosocial issues. The student is evaluated on communication skills, subjective history taking, assessment, physical examination, and a plan that includes patient education and follow-up plans.

  The student writes up the encounter and presents the patient to the faculty, who then spend over one hour reviewing and evaluating the student. The tape is then reviewed by the student and behavioral science faculty. The student is encouraged to self-report and monitor and is also tutored by the faculty at this time. The practicum in this complete form is used at the end of second, third, and fourth quarters. At the end of the first quarter, a practicum that addresses a psychosocial problem alone is used.
- Three site visits.
- One audiotape review—tape of interview of patient in your practice.

Since a large portion of the course is process as opposed to content, students need to attend all classroom sessions. The curriculum is presented with goals, references, objectives, and relevant reading materials.

Quarter I—Basic Communication Skills

Goals

I.   The student will be able to demonstrate clear values about his/her role as a helper and attitudes about his/her own health and about his/her relationship to him/herself and to others.

II. The student will understand the clinician/patient relationship and the interaction of emotions and expectations of both parties.

III. The student will understand the theoretical aspects of good communication and demonstrate sensitivity to the feelings of both him/herself and others.

IV. The student will be able to project his/her concern, sincerity, respect, and integrity.

Objectives—Communication

1. Discuss his/her personal needs and role as a helper.
2. Describe and demonstrate the ability to introduce him/herself and describe his/her role as a student F.N.P./P.A.
3. Describe, discuss, and demonstrate attending behaviors.
4. Describe and demonstrate beginning proficiency in listening and paraphrasing skills and responding to affective material.
5. Demonstrate high-level skills in structuring the interview, utilization of open-ended questions, directive questions, and recognition and avoidance of leading questions.

6. Describe and be able to demonstrate beginning level skills in direct forms of communication (i.e., congruence, negotiation, relabeling, recognizing hidden agendas).

Level of competency required

1. Demonstrate an understanding of their own feelings and values.
2. Demonstrate an ability to generate acceptance, trust, safety, and empathy with patients.
3. Integrate his/her own values and beliefs with a personal style of helping.
4. Display the following specific skills competently and appropriately:
   a. Structuring the interview.
   b. Introducing him/herself and describing his/her role.

    c. Use open-ended (exploratory), graduated open, and directive questions.
      1. Avoid very leading questions.
      2. Use appropriate language—minimal medical jargon.
    d. Take notes in a nondisruptive manner.
    e. Be adept at transitions and closing.
    f. Use excellent active listening skills.

Format

Readings, didactic presentations, and group work using theme-centered interation techniques.

Evaluation

—Attendance and participation at all sessions.
—Site visit evaluation of communication section.
—Written paper-and-pencil quarterly examination.
—Participation in and audio recording of patient encounters.

Quarter II—Communication, Sexuality, and Holistic Perspectives

Goals

I. The student will continue to practice and expand his/her communication skills with emphasis on understanding the helper role and increasing self-awareness and awareness of others.

II. The student will explore various aspects of health and wellness and entertain a variety of viewpoints and influences that are approached from multiple orientations, i.e., personal, social, and environmental.

III. The student will understand his/her own sexuality and that of his/her patients. He will increase his counseling and history-taking abilities and explore personal and social attitudes about sexual and sensual matters.

Objectives—Communication

1. Explore his/her own feelings and those of patients.
2. Record two patient interviews, the tape of which will be reviewed

and criticized, first by the student alone and then with a student peer or faculty person for further observations.

3. Perform the following with increasing skill:
   a. Conduct a smooth interview.
   b. Mirror, attend, pace, and lead.
   c. Utilize a balance of open and directive questions, explanation of both content and affective information.
   d. Effectively summarize, reflect, make transitions, and close the interview.

Objectives—Sexuality

1. Elicit an appropriate sexual history including starting the sexual interview with an open, nonintrusive question about sexual relations; obtaining a detailed sexual history; discuss the sexual stimulation and arousal patterns; and describe the sexual response cycle in men and women.
2. Describe the following sexual dysfunctions, including the common presenting indications and relative information regarding the causes and occurrences:
   a. Impotence (primary and secondary)
   b. Premature ejaculation
   c. Orgasmic dysfunction
   d. Difficulty lubricating
   e. Vaginismus
   f. Retarded ejaculation
   g. Dyspareunia
3. Identify areas of sexual concern with patients and develop an appropriate treatment plan utilizing the P-LI-SS-IT (Permission –Limited Information–Specific Suggestions–Intensive Therapy) model.
4. Identify medications that commonly alter sexual function and utilize a framework for differential diagnosis of sexual dysfunctions.
5. Clarify his/her own values and provide patient education regarding common sexual concerns:
   a. Size of penis
   b. Size and shape of breast
   c. Size and shape of female genitalia
   d. Masturbation
   e. Duration and frequency of intercourse
   f. Intercourse during menstruation

g. Oral-genital sexual contact

h. Premarital intercourse

i. Homosexuality

6. The student will discuss the following topics related to childhood sexuality:

a. Sexual abuse

b. Sexual play

c. Masturbation

d. "Dirty" words

e. Genital exhibition

f. Pornography

g. Observing parents having sex

7. The student will clarify their own feelings about abortion and be able to offer support to a woman/couple through the abortion process.

Objectives—Holistic Perspective

1. Discuss the paradigm shift in health care.

2. Discuss and explore aspects and notions of holistic health to include the following areas:

a. Biomedicine and bioethics

b. Characteristics of holistic health

c. Qualities of the practitioner, self-responsibility

d. Wellness as a continuum

3. Discuss and explain concepts regarding psychosomatics:

a. Autonomic nervous system

b. Mind-body connection-disconnection

1) Self-regulation

2) Feedback systems

3) Placebo effect

4) Biofeedback, acupuncture, endorphins

4. Discuss and explain theories about healing:

a. Relaxation

b. Pain

c. Touch

5. Discuss and describe major concepts of the study of consciousness and brain functions:

a. Reticular activating system

b. Limbic system

c. Neocortex

   d. Learning
6. Discuss and describe the nature of stress:
   a. Concepts of fight or flight
   b. Immune system
   c. What makes stress
   d. Psychological response to stress
   e. Physiology and philosophy of stress reduction
   f. Neurophysiological stress profile
   g. Impact of life events
   h. Utilize tools to measure their own patients' stress levels
   i. Utilize knowledge to identify stress in clients and be able to
      advise them and teach stress reduction, e.g., relaxation response

Choose one of the modalities for relaxation promotion. Become familiar
with your modality of choice by practicing it yourself and reading about it.
Practice teaching it to two other individuals—a classmate or a friend and one
patient. A videotaped interview will be reviewed and evaluated by the faculty.
Particular attention will be paid to skills in the following:

   a. Conducting a smooth interview
   b. Mirroring, attending, leading, and pacing
   c. Proper utilization of open-directive questions
   d. Exploration of content and affective material
   e. Effective summarizing, reflection, transition, and closing of the in-
      terview

Level of competency required

   Students not meeting minimum requirements are tutored individually
by a faculty member or psychologist.

Evaluation

   —Take-home examination on holistic health perspective
   —Self and faculty evaluation of audiotape encounters
   —Two to three site visits to evaluate communication skills

Quarter III—Human Life Cycle and Assertion

Goals

   I.   To provide the student with a basic overview of normal human
        development and to aid the student in cultivating an understanding

that his/her own personal experiences and those of patients occur within a developmental framework. To develop an awareness of problematic areas in development as they relate to health and illness behavior.

II. To teach the student the difference between assertion and aggression and between nonassertion and politeness. To help the student identify and accept both his own personal rights and the rights of others. To develop assertive skills through practice and to be able to assist others, clients, etc., to develop assertive skills.

Objectives—Human development/life cycle

1. Discuss and compare several theories and viewpoints pertaining to adult development.
2. Describe the adolescent development tasks of:
   a. Establishing a self-image
   b. Resolving conflicts
   c. Developing a capacity for tenderness toward others
   d. Competency and achievement
   e. Sexuality
3. Describe the common issues that arise between parents and adolescents in the following areas:
   a. Sexual activity
   b. Conflicts
   c. Limits
   d. Parents' rights
   e. Privileges
   f. Parents' ambivalence regarding certain issues
4. Discuss the meaning of illness behavior, death and dying, and grieving for different patients.
   a. Understand illness and health behavior
   b. Understand the reasons for and functions of denial
   c. Discuss how to reduce anxiety
   d. Discuss and initiate appropriate treatment plans for specific concerns patients may experience, e.g., fear of dependency and closeness
   e. Describe six crucial psychological tasks imposed on the dying person
5. Describe the six common reactions that appear as one adapts to the prospect of death:
   a. Death

    b. Anger

    c. Depression

    d. Anxiety

    e. Dehumanization

    f. Detachment

6. Describe the three stages of acute grief:

    a. Disbelief

    b. Working through

    c. Resolution and resumption of normal functions

7. Describe the pathological forms of grief and identify the factors that place a survivor at higher risk for the development of pathological grief.

8. Develop a family tree—to be completed in the fourth quarter.

Objectives—Assertion

1. Distinguish between assertion, aggression, nonassertion, and politeness and be able to describe behaviors that reflect these concepts.

2. Describe why someone might act in an assertive, aggressive, nonassertive, or polite manner.

3. Demonstrate the above responses to various situations, verbally and in written form.

4. Risk looking at your own behavior patterns, and in the class, practice changes you would like to effect.

5. Describe common socialization messages for both men and women and their effects on rights and assertive behavior. What would a "healthy" socialization message be?

Level of competency required

The students will demonstrate assertive behavior while observed at clinical site visits and in role plays designed to practice assertion skills.

The students will demonstrate knowledge of the theories of assertive behavior and distinguish assertion from passive aggression and nonassertive and aggressive behavior on a written examination.

Evaluation

The student's knowledge of assertive behavior will be evaluated by a written examination.

Quarter IV—Psychiatric Approaches, The Family in Health and Illness and Role Changes

Goals

I.   The student will be able to evaluate and assess common psychosocial conditions, including the healthy person and persons with conditions requiring referral or secondary care.

II. To assist the student in gaining a practical understanding of family dynamics and their role in health and illness and examine how family therapy approaches can be used in the context of providing health care.

III. To assist the student in exploring and expanding the contemporary role of the nurse practitioner and physician assistant; to assist the student in role formation and transition; to explore the historical development of the nurse practitioner and physician assistant movement; and to increase knowledge regarding current issues that are relevant to present and future professional development.

Objectives—Psychiatric approaches

1. The student will state the basic pathophysiology, etiological agents, and/or risk factors, preventive measures, signs and symptoms, differential diagnoses, investigative measures, management, and patient education for the following diagnoses:
   a. Hypochondriasis
   b. Depression
   c. Anxiety
   d. Organic brain syndrome
   e. Hyperventilation
2. The student will know the basic signs and symptoms of the following diseases but will not need an in-depth understanding:
   a. Manic-depressive illness
   b. Schizophrenia
3. The student will have sufficient knowledge to recognize these disorders and initiate treatment. As well, they should have a working knowledge of the basic pathophysiology, risk factors, preventive measures, and patient education for the following patients:
   a. Patients who are a danger to themselves, i.e., suicidal or unable to care for themselves
   b. Patients who are a danger to others

4. The student will be able to perform a focused history and physical, know the possible etiological agents and/or risk factors, preventive measures, signs and symptoms, generate a differential diagnosis, and order appropriate examinations or tests. The student will be able to present the problem orally, do a write-up in SOAP (Subjective–Objective–Assessment–Plan) format, and manage diagnosis for the following conditions:
   a. Organic brain syndrome
   b. Substance abuse
   c. Chronic pain
   d. Family problems (see references to the normal family, family development)
   e. Sexual dysfunction (see second-quarter references to sexuality and concerns)
   f. Psychosomatic presentations (state the difference between psychosomatic disease and psychosomatic symptoms)
5. The student will be able to perform basic skills in assessment, including the mental status examination, as follows:
   a. Behavior and appearance
   b. Sensorium—level of consciousness, orientation
   c. Intellectual function—attention and distractibility, concentration, memory, general information, numerical ability
   d. Speech and thinking—progression and speed, form, content, abstraction
   e. Affect—mood, anxiety level, congruence, appropriateness, lability
   f. Insight
   g. Judgment
   h. Reliability
6. Students will be familiar with those organic diseases that may contribute to or cause problems which are more often of a psychosocial nature; e.g., in anxious persons, consider hyperthyroidism; in persons with psychosis, consider drug intoxication, thyroid dysfunction, etc. All patients with problems considered to be of a psychosocial nature or with a psychiatric label should have at least a focused history and physical. Further evaluation will then depend on clinical judgment.

Objectives—Family

1. Understand the concept of the ongoing progression or development of the family from inception (courtship and marriage) to passing of the family (death of parents onto the next generation).

2. Be able to describe and understand family systems theory, family dynamics, and contemporary family structures.
3. Understand areas of family function that include recognition of roles within the family, the family tasks, functional and dysfunctional patterns (i.e., situations at high risk for child abuse), and recognize normative and nonnormative crises.
4. The student will be able to identify problems manageable in the practice and have referral plans for those needing community referral.
5. Understand some of the specific issues involving families such as divorce, the family with chronic illness, old age, single parent families.
6. Understand and identify illness behaviors and recognize the impact of illness and the various roles of illness in the family.
7. Be able to identify the individual's role within the family and evaluate the individual from a personal and family developmental standpoint.

Objectives—Role changes

1. Understand the history of the nurse practitioner and physician assistant (N.P./P.A.) movement and be able to discuss these and relevant current issues such as political, legal, role, reimbursement, licensure.
2. Participate in peer group discussions of their N.P./P.A. role development as a student and be able to critically examine their professional development as it relates to areas of professional relationship and adjustment to medicine, nursing, decision making, patient care, changing responsibility, and other key issues that develop from the evolution of the expanded N.P./P.A. role.
3. Examine the function of the N.P./P.A. in relationship to educating other health professionals, balancing dependence, independence, and interdependence, and joint decision making as they construct their own N.P./P.A. practice in clinical patient care.
4. Develop a personal plan for negotiating entering practice.

Evaluation—Family

The students will develop a family-problem-oriented record that will facilitate the analysis of a family in their practice. They will systematically evaluate the family status with the Beavers-Timberlawn family evaluation scale. This family will be followed for a six-month period. During this time, a health and psychosocial database will be developed for each family member.

Appropriate identification of health problems will be ascertained and appropriate education and intervention will be undertaken with the family. During the six-month project, two family interviews will be conducted. The outcome will be reported in a final written paper and an oral small-group presentation.

Each student will understand the relationship of family to health and illness behavior by examining his own family genogram and exploring certain pertinent questions.

Evaluation—Role

Each student will role play adequate job negotiating skills and develop a written resume.

Oral Practicum

At the end of each quarter, the students are given an oral examination which incorporates the entire behavioral science curriculum as well as the medicine curriculum. This process entails a well-developed clinical problem that encompasses a medical and psychosocial history, physical examination, assessment, and plan. The programmed patient presents both a medical and psychosocial problem.

The interview and examination is evaluated by the faculty during the taping; the student then writes up the encounter and presents it orally to the faculty who give them feedback in the following areas:

—Communication skills
—History taking
—Physical examination
—Assessment
—Plan—to include patient education

Then the tape is reviewed for one hour with the student and faculty reviewing the communication and interaction.

These oral practicums are evaluated by the student and have constantly been described as an excellent learning activity.

REFERENCES

Davidson, R. C. (1980). Family practice physicians: Their impact on improving family and community health. *Journal of Family and Community Health, Special Edition: Primary Care at the Crossroads*. Rockville, MD: Aspen Publications, pp. 1–20.

Rakel, D. C. (1977). *The principles of family medicine*. Philadelphia: Saunders, pp. 1–106.

Schumacher, E. F. (1973). *Small is beautiful*. New York: Harper & Row.

APPENDIX

UNIVERSITY OF CALIFORNIA, DAVIS
F.N.P./P.A. PROGRAM
COMMUNICATIONS SKILLS CHECKLIST

Student's name: _____ Date: _____

Evaluator's name: _____

Opening   *Comments*

1. Introduces self and
   role   4 - 3 - 2 - 1 - 0 - N/A _____
2. Appropriate physical
   contact, i.e., shakes
   hands with patient,
   touches shoulder, etc.   4 - 3 - 2 - 1 - 0 - N/A _____
3. Asks patient how
   he/she wishes to be
   addressed   4 - 3 - 2 - 1 - 0 - N/A _____
4. Sets expectations for
   interview   4 - 3 - 2 - 1 - 0 - N/A _____
5. Asks for patient's
   reason for visit   4 - 3 - 2 - 1 - 0 - N/A _____

Questioning process

Open-ended questions

6. Moves within each
   topic from general to
   specific   4 - 3 - 2 - 1 - 0 - N/A _____
7. Encourages more than
   a "yes" or "no"
   response   4 - 3 - 2 - 1 - 0 - N/A _____
8. Allows patient to
   respond in own terms   4 - 3 - 2 - 1 - 0 - N/A _____

Closed questions

9. Appropriately directs
   patient's attention to
   specified area of
   concern   4 - 3 - 2 - 1 - 0 - N/A _____
10. Asks one question at a
    time   4 - 3 - 2 - 1 - 0 - N/A _____
11. Does not "lead"
    patient   4 - 3 - 2 - 1 - 0 - N/A _____

Facilitative responses

Encourages patient by use of

12. Verbal facilitation (i.e.,
    "go on")   4 - 3 - 2 - 1 - 0 - N/A _____
13. Nonverbal facilitation
    (i.e., nod)   4 - 3 - 2 - 1 - 0 - N/A _____
14. Attentive silence   4 - 3 - 2 - 1 - 0 - N/A _____
15. Paraphrases or restates
    what patient has said   4 - 3 - 2 - 1 - 0 - N/A _____
16. Does not interrupt
    patient   4 - 3 - 2 - 1 - 0 - N/A _____

Reflection of feelings

17. Identifies, labels, and
    reflects feelings (i.e.,
    "You seem *worried*
    that the *pain in your
    chest* might be
    something serious—
    like a *heart attack.*")   4 - 3 - 2 - 1 - 0 - N/A _____
18. Responds
    nonjudgmentally to
    patient's feelings,
    attitudes, and beliefs   4 - 3 - 2 - 1 - 0 - N/A _____
19. Is able to assist patient
    with identifying and
    exploring feelings   4 - 3 - 2 - 1 - 0 - N/A _____

Language is personalized

20. Uses terms patient can
    understand   4 - 3 - 2 - 1 - 0 - N/A _____
21. Asks patient to clarify
    any confusing or
    idiosyncratic
    information   4 - 3 - 2 - 1 - 0 - N/A _____

Transitions

22. Makes explicit
    transitions from one
    area to another   4 - 3 - 2 - 1 - 0 - N/A _____

Nonverbal behavior

23. Maintains eye contact   4 - 3 - 2 - 1 - 0 - N/A _____
24. Posture open   4 - 3 - 2 - 1 - 0 - N/A _____
25. Paces appropriately   4 - 3 - 2 - 1 - 0 - N/A _____
26. Mirrors   4 - 3 - 2 - 1 - 0 - N/A _____
27. Writes or uses chart
    appropriately   4 - 3 - 2 - 1 - 0 - N/A _____
28. Awareness of
    nonverbal cues in
    patient (posture,
    mood)   4 - 3 - 2 - 1 - 0 - N/A _____
29. Awareness of own
    feelings and throughts
    during interview   4 - 3 - 2 - 1 - 0 - N/A _____

Summary

30. Internal summaries
    when needed   4 - 3 - 2 - 1 - 0 - N/A _____
31. Gives patient
    opportunity to correct
    or add information   4 - 3 - 2 - 1 - 0 - N/A _____

Closing

32. Summarizes what's
    been covered and/or
    what is meant   4 - 3 - 2 - 1 - 0 - N/A _____
33. Asks patient if he/she
    has further
    comments/questions   4 - 3 - 2 - 1 - 0 - N/A _____
34. Develops a plan and
    patient education *with*
    the patient as a full
    partner   4 - 3 - 2 - 1 - 0 - N/A _____

Feedback

35. Student is able to
    receive feedback
    without becoming
    defensive   4 - 3 - 2 - 1 - 0 - N/A _____
36. Student shows
    willingness to accept
    and use feedback   4 - 3 - 2 - 1 - 0 - N/A _____

37. Student communicates
    with faculty in an
    open, cooperative
    manner   4 - 3 - 2 - 1 - 0 - N/A _____

Strengths   *Areas for improvement*

Key

  4 = Excellent throughout
  3 = Good, allowed progress, most of time
  2 = Fair, awkward, rarely done
  1 = Inadequate or distracting
  0 = Missed, negative effect
N/A = Not necessary, would not be helpful,
       not expected this level of student

Chapter 18

Caring for the Health and Wellness of the Healer Within the Health Care Institution

Esther M. Orioli, M.S.

> To ward off disease or recover health, men as a rule find it easier to depend on healers than to attempt the more difficult task of living wisely. —Dubos, *The Mirage of Health*, 1959, p. 114

Hospitals have a great opportunity to be innovative and pioneering in meeting the need and demand for services that promote health and wellness. Meeting this challenge lies in the willingness of hospitals to utilize wellness opportunities within their own institutional walls, and to create an internal shift in their "consciousness" to become models of good health practices.

Economically, hospitals and health care institutions have actively entered the health promotion/disease prevention marketplace for several reasons: to improve community relations; to enhance hospital relations with local businesses; and to develop long-term revenue sources (Jones, 1981). But what of the hospital employee, the healing professional, within their institutions. Are they the recipients of innovative state-of-the-art stress reduction and health care technology, or are they the cobbler's children with no shoes?

Studies have revealed that some of the most stressful occupations are in the health care system and that the problems associated with stress may not be dealt with appropriately for those closest to professional help (Schulz & Johnson, 1971; Weiman, 1977). Health care settings have been subject to intense scrutiny for many reasons. Among them are the soaring cost of medical technology and hospitalization, the singular focus of allopathic, disease-oriented thinking, and a questionable interest in the health and well-being of the community at large. It would also seem appropriate to ask what efforts the hospital has taken to help individuals within their walls. Robert Cunningham (1978), one of the country's leading journalists, asks the question this way: "Is the (hospitals') mission to make a positive contribution to the health of the population or is it basically to find a body for every bed?" (p. 20).

Hospital administrators are being compelled to focus not only on the issues of medical/health care delivery, but also on organizational productivity, fiscal stability, and business acumen in order to remain competitive and profitable in the business world. Hospitals and health care settings must develop and implement innovative workplace programs if they are to assume leadership roles within the health promotion field, as well as within the community at large. Perhaps we need only look at the response of hospitals to the personal problems (high distress, burnout, alcoholism, drug abuse, and mental, emotional, and behavioral problems) of their own staff to gauge their commitment to the promotion of health and wellness to the community they seek to serve.

MEETING THE CHALLENGE

The health care industry can learn much from a review of the private sector's response to some of these issues. For example, employee assistance programs, the first generation of worksite wellness models, are an effective way to contain deteriorating performance and to minimize the cost of distress and illness in the workplace.

Employee assistance programs (EAPs) are uniquely suited to the hospital setting as centers of healing and health care. Once such a program is functional within the organization, the EAP can serve as both a model and a delivery base for local industry and business. To understand the unique challenges of implementing EAPs in the hospital setting, it is important to examine existing private sector EAP models as a basis for comparison and discussion.

EMPLOYEE ASSISTANCE PROGRAMS AND THE HOSPITAL SETTING

Hospitals Are High Stress Employers

Employee health and productivity are intricately interconnected. The impact of dysfunctional stress is often manifested in higher absenteeism, lost time due to illness and disease, increased accident rates, higher turnover rates, higher medical-health care utilization, and so forth (Calhoun, 1980). Although hospitals would like to project a public image that shows them as islands of comfort and healing in a chaotic and uncertain world, they can, in fact, be particularly stressful employers. Some of the hazards of hospital work are obvious, like the stress of dealing with people in pain, risk of infectious disease, and increasing workloads with decreasing staffs. Other hazards are invisible and insidious, often inherent in the hospital system itself: multiple levels of authority; heterogeneity of personnel; work interdependence; and specialization (Schulz & Johnson, 1971). The National Institute for Occupational Safety and Health (NIOSH) studied the relative incidence of mental health disorders in 130 major occupational categories. When the major occupations were rank-ordered in terms of the relative incidence of mental disorders, seven of the top 27 occupations related to health care operations: health technologists; licensed practical nurses; clinical laboratory technicians; nursing aides; health aides; registered nurses; and dental assistants. If the list of health care occupations were expanded to include those not exclusively involved in health care delivery (dishwashers, warehouse personnel, laborers, research workers, telephone operators, chemists, social workers, secretaries, and other support staff), 15 of the top 27 occupations with the highest evidence of mental health disorders would come from hospitals (Colligan, 1977).

ESTABLISHING A FIELD

Background History

For over a decade, private sector corporations and companies have utilized innovative employee programs to minimize the effects of stress and illness in the workplace. It has been important for managers to be aware of productivity factors and the level of employee performance, and to provide themselves and their employees with improvement opportunities.

Historically, EAPs have grown out of industrial alcoholism programs. First started to address personal problems in the workplace, industrial programs focused largely on the disease of alcoholism in the male manufacturing worker. For over 20 years, from the mid–1940s to the mid–1960s, alcoholism programs were slowly breaking ground in American corporations because of two factors: an increased awareness of the serious impact of alcohol problems on productivity and profit; and the advent of successful treatment methods for alcoholism recovery, i.e., Alcoholics Anonymous (A.A.).

Early pioneers of EAPs were hard pressed for statistics that could validate their services' existence in the workplace, and could be easily faulted for vague estimates of cost impact as rationale for any corporate obligation or benefit. Indirect societal costs were the main vehicle for legitimizing these workplace efforts.

Increasingly, industry has been encouraged to calculate the impact of alcoholism on their workers, with discernible results. In 1950 an estimated 50 companies had some form of alcoholism programming. By 1973, 500 companies had installed assistance programs. By 1977, nearly 2400 organizations countrywide had established some form of EAP.

The tradition of these early alcohol programs has laid the groundwork for the development of current day worksite wellness programs: EAPs. Increasingly sophisticated methods of service delivery and valid life-style change studies (Bauer, 1980) have encouraged the redefinition of many alcoholism programs to embrace a full range of medical-behavioral dysfunctions affecting workers and their families. Now most commonly referred to as a broad-brush approach, EAPs often include marital, family, emotional, stress, and personal problem areas. Most corporate-based programs also offer legal and financial assitance in the form of resource referral.

Quite simply, an EAP is a system for identifying and treating medical-behavioral dysfunction in an employee or dependent, using the structured characteristics of the work world as an environment for early identification and treatment.

Next Steps

With more than a decade of study behind it, the EAP field has statistical support for the cost-benefit of programs, and some of the strongest advocates in the 1980s come from within corporate America itself:

> Current estimates indicate that over $1 billion each year is lost on stress-related problems through loss of time, productivity, accidents, doctor and hospital bills, medicines and drugs. Add to this the $42 billion lost each year on alcoholism and chemical dependency, and you have a very high cost. Obviously, it is in the best interest of all businesses to provide help for our employees. . . . As business people we must be concerned with our bottom line, and it is a proven fact that healthy people make a stronger contribution to their companies and communities. (Kinney, 1981, p. 3.)

Currently, corporations attempting to increase profitability and decrease direct and indirect cost losses due to stress and illness have been implementing a variety of health promotion and wellness programs: 1) risk and disease identification for early intervention and treatment; 2) broad-brush EAPs for confidential counseling of troubled employees; and 3) full-scale, voluntary life-style change programs. All of these programs address the cost of stress and its impact on the company goals and mission. New and innovative approaches have been designed to assist individuals and groups to adopt wellness life-styles and create healthful environments.

Health Care Settings Participate

The one industry that has fallen behind the pace of wellness is the very one to whom employers have turned for leadership in the wellness movement: health care institutions and hospitals. It is paradoxical that physicians and hospitals should be called upon to counsel employees to lead less stressful life-styles when they themselves engage in tremendously stressful practices. Studies reveal that some of the most stressful occupations are in the health care delivery system and for the most part, are left unaddressed by their administrations (Pelletier, 1984).

PLANNING AND DESIGN

There are several phases leading to implementation in a hospital setting.

Phase I—Assessment of Hospital Need

Most effective cost-efficient EAPs begin with clear pictures of goal and outcome expectations. Depending on the environment, the population, and the desired impact, the hospital EAP should be designed specifically to address the greatest need first, progressing from renewal of health for the most distressed employees to maintaining and maximizing healthy and productive employees for peak performance.

To determine the EAP type and model, it is important to define the workforce in terms of present performance and health levels. Doctors, nurses, technicians, aides, and assistants in health care institutions, although healers by profession, are still employees of hospitals—institutions with layers of authority, and varying levels of accountability.

There are classifications (see Table 1) of work performance and health that we must keep in mind in determining the level of EAP need. The first classification is *productive/untroubled* employees, those who successfully fulfill the requirements of their work and deal effectively with job and life stress.

The second classification is the *productive/troubled* employee. This individ-

Table 1

Classifying EAP Target Populations

Work Performance Level	Medical/Behavioral State
Productive	Untroubled
Productive	Troubled
Unproductive	Troubled
Unproductive	Untroubled

ual's work performance, although definitely affected by distress or a medical or behavior problem, has not yet deteriorated sufficiently to attract the attention or correction efforts of a superior. Classification three is the *unproductive/troubled* employee who is typically the target of EAPs, regardless of the nature or type of dysfunction. Supervisors and administrators can easily identify this productivity level since it is common to have one or more dissatisfactions with work task performance or quality. The fourth classification is the *unproductive/untroubled* worker. This group comprises those who are over-trained and under-utilized, or mismatched for the job by training or attitude.

The *unproductive/troubled* employees have the greatest need for treatment. They also account for the highest direct and indirect losses in hospital employment and quality of patient care. Typically, between 8% and 15% of any worksite population can fall into this category and represents the most distressed group manifesting the greatest dysfunction.

The *productive/troubled* employee also falls within the direct service range of EAPs. These employees often utilize the program option that encourages voluntary self-referral for program assistance. Approximately 10% of any workforce comprises this group.

Phase II—Program Development

The four major components of an EAP in hospitals are: policy review; training; orientation of employees and dependents; and assessment and referral. Each of these components is necessary to build a strong, cost-effective program.

Policy review

One of the first considerations in EAP planning is a review of existing hospital/clinic policies that may influence EAP effectiveness. Health insurance and medical coverage plans need to be compatible with the treatment offerings of the program. Alcoholism, substance abuse, and psychotherapy services should be covered. While many insurance carriers have expanded coverage for alcoholism and drug dependence, the types and kinds of limitations need careful review to ensure EAP utilization. Prime issues to review in planning include: the nature and extent of detoxification programs; comprehensive medical health assessment and treatment policy on covered illness; ongoing case review; outpatient counseling services; and amount of times employee can use benefits.

Personnel policies. One way to utilize EAPs involves using work performance as a criterion for referral by supervisors and administrators. Personnel policies should provide consistent documentation procedures for employee performance appraisal and correction. This will serve as a guideline to managers and supervisors when confronting employees with impaired or troubled performance work records. Referral to the EAP for poor work performance must be accompanied by detailed records of correction attempts and specific delineation of work improvements required. Clear personnel policy and guideline procedures should enhance the overall EAP function. The following areas should be checked for congruence: job descriptions, performance review system, corrective discipline, and union agreements in regard to employee grievance procedures.

Accident and safety policies. Statistics report that unproductive/troubled employees experience three to four times more accidents and injuries than untroubled employees. Many companies have tied EAPs into their accident and safety policies by requiring medical/behavioral dysfunction assessment for employees showing high accident levels. The accident repeater policy becomes a vehicle for early identification of employee problems, and can be used consistently by supervisory and management personnel to control costs and losses due to accidents.

Hospital settings can easily incorporate such policies by focusing on employee errors, mistakes with medical equipment, inattention to tasks, missed routines, injury accidents or patient neglect.

Union and labor policies and agreements. Most hospitals have negotiated agreements with one or more unions or labor groups. From the onset, these arrangements should be reviewed with regard to corrective discipline and union steward involvement in grieving employee cases. Care should be taken to invest the union or labor leadership in the EAP planning process, focusing on the benefit of such steps as an employment enhancing vehicle, as well as an employment retention tool.

The employee assistance policy statement. The purpose of any policy statement is to ensure consistency of organization standards and operating procedures. The EAP policy is no exception and needs to be widely distributed to hospital employees, professional staffs, and administrators; it should address those issues that are most likely to be obstacles to utilization. If an organization has never had a service of this type, employee distrust or confusion may hinder any widespread acceptance, regardless of assurances from administrative or program staff. Fear is the predominant reaction of employees when there is no policy statement preceding the start-up of an EAP.

One of the prime issues for clarification in any EAP policy statement is the hospital's view of alcoholism, drug dependence, or psychological distress. In addition, such a statement must address communication and reporting mechanisms with licensing bodies; confidentiality of employee treatment records; and any incidence requiring restriction of patient care duties.

Training

The key to successful program start-up and utilization lies with the supervisor, since he or she can become a strong advocate of the effort. Policy and procedure training enhances supervisor involvement and lays the groundwork for effective utilization of the program. An employee referred to the EAP for patterns of poor work performance, which is pending disciplinary action, has rights and administrative remedies under local, state, and federal laws. It is imperative that all supervisory personnel be knowledgeable and capable of fulfilling the intent of the law, in order to protect the organization from potential employment practice suits or grievances and to legitimize fair and equitable treatment of all employee groups.

Hospitals should develop a two-channel referral system for employee access to EAP services. The first channel is a management referral system, where the supervisor initiates a request for assistance because of an employee's continued poor performance. The second channel is a voluntary self-referral system, which does not include supervisory intervention. The two-channel system has yielded the most effective utilization of program services in other organizations and could be easily implemented in hospitals.

In essence, the management referral model identifies those employees most distressed and in need of intensive tertiary approaches for recovery. The drawbacks of this system are that it does little to identify secondary treatment needs and has no focus on early identification of problem performance. The voluntary self-referral system will focus on the productive employee, who identifies himself or herself as one who is in need of assistance. The voluntary system does little for the employee for whom job confrontation may be the only motivator for seeking treatment. In either case, one set of needs will be neglected to the detriment of the other.

Supervisory training, therefore, becomes the foundation block for sharing EAP information, expectations, and procedures, which can then assure successful outcomes and cost-effective implementation.

ORIENTATION OF EMPLOYEES AND THEIR DEPENDENTS

The orientation of employees for promotion of the EAP can take several forms. The number of people within the organization and their time availability will determine the most suitable approach.

Whether orientation meetings are conducted in large groups or in smaller departmental groups, these meetings set the tone and spirit for EAP acceptance, explain the policy statement, introduce the program personnel, and address outstanding concerns of the workforce. As such, they then become the kick-off for any hospital-wide implementation.

Ideally, representatives from the highest levels of management, and the Union Leadership should accompany the program personnel when they introduce the mission and intent of the EAP. This will strengthen the perceived support and commitment for the program, through a demonstrated alignment in goals. Policy statements should be distributed with any explanatory or promotional literature to detail the type and kinds of services and ways to use the system.

Direct mailing of this information to the employees' residence will aid in announcing the service to dependents and covered household members. Many organizations use internal house organs and newsletters, others hold an "open house" or feature a special event to draw attention to inception of the Program.

Regardless of the initial steps taken to promote the Program, the best results will come from exposure and visibility on an ongoing basis.

Assessment and Referral

The point of employee entry into the EAP, whether through the management referral system or the voluntary system, begins with an intake process and medical-behavioral assessment of need. It is at this stage that the nature and type of problem area will be determined for referral to appropriate treatment or attention. Two of the most vital elements of this component of the EAP are the intake/assessment interview and treatment referral management. Experience has shown that without careful attention to these issues, the EAP can be tremendously ineffective or nonproductive. The intake/

assessment interview process is primary to accurate diagnosis and subsequent referral for treatment or assistance. Since many an employee will approach the program with a presenting problem, the EAP professional is ill-advised to make a referral based solely on the concern as presented. A comprehensive, one-on-one medical-personal history should accompany any EAP intake process, to assure a total perspective on the nature of the concern, and any variables that are likely to influence the potential treatment plan or selection of a provider. For example, a 29-year-old female lab technician for a small privately owned hospital approached the EAP, seeking help with her eight-year-old daughter who was having problems in school. The mother was attributing these difficulties to her sporadic time schedule, since she was a full-time student, in addition to her job at the hospital. Upon completion of a comprehensive medical-personal assessment, it was obvious that this woman was also dealing with the alcoholism of her spouse, which clearly affected the child's ability to function in school.

Had the presenting problem been taken at face value without consideration for the family situation as a whole, the treatment plan would have failed to identify the most significant issues in need of attention.

INTERNAL VS. EXTERNAL EAP PROGRAMMING

Typically, there are several options available for determining staffing and implementation of the assessment and referral component. Two of the most commonly used are: 1) the external contract for delivery of assessment and case management; and 2) hiring and training staff for in-house delivery.

Some considerations in selecting the most appropriate avenue for any organization include: (a) the size of the organization; (b) the targeted medical-behavioral areas most in need of attention; and (c) the protection of individual confidentiality and treatment records.

If the hospital or health care institution's total population numbers 1500 or more, cost implications may warrant the selection of an in-house EAP coordinator, on a full- or part-time basis. The EAP should be housed and administered with as much independence from management as possible, to decrease the fear of jeopardizing professional or staff positions. Treatment referral resources must be examined to ensure confidentiality of the EAP user and the nature of the medical-behavioral problem.

Confidentiality cannot be taken seriously enough as a primary element for successful utilization. Take, for example, the case of a small independent hospital seeking to implement a program with a major emphasis on alcohol and drug treatment. It was reasoned that the internal alcohol and chemical dependency unit of this hospital could be appropriately utilized to care for its own treatment needs. The EAP could refer to the unit as a cost-saving device, and it seemed a natural alternative to external referral. After several months of active promotion of the EAP, utilization reports were falling far below their expectations. The problem quite simply was one of employee unwillingness to risk real or imagined repercussions from lack of confidentiality and the availability of records to the hospital administration as a patient within the institution. Unfortunately, when the EAP could not produce the kind of results to justify its operation, the program was cut from the hospital budget; however, the needs remained.

Although the arguments strongly favor an external model, hospitals interested in successful programming can take precautions and anticipate obstacles. Housing the EAP off-site or establishing a policy to guarantee external treatment availability will greatly enhance the situation.

SUMMARY

Employee Assistance Programs provide hospitals with the means by which the troubled employee or professional is identified at an early stage and is motivated to seek rehabilitation. Altruism may initially motivate the employer's concern with the troubled employee's personal problem, and rehabilitation may be a humane and desirable goal, but the rewards for employers lie within both financial considerations and the interest of operational efficiency.

The key to successful programming, more than any other single element, falls heavily on the pre-implementation and planning functions. Without an accurate picture of the service needs of the population, and a well-designed, fully responsive mechanism to address resistances, the best of intentions will not yield the results possible. Employee Assistance Programs offer a structured management alternative for addressing troubled performance in the workplace in a prudent and efficient manner that ultimately benefits both the employer and the employee.

REFERENCES

Bauer, K. G. (1980). Improving the chances for health lifestyle change and health evolution. *US Department of Health and Human Services, Center for Health Statistics*, p. 414.

Calhoun, G. L. (1980). Hospitals are high stress employers. *Hospital*, June 16, p. 171.

Colligan, M. J. (1977). Occupational incidence rates of mental health disorders, *Journal of Human Stress, 3*, 34.

Cunningham, R. M.(1978). Who's minding the store? *Hospital*, March 16, p. 20.

Dubos, R. (1959). *The mirage of health*, Garden City, N.J.: Anchor Press, p. 114.

Jones, L. (1981). *AHA special selected topic survey data on employee health*. Unpublished report.

Kinney, R. E.(1981). Mental health, the essential benefit, as presented by Willis Goldbeck to U.S. House of Representatives Subcommittee on Compensation, p. 3.

McNerney, W. J.(1977). As health costs soar. *U.S. News & World Report*, March 28, pp. 39–45.

Pelletier, K.(1984). *Healthy people in unhealthy places: Stress and fitness at work.* New York: Delacort Press.

Schulz, R., & Johnson, A. C. (1971). Conflict in hospitals. *Hospital Administration Canada, 16,* 36.

Weiman, C. G.(1977). A study of occupational stresses and the incidence of disease/risk. *Journal of Occupational Medicine, 19,* 119.

Chapter 19

A Health Awareness Workshop: Enhancing Coping Skills in Medical Students

Leah J. Dickstein, M.D.,
and Joel Elkes, M.D.

There is a welcome resurgence of interest in the health risks attendant upon becoming and being a physician. The health of the healer is no longer being taken for granted. Whether the rigors of medical training and practice present a higher health risk than those prevailing in other demanding professions is a question that only more data can answer. However, within the profession, there is good cause for concern.

A mounting literature attests to professional and personal dysfunction in the "impaired physician" (Scheiber & Doyle, 1976). The incidence and prevalence of depression, alcohol and substance abuse, marital difficulties, professional burnout, and attempted and completed suicide among physicians are by now well documented (Scheiber & Doyle, 1976). In a pathbreaking prospective study, Caroline B. Thomas followed the careers of 1,337 Johns Hopkins medical students in the classes from 1946 to 1964. This group became the core of the Hopkins Precursors Study, which clearly demon-

We are deeply grateful to the McLean Foundation, Louisville, for support of the videotaping of the workshop.

strated that medical students and physicians are at considerable health risk, that hypertension, coronary artery occlusion, depression (including suicide), marital discord, substance abuse, and cancer represent what she called "the dark side" of medicine (Thomas, 1976). Thomas and Betz developed the "Habits of Nervous Tension Scale" as a possible predictor of illness or premature death some 10 to 15 years after graduation (Thomas, 1971). This work is now fully documented in more than 100 papers and represents a courageous attempt—far ahead of its time—to understand the genesis of the so-called "impaired physician" (Thomas, 1983).

Other authors have borne out these broad conclusions. Vaillant, Sobowale, and McArthur (1972) studied physicians' earlier lives and found that vulnerability to impairment antedates entry into medical school. Breiner (1979) surveyed psychiatrists who had worked with impaired physicians and found that prodromal warning signs commonly appear during medical school. Gardner and Hall (1980) reported that protracted stress syndromes, usually self-imposed, are seen in medical students. Linn and Zeppa (1984) examined stress in junior medical students, attempting to define unfavorable and favorable responses to stress. The study involved 169 medical students before and after clinical clerkships and measured their degree of stress—judged "favorable" or "unfavorable"—using locus of control and self-esteem scales to measure personality function. They found that students likely to experience stress unfavorably were more externally controlled and lower in self-esteem than other students. Cognitive performance was evaluated by two written and two oral examinations, and attitudes and skills were assessed by a behavioral scale completed by faculty members and residents. The authors conclude that "since stress predictably will increase in residency and in the practice years, students should be exposed to stress management techniques to help prevent the known high consequences of stress such as substance abuse and suicide among practicing physicians."

Small and co-workers (1969) studied the vulnerability of residents to stress and described the "house officer stress syndrome," marked by episodic cognitive impairment, chronic anger, pervasive cynicism, and family discord. Severely affected house officers were found to suffer from major depression, suicidal ideation, and substance abuse. Possible contributing stresses include sleep deprivation, excessive work load, responsibility for patient care, perpetually changing work conditions, and competition. Their approach to prevention and management includes improved work conditions, increased group responsibility, and psychiatric referral.

In a sensitive essay Bogdonoff (1983) comments on the nagging sense of dissatisfaction inherent in current medical education. Though "most of these very same students and faculty members believe that medical education in the United States ranks with the finest in the world," they "hold persistent doubt that perhaps all is not quite right with the process," that ". . . it is a singular paradox that an educational realm which recruits its students from the scholastic top ten percent of college graduates and that promises a life-long career of economic surety, societal prestige and emotional gratification should be in any way significantly disquieted." Trying to define this sense of malaise Bogdonoff focuses on the *lack of collegiality* among students and faculty and the lack of awareness of common purpose and mutual interest in each other's work. Students are too busy to be aware of each other, and competition creates distance. Bogdonoff does not recommend student-faculty dialogues, "sensitivity seminars," or adding students to curriculum and administrative committees, but instead argues cogently for a continued sense of awareness of self and others and for continuity of contact with faculty and peers rather than the "staccato encounter of lectures, classes, shifting clerk-ships and the like." Yet, the opposite is still sadly true: the medical student is mired down in an overwhelming atmosphere of fierce competitiveness, unseemly haste, fragmentation, overscheduling, rote learning, overwork, examination pressure, insensitivity, unawareness, and the inappropriate use of denial. Despite many well-meant attempts, the problem has clearly not gone away.

The two steps recommended by the AMA for long-term prevention of impaired physicians are to "humanize medical training" and to "teach coping skills" (Robertson, 1980). Many schools are trying to do just that. Goldstein (1975) suggested that medical schools should rate personal growth equally with knowledge of medicine, and Lief (1971) argues that *developing attitudes* is as important as acquiring information and skills. Stephens and Kitchen (1978) began a course at the University of Southern California, Introduction to Clinical Medicine, whose specific purpose is professionalization. The course encourages students to believe that psychosocial factors *are* science. To clarify this point Stephens and Kitchen recommend that any program to broaden students' definition of medicine should *not* be run by the psychiatry department. If information comes from professors of all subjects, the message is much clearer. Humanity is the province of all physicians, a message that students will find harder to dismiss.

There are a number of programs to support students through their career in medical school. Some have selected high-risk students for attention, others have experimented with random samples. Flach and co-workers (1982) constructed a mentor program designed to help students move from child-adult to peer-adult relationships. Hilberman and co-workers (1975), Cadden and co-workers (1969), and Rosenberg (1971) favor small discussion groups. These programs work. Rosenberg reported "observable lessening of tension and growth of mutual respect between students and faculty." Our own Student Hour at the University of Louisville (Dickstein, 1982) has met with similar success. Sharing concerns, hassles, professional ambiguities, and worries and getting to know other students and faculty can improve medical students' attitudes and performance and can reduce the sense of isolation and the risk of a student's failing or dropping out.

All the above programs take up the problem while the student is *in* medical school. Our modest aim has been to impart to the student a *sense of self-awareness and some coping skills* (based on solid information) *before actual enrollment*, and to make the offering a *voluntary* one, rather than one required. Our program, presented below, combines large presentations with small-group discussions; it makes use of sophomore "health tutors" as group leaders and resource persons; it emphasizes positive student-student and student-faculty interaction at a very early stage in the student's career; it mixes didactic teaching with experiential exercises; it also shows students creative aspects of physicians' lives (art, music, literature) of which they may not necessarily be aware. However, the first and last aim of the Health Awareness Workshop is to be *useful* and to emphasize effective functioning, coping, and competence rather than pathology and disease.

We feel that in this respect, medical education may still be following rather than leading. "Self-care" and responsibility for personal health are clearly more than a fad. They reflect an increasing awareness and concurrence by the general public that *mode of life* and *behavior* are emerging as powerful pathogens. Medical schools cannot let the concept of well-being go by default, particularly since there is a body of knowledge that is slowly defining a Science of Health complementary to the great traditions of the Sciences of Medicine. This complementarity will grow as the scientific base deepens. Neurochemistry, neuroendocrinology, neuropsychoimmunology; cognitive and developmental psychology; learning theory; the increasing understanding of the physiology of eating, exercise, sexuality, sleep, and relaxation; and the psychology of work satisfaction, social play, and social support are steadily laying the foundation for what might be called a "psychobiology of positive states of being." Interestingly enough, the methods of investigation are the very same methods that have given us a Science of Medicine. Applied to health, they may well enlarge the terrain of medicine itself.

THE UNIVERSITY OF LOUISVILLE HEALTH AWARENESS WORKSHOP

Genesis of the Approach

While one of us (J.E.) was at Johns Hopkins, he introduced in 1964, with several colleagues, a Behavioral Sciences course during the first year, which involved the Departments of Psychiatry and Behavioral Sciences, Medicine, Pediatrics, and Obstetrics and Gynecology in joint presentations of the behavioral sciences inasmuch as they related to medicine as a whole (Elkes, 1965). A core message of the course was an opportunity for the student to *meet him/herself*. As the author put it at the time:

THE STUDENT MEETS HIMSELF

As he meets psychiatry, the student is prepared for yet another specialty. In this he is wrong. Psychiatry cannot compartmentalize: it deals in patterns and not pieces, in people and not organ systems. In making contact with the subject the student brings to it his most important piece of portable equipment, namely himself. In his skull he carries a vast and fascinating laboratory, of which he may be only dimly aware.

Yet somehow he must be made aware, before he moves too far into his clinical training, that behavior and subjective experience are not only phenomena but also instruments of high inferential value; that skill in observation of behavior, including his own behavior, though more native to some than to others, can be both taught and learned; that such learning requires conceptual tools of its own; that it can never be didactic and always has to be experiential; and that relative absence of hardware in clinical psychiatry and human psychology in no way reflect in its ability to measure, conceptualize, and predict.

In short, the student must learn to respect the use of himself as much as of his slide rule and statistical tables. In this self-acceptance and growing self-knowledge there can be a source of much power. If acquired early, it will serve him well with his patients and equally well should he choose a life in the laboratory rather than a life in the clinic. Adolf Meyer, in requiring autobiographies of his students, saw this clearly.

This course, one of the first of its kind offered in a medical school, was built around four elements: Human Development, Human Learning, Human Communication, and the operation of the Social Field. It also comprised key concepts in psychobiology and included didactic as well as experiential exercises. A workbook accompanied the course. It continues to this day, with a number of modifications and improvements.

Also while at Johns Hopkins, one of us (J.E.) discussed with Dr. Caroline B. Thomas the desirability of taking her study one step further and moving it from a purely observational/epidemiological to an active, interventive approach. The opportunity arose when he came to Louisville, upon retirement from Johns Hopkins. Here, one of us (L.J.D.), in her capacity as Medical Director of the Student Mental Health Service (where, since 1977, she had treated some 300 impaired medical students) and subsequently as Associate Dean for Student Affairs, had introduced the Student Hour (Dickstein, 1982), a support program for freshmen, staffed by sophomores and faculty members, chosen by students, who were trained each spring and met with the freshmen in a series of meetings during the school year. Thus the template for a Health Awareness Workshop already existed in Louisville. Not only was there a ready acceptance of this central idea, but there was a group of colleagues dedicated to conveying to freshmen a very practical message, namely, that both faculty and students *cared* about students' well-being. It remained to devise an approach that was nonintrusive to an already over-loaded curriculum, nonthreatening, and one which would mobilize student initiative and make the effort—on both sides—its own reward. We opted for a *voluntary* approach *before* students entered medical school. Out of many preparatory discussions and training sessions there grew a program for a Health Awareness Workshop, which was begun in 1981 and which has since been offered yearly to incoming students.

Structure of the Program

The program lasts four days and is offered to students in the week immediately preceding formal enrollment. It is open to the students themselves, their spouses, and significant others. Since the second workshop, mothers have attended every year. In 1984 a special program was initiated for children.

The offering is made in a letter of invitation from the Dean's office, sent during the spring semester to all students accepted to medical school during that year. The first letter, sent in 1981, reads:

> To: All Incoming Freshman Medical Students
> Re: Health Awareness Workshop for Freshman Students
>
> We congratulate you on being accepted to the University of Louisville School of Medicine and look forward to seeing you in a few weeks.
> This letter is a personal invitation for you to attend a Health Awareness Workshop, August 10–13, 1981, which has been designed specifically for all incoming freshman medical students and spouses.
> It has been documented that many freshmen students experience a great deal of stress in the transition from college to medical school. Therefore, the objective of the Health Awareness Workshop is to focus on *preserving* health and *preventing* illness. The Workshop will offer

you various skills to develop competence in dealing with stress; relaxation techniques; practical nutrition; time management.

The Health Awareness Workshop will also offer you an opportunity to become acquainted with your classmates, sophomore students, and faculty members.

We encourage you to make arrangements to attend the Workshop and look forward to meeting you.

During the year preceding the workshop sophomore students are instructed in skills pertaining to their future role as "health tutors," group leaders, and resource persons to 16-member freshmen groups designated as "unit labs." Faculty members, usually selected by students, play a similar role. These small-group "unit labs" provide an important counterpoint and "practicum" to the larger presentations that are given in the Freshman Lecture Hall of the School of Medicine. One of the most heartening and surprising aspects of the exercise was the degree of voluntary participation by freshmen. Despite the inconvenience of an early start (one week before formal enrollment), the extra cost of lodgings, etc., 95 students of a class of 138 (69%) and eight significant others attended in 1981; 112 students (90%) and 15 others in 1982; and 95 students (68%) and 15 others in 1983. In 1984 the attendance was 113 of a class of 124 (91%) plus 37 significant others. A special program was also arranged for 10 children. In 1985 the attendance was 115 of a class of 124 (93%) plus 20 significant others and eight children.

On the afternoon before the beginning of the workshop there is a final planning session of student, faculty, and health tutor staff. Registration takes place on the morning of the first day. At this time students are given handouts, including a cookbook, and the tutors wear a T shirt stenciled with the emblem of the workshop. During the practicum, faculty wear these shirts as well. There are muffins and juice, and the group then adjourns to the auditorium for the introductory presentations.

These center on up-to-date evidence linking mode of life with illness and disability ("On Being Ill and Being Well: Awareness and Personal Responsibility;" "The Psychobiology of Stress and the Stress Response"). There follow, over the next few days, presentations on the physiology and role of exercise, the physiology of relaxation, practical nutrition, effective coping in relationships, and listening skills. The elements of efficient time management are presented, complemented by a presentation by sophomores on study skills. A convention bureau film introduces the out-of-town student to the city of Louisville, and an archivist presents the unique history of the medical school. Substance abuse is presented by way of showing the film "Our Brothers' Keeper," followed by a panel discussion led by physicians from the state medical society's Committee on Impaired Physicians. There are presentations by senior colleagues on "The Importance of Medical Ethics" and on "The Role of Belief in Healing."

Yet, the most significant aspect of the workshop is that, throughout, it attempts to maintain a balance between scientific presentations of evidence and a participatory, experiential "fun" approach to the exercise. The nutrition component, for example, includes the preparation of nutritious (and delicious) meals by sophomore students, under the guidance of an expert nutritionist, and the serving and eating of these meals in the form of a lecture-demonstration in the auditorium—a possible "first" in the annals of a medical school. Relaxation techniques are taught by faculty members to the class in two separate sessions; the "do's and don'ts" of study skills are imparted by sophomores to their newcomer colleagues in lifelike small satirical sketches and vignettes; a jazz band, which includes prominent physicians, plays for the students one evening, along with a small art show to make the point that there is room for leisure and recreation in the life of a physician; there is a river cruise on the Belle of Louisville, and on the last evening before formal enrollment, a picnic-fair in a public park (complete with student folk music) welcomes the students to their medical school. In all these activities faculty and significant others participate freely. Strangers get acquainted, and some become friends. A sense of "welcome" and "feeling at home" is nurtured. This "feeling at home" requires more than a quick tour of the Medical Sciences Center.

Handouts, Health Checks, Scales: The Role of the Health Tutor and of Small Groups

Each student receives a handbook which includes a statement of the basic philosophy of the workshop; rankings of various medical school stresses; 15 ways to substitute exercise for sedentary activities; a game to evaluate one's risk of heart attack; instruction for relaxation exercises; advice and bibliography about accepting other life-styles; a time management chart; study pointers from upper classmen; advice and bibliography about married students' stresses; advice from senior medical students; charts listing fat, sodium, and calorie contents of food; recipes for protein-rich vegetarian foods; a menu-planning guide with sample menus; and grocery-shopping tips with instructions for evaluating food labels. Along with the handbook students receive copies of "The Longevity Game" (donated by Northwestern Mutual Life), information about Louisville from the Visitors' Bureau, a list of university resources, a list of reasonably priced restaurants recommended by students, and the Group for the Advancement of Psychiatry's *A Survival Manual for Medical Students* (1982).

The health check, carried out in the outer office of the Associate Dean for Student Affairs, includes recordings of height, weight, blood pressure, and skinfold measurement by senior students and sophomore health tutors. All students complete four instruments to assess their response to stress: the Habits of Nervous Tension Scale (Thomas, 1980), the Lorr Mood Scale (Lorr et al., 1967), the Katz Social Adjustment Scale (Katz & Lyerly, 1963), and a questionnaire about drinking problems and art form activities. In all these activities the role of the sophomore health tutors is crucially important. These students (who earn elective credit in the previous spring for their workshop training) become very important resource persons during the exercise and thereafter. They do most of the legwork in the preparatory phase and during the workshop. They become attached to "their" freshmen, maintain contact, and check up on them during the year. They prepare a practical version of the Convention Bureau's introduction to Louisville. They conduct surveys of facilities, publish a list of medical students' favorite restaurants, of banks with inexpensive checking accounts, of available apartments, etc. To their particular group they become a friend in need and in deed.

The further development of this human network of self-help support seems to us of crucial importance for the future. A medical school supporting kindness and mutual concern can hope to have this attitude reflected in the physicians it trains.

FIRST IMPRESSIONS: NEED FOR LONG-TERM FOLLOW-UP

The above experiment, essentially a pilot study, was carried out on a minute budget. Fortunately, support for the videotaping of the actual workshop provided us with some material by which we can in retrospect decide how to improve the planning and content of the workshop. The crucial question of long-term impact must remain unanswered for the time being. Some data are being gathered and will be analyzed and reported when funds for such analysis are available. The next phase will include much more extensive use of health risk appraisal instruments and long-term (10 to 15 years) follow-up, similar to the study carried out by Caroline B. Thomas: only such a program could give us the true measure of effectiveness. Nevertheless, such data as are in our possession from the students' feedback forms are highly encouraging. Students' comments were consistently positive. They found the relaxation exercises particularly helpful. They felt closer to classmates whose families they had met. They acknowledged attention to eating habits and were grateful for sophomore study hints.

In all workshops, participants found the information interesting and useful, and none, boring. Their comments on scheduling varied widely—too concentrated, not concentrated enough, too long, too short. We changed format from four whole days to four half days in 1982, and 84 of 95 evaluations reported that the length now was optimal. We also took students' advice about food, eating, exercise, and additional activities; for example, we turned over much of the introduction to the city to the sophomores, cutting down on the public image and presenting insiders' views instead. Only one student said that all the advice and warnings made him more nervous than before, a possible hazard of any program that calls attention to anxiety. Everyone else was pleased with the positive emphasis on actively preventing and coping with anxiety.

The one feature students mentioned most often, both spontaneously and in writing, was the chance to meet friends before school started. The immediate effect of the workshop is to form a social network. The freshmen were glad to have begun relationships with faculty and upperclassmen as well as with each other in the relative calm before the first term. We hope these relationships will further a sense of community in the years to come. There is always the hazard of students forming tight little groups of companions in misery, trying to outwit the "faculty." We try to convey to students that faculty are their allies, that they are "there," and that they care and are available.

Some anecdotal evidence supports the positive written evaluations. In the freshmen photographs of previous years, students looked rather somber and severe. The class pictures taken at orientation since 1981 and 1982 show smiling faces. Students drop by the Student Affairs Office more than ever, and they are watching out for each other as well as for themselves. For example, two students this year reported that two members of their unit labs were considering dropping out of school, and one was in danger of suicide. They asked how to help and persuaded their friends to seek help. Other students and a sophomore tutor, disturbed by seeing a classmate on a psychiatric ward, wanted to know how to respond to him when he was discharged. These are dramatic incidents. It is probable that students are helping each other in many less dramatic ways that we cannot see or do not even hear about.

A week is long enough to learn names and faces, to befriend one or two, to begin a social network, and to become aware of the importance of one's well-being. We hope that the information we share with students and the experiences we go through may affect these students' self-management effectiveness. It will take much rigorous design and long-term effort and funding to test this hypothesis. So far, we and the students agree that information conveyed in the way we have described, taken at its simplest, is useful.

COMMENT AND CONCLUSION: THE NEED FOR LABORATORIES OF STUDENT HEALTH

The Health Awareness Workshop differs from support groups and "orientation" sessions in several important respects. First, it is a *voluntary* exercise, offered before the formal beginning of the academic year. Second, it mixes didactic and experiential programs. Third, the material offered goes beyond mere "survival"; it presents an introduction to some basic life skills (in terms of theory and practice), which we hope may "carry over" into the students' subsequent life and the way he/she views patients and practices medicine. We offer an opportunity to *learn*, knowing full well that changes in life-styles cannot really be taught. The best one can do is to present adequate information and the option of change through personal choice.

A large body of data concerning the stressors of everyday life is available. The epidemiology of psychosomatic disorders has provided new insights into the health risk factors endemic in Western society. Of all people, medical students especially deserve an early acquaintance with this information. We cannot leave the important concepts of health prevention to accidents of the students' spare time. Preventive medicine, through personal awareness, initiative, and responsibility, is likely to emerge as a powerful force in public health and in the shape of future medical practice; future physicians need to know about this trend. Moreover, the Health Awareness Workshop is *pro* active. It avoids the pitfalls of administrative supervision to identify impairment among students which can make an ostensibly helpful program just one more threat from "above" (Knott & Whitfield, 1977). The Health Awareness Workshop treats all students equally: there is no focusing on "impairment." The social network starts from the first encounters and strengthens visibly during the four days of the exercise. The health tutors become resource persons and, in some instances, personal friends. There is throughout a spirit of cooperation, sharing, and in the best sense, an "ethic of commitment" (Yankelovich, 1981).

There is, however, one other aspect to which we wish to draw attention, namely, the research potential of such a workshop in terms of follow-up data. A medical student who appreciates the effort spent on his/her behalf by faculty and students may be willing to return the compliment by furnishing data to questionnaires as he/she goes through medical school and beyond. This was the core of Caroline Thomas' study (1983). The difference in our experiment is that we intend to *monitor* the effectiveness of an intervention. We are the first to acknowledge (despite the encouragement and feedback we have received) our own dissatisfaction with our data to date.

What could emerge out of this workshop is the concept of a *Laboratory (or Center) for Student Health*, engaged in long-term studies to assess effectiveness of the intervention procedures and to improve them whenever appropriate. Such studies, while drawing on established methodologies, could expand and codify new procedures using modern data retrieval systems and lead to the establishment of a long-term *scientific estate* capable of being carried on beyond the lifetime of principal investigators. More specifically, such studies could do the following:

1. Appraise life-style and health risk in the incoming medical student.
2. Identify and codify the stresses operating throughout a student's career in medical school.
3. Equip students with coping skills in the face of identified stresses.
4. Develop a schema for successive learning and training opportunities offered at career transition points (junior-to-senior; student-to-internship; internship-to-residency; residency-to-active practice, etc.).
5. Create student/student and faculty/student social support groups to enhance coping skills.
6. Provide students with skills that could be carried over from their personal lives into the practice of their profession—a "pharmacopoeia of skills" (Elkes, 1978).
7. Initiate experiential educational experiments for other health care personnel in the institution.
8. On the basis of data, and by osmosis and example, influence teaching methods and curriculum design and introduce the principles of "health behavior" and "behavioral medicine" into the institution.

In sum, we feel that a personal and practical concern for the health of the health provider-to-be is a timely and appropriate response to the mounting problem of the impaired physician.

REFERENCES

Bogdonoff, M.D. (1983, Fall). The sense of transcience as it contributes to medical student unease. *Pharos*, 11–14.

Breiner, S.J. (1979). The impaired physician. *Journal of Medical Education, 54*, 673.

Cadden, J.J., Flach, F.F., Blakeslee, S., et al. (1969). Growth in medical students through group process. *American Journal of Psychiatry, 126*, 862–868.

Committee on Medical Education/Group for the Advancement of Psychiatry (1982). *A survival manual for medical students*. New York: Mental Health Materials Center.

Dickstein, L.J. (1982). The student hour: A support system for freshmen medical students. *Journal of the American College Health Association, 31*, 131–132.

Elkes, J. (1965). On meeting psychiatry: A note on the student's first year. *American Journal of Psychiatry*, 121–128.

Elkes, J. (1978). Education for health enhancement. B.M.A. Audio Cassette Publications, Master Lectures Series #T-233.

Flach, D.H., Smith, M.F., Smith, W.G., et al. (1982). Faculty mentors for medical students. *Journal of Medical Education, 57*, 514–520.

Gardner, E.R., & Hall, R.C.W. (1980). Protracted stress syndrome in health care providers. *Texas Medical, 73*, 63–65.

Goldstein, M.Z. (1975). Preventive mental health methods for women medical students. *Journal of Medical Education, 50*, 289–291.

Hilberman, E., Konanc, J., Perez-Reyes, M., et al. (1975). Support groups for women in medical school: A first year program. *Journal of Medical Education, 50*, 867–875.

Katz M.M., & Lyerly, S.B. (1963). Methods for measuring adjustment and social behavior in the community: I. Rationale, description, discriminative validity, and scale development. *Psychology Report Monogram, 13*, 503–535.

Knott, D.H. & Whitfield, C.L. (1977). Medical students—Opportunities for prevention. *Impaired physician* (Proceedings of AMA Conference on the Impaired Physician: Answering the Challenge. M.B. Hugunin (Ed.). Feb. 4–6, 1977). Chicago: Department of Mental Health, American Medical Association, pp. 63–66.

Lief, H.I. (1971). Personality characteristics of medical students. In R.H. Coombs and C.E. Vincent (Eds.), *Psychosocial aspects of medical training*. Springfield, Ill.: Charles C Thomas, 44–48.

Linn, B.S., Zeppa, R. (1984). Stress in junior medical students: Relationship to personality and performance. *Journal of Medical Education, 59*, 7–12.

Lorr, M., Daston, P., & Smith, I.R. (1967). An analysis of mood states. *Educational Psychology Measure, 27*, 80–96.

Robertson, J.J. (Ed.) (1980). Proceedings of the third AMA conference on the impaired physician. September 29–October 1, 1978. No. 55. Chicago: Department of Mental Health, American Medical Association.

Rosenberg, P.P. (1971). Students' perceptions and concerns during their first year in medical school. *Journal of Medical Education, 46*, 211–218.

Scheiber, S.C., & Doyle, B.B. (Eds.) (1976). Emotional problems of physicians; nature and extent of problems. *The impaired physician*. New York: Plenum, pp. 3–10.

Small, I.F., Small, J.G., Assue, C.M., & Moore, D.F. (1969). Fate of the mentally ill physician. *American Journal of Psychiatry, 125*, 1333–1342.

Stephens, L.L., & Kitchen, L.W. (1978). Suicide among medical students. *Western Journal of Medicine, 129*, 441–442.

Thomas, C.B. (1971). Suicide among us:II. Habits of nervous tension as potential predictors. *Johns Hopkins Medical Journal, 129*, 190–201.

Thomas, C.B. (1976). What becomes of medical students: The dark side. *Johns Hopkins Medical Journal, 138*, 185–195.

Thomas, C.B. (1980). Precursors of premature disease and death: Habits of nervous tension. *Johns Hopkins Medical Journal, 147*, 137–145.

Thomas, C.B. (1983). *The precursors study, a prospective study of a cohort of medical students*. Vol. V, 1977–1982. Baltimore: Johns Hopkins University School of Medicine.

Vaillant, G.E., Sobowale, N.C., & McArthur, C. (1972). Some psychologic vulnerabilities of physicians. *New England Journal of Medicine, 287*, 372–375.

Yankelovich, D. (1981). *New rules: Search for self-fulfillment in a world turned upside down*. New York: Bantam, p. 247.

Chapter 20

Developing a School of Dentistry Wellness Program at the University of California, San Francisco

Lewis E. Graham II, Ph.D., Cary E. Howard, Ph.D., Jared I. Fine, D.D.S., M.P.H., Larry Scherwitz, Ph.D., and Samuel J. Wycoff, D.M.D., M.P.H.

The problems of stress and life-style risk factors in a highly technological, affluent society have received increasing attention from health professionals, the lay public, and the media. In fact, both psychosocial factors and life-style patterns have been related to general malaise in the mind and body as well as specific disease manifestations. Stress and life-style risk factors are a silent partner in everyday life. A fairly recent development is that these are specifically addressed as a problem on university campuses.

The activities of the U.C.S.F. wellness program were supported in part by a generous grant from the Ichinose Family Foundation. We express special appreciation to Benjamin Ichinose, D.D.S.; the Ichinose Family Foundation; Dean John C. Greene, D.M.D. of the U.C.S.F. School of Dentistry; and Philip R. Lee, M.D., former U.C.S.F. Chancellor who now serves as director of the Age and Health Policy Center.

In early 1983, the School of Dentistry at the University of California, San Francisco, began developing a wellness and health promotion program for students, faculty, and staff. The first step in this process was defining the wellness program's scope and substance. The second, considerably more challenging step was to effectively communicate the rationale and substance for such an endeavor and to credibly integrate it into the existing academic structure.

The U.C.S.F. School of Dentistry wellness program was primarily conceptualized and implemented by the five authors of this chapter. We believe we succeeded in all these respects. In fact, our program evaluation measures consistently have indicated that the U.C.S.F. wellness program has been highly successful, and this chapter is a synopsis of our efforts. We have consciously chosen to provide the reader with a brief anecdotal account rather than statistical data. We hope that those interested in health promotion on university campuses and other settings will find our account useful as they consider how to plan and implement similar programs.

PROGRAM DEVELOPMENT

The Importance of Timing

We recognized from the outset that taking the right steps in an effective manner at an appropriate time is essential to success in any institutional effort. Accordingly, we believed that this program should be carried out with timing considerations clearly in mind.

We reasoned that preparing to implement such a program would require two to three quarters of planning and program design. Since the program was scheduled to begin in the fall quarter (September), which began a new academic year, our planning and background research efforts were initiated in January of that same year. This permitted us nine months' planning time before the official program kickoff.

Background Research

Our overall goal was to develop the best intervention program possible for promoting health among dental students, staff, and faculty. We wanted to develop a program with campus-wide applicability that had potential for being a model for other campuses and settings. To define program content and scope, we took several important steps intended to ensure both quality and relevance.

1. Wellness program faculty members interviewed selected students,

faculty, and staff at U.C.S.F., within and outside the School of Dentistry.

2. We reviewed existing literature in the fields of stress, preventive medicine, and health promotion programs.

3. We reviewed many existing health promotion programs from all parts of the country. In doing so, we frequently traveled to other institutions for site reviews of various components in existing programs (e.g., the Swedish Wellness Center in Englewood, Colorado; the Institute for Advancement of Health in New York City; and the American Institute of Stress in Yonkers, New York).

4. We contacted and visited many established health promotion professionals and opinion leaders (e.g., William Hettler, M.D.; Kenneth Pelletier, Ph.D.; Joel Elkes, M.D.; Paul Rosch, M.D.; David Sobel, M.D.; and Richard Disraili, D.D.S.). This process of networking with those in the field was enhanced through attending national and regional annual conferences such as the annual Wellness Promotion Strategies Conference (in Stevens Point, Wisconsin) and those sponsored by the National OD Network, the Society for Psychophysiological Research, and the Society for Behavioral Medicine.

5. Student and staff/faculty input was specifically solicited in a variety of ways. For example, we assessed stress, psychosocial factors, and life-style patterns among the entire second-year dental school class. In doing so we used the state-trait anxiety inventory, a modified version of the work environment survey, and the stress questionnaire from the Stanford Heart Disease Prevention Program's Five Cities Project.

Also, we polled students with open-ended questions to determine which human interest or life-style topics they were most interested in or most wanted to discuss. This information was then used to tailor program elements to meet authentic personal needs. (The most frequently cited topics were physical fitness, nutrition, learning skills, and visualization/affirmations; communication skills; meditation/ relaxation; and life stages, death, and dying.)

6. Finally, a background planning report was prepared, summarizing the current status and components of representative wellness programs, and information gained from interviews with students, faculty, and practicing dentists.

Program Focus

Although we found wellness programs to vary widely, we also found that, in general, wellness efforts involved health promotion through improving one's life-style with stress reduction as a primary focus. (We also determined that, depending on the program, wellness programs may further include focus on physical fitness; nutrition; weight control; smoking cessation; alcohol and drug abuse assistance; safety; mental health; interpersonal and group communication skills training; human sexuality; realizing our potential through life planning and goal setting; learning skills; time management; self-care and social support/networking.)

Furthermore, consistent with our survey of the health promotion field, the planning report identified "stress management" as the most pressing perceived need *among those on campus*. Accordingly, we began to structure a program based on stress management as a centerpiece. In addition, our report identified four primary stress triggers experienced by members of the U.C.S.F. Dental School community:

- A general feeling of uncertainty about the future of the profession.
- The increasing need to develop nontraditional business and people skills: Although technically proficient, most dental professionals have little knowledge or training in the business practices or the motivational/managerial principles so essential for dealing effectively with staff and patients.
- The demanding combination of academic and technical training: Besides needing a tremendous amount of knowledge, dentists must also learn to be "super mechanics in a tiny little space."
- The push for perfection: The emphasis on producing perfect work is a highly stressful training orientation for students and instructors. It results in a negative atmosphere that leads to "seeing what's wrong rather than what's right" in most situations. Moreover, students were seldom treated as professional equals until the day of graduation. Their self-image suffers in a learning environment that is short on positive reinforcement and long on criticism.

OVERVIEW OF KEY PROGRAM ELEMENTS

Our planning report had concluded that the most effective stress management programs address the broader concept of wellness. We took the position that a stress program must empower the individual with knowledge, attitudes, and skills and must work to change the structure of the individual's social environment. Therefore, our report described the need for the University to develop a new model of health care and provider training as a long-term solution to the campus-wide problems of stress in health professionals' education. In addition to long-term recommendations, we targeted our immediate efforts on the design and implementation of a visible, multifaceted stress reduction program that could be integrated with current dental school efforts.

During its first year of operation the U.C.S.F. School of Dentistry wellness program undertook a number of program implementation steps. Among these were the following:

- sponsoring workshops, forums, and classes in health promotion
- providing consultation services to students, faculty, and staff
- maintaining a current referral list of key campus and community health promotion resource groups
- providing intensive small-group stress reduction therapy for select individuals (eight two-hour sessions)
- networking with other universities and health promotion programs
- broadening student education in applying behavioral science to problems in dentistry by revising an existing second-year course
- engaging in ongoing research evaluating the effects of current programs
- conducting behavioral science research relevant to dentistry in such areas as student stress, self-involvement and disease risk, pain and anxiety control, and characteristics of successful dental practices

The entire wellness program was implemented on a stepwise basis with each component designed to follow from and build on preceding activities. In particular, the program included eight key activities described below.

Stress Inoculation Course for New Students

We assumed that one key program step should involve preparing incoming students for the rigors they would experience in dental school and providing them with tools for self-awareness and more effective coping. Accordingly, a four-week stress inoculation/management course was designed and given in the fall quarter as a part of the orientation program for incoming first-year dental students. The entire course comprised eight one-hour group meetings.

This stress inoculation/management course included an overview of the concept of stress and its effects on physical and mental functioning; attitudes and the stress response; a demonstration of biofeedback technology as an aid to reducing stress; and experiential work with representative stress reduction techniques such as autogenic training, progressive relaxation, meditation, paced respiration, the relaxation response, self-hypnosis, visualization, learning skills, and time management.

Response to the program was highly favorable from students and faculty. Students participating in the program completed questionnaires indicating immediate interest in follow-up seminars in health promotion. Major areas of interest included nutrition, learning skills, physical fitness, communication skills, visualization, meditation, and death and dying. (These were later expanded upon in the Issues in Wellness Forum Series described on p. 288.) Moreover, the program was so well received that it was repeated later in the year for interested second-, third-, and fourth-year students and was adopted as a part of the summer orientation program for incoming dental students.

Networking on Campus and Achieving Campus Visibility

The dean of the School of Dentistry arranged a miniconference on stress/wellness early in the academic year. This meeting was attended by selected interested persons on campus and in the wider community and helped to build a consensus of support for our program's goals and planned activities.

Beyond such events, program faculty presented the wellness program and taught stress management/health promotion to students in classes and to university staff through in-service workshops. In addition, the university Office of Public Service was continually updated on all health promotion and wellness activities available to students and faculty on campus and in the community. A resource list of faculty and staff interested in promoting wellness activities was maintained for possible future support and reference.

Networking with Other Schools

To increase the visibility of program efforts and to gain insight and information, networking was begun by sending descriptive letters and brochures about our program to all accredited dental schools in the United States, Canada, and other selected countries, and to other health organizations. We thereby assessed the level of development of health promotion programs in dental education.

Establishing Program Identity and Mission

Once our orientation program was complete and political support had coalesced, we acted swiftly to communicate publicly our identity and mission. Since allocation of physical space is so often synonymous with support in academic settings, office space was established for the wellness program in the Department of Dental Public Health and Hygiene. We designed and decorated program offices to appear both professional and warm.

We then produced a health promotion brochure that described and defined the wellness program (see Figure 1). We also designed and produced a brochure describing the Issues in Wellness Forum Series (see Figure 2), which is discussed below. These brochures were widely distributed to campus personnel, to community groups, and directly to students in many classes along with brief presentations on the program's focus and goals. In addition, pamphlets and existing communication channels (closed-circuit television announcements, special flyers, bulletin boards, campus mailboxes, etc.) were used to spread word of the program and its activities.

Forum Series

A highly publicized public forum series was established to increase campus awareness of healthy life-style factors, to enhance wellness program visibility, and to provide students with opportunities to explore broader human issues than those discussed in their classes and textbooks. We recognized that the forum series would play a significant role in promoting campus-wide acceptance of the program, so we took a number of steps to ensure success. In particular, we invited well-known national figures to chair each of five sessions, which were extensively advertised in advance. Two-hour sessions included refreshments, practice of experiential techniques, discussion periods, and distribution of a resource list for those with special interest in the topics.

The five-part Issues in Wellness Forum Series was held during the second and third quarters of the academic year, with attendance open to the entire university community as well as the public. The forum series featured in-depth discussion of wellness topics that students had previously identified as being of particular interest:

- Health awareness for health professionals: Life-style and well-being, chaired by the immediate past president of the American Dental Association (Burton Press, D.D.S.)
- Health awareness for health professionals: Life stages, death, and dying, chaired by a professor of medical ethics (Al Jonsen, Ph.D.)
- Learning and health: Memory, recall, and mental efficiency, chaired by a professor of psychology (Martin Covington, Ph.D.)
- Personal wellness through meditation and cognitive imagery, chaired by a well-known author in this area (Kenneth Pelletier, Ph.D.)
- Personal wellness: Nutrition and physical activity, chaired by another well-known author in the field (Peter D. Wood, D.Sc.)

Intensive Stress Groups

In addition to large-group presentations, we recognized the need for additional, more intensive work with a subgroup of students. Accordingly, we purchased usage rights for a comprehensive, small-group stress management program from the Stanford Behavioral Medicine Group. The program we chose was based on eight years of research on teaching stress reduction in groups and had been tested in academic, medical, government, and business settings with documented therapeutic efficacy and cost effectiveness. It was a flexible and adaptable program that provided slides, an instructor's manual, and participant handouts. The program's text was available on computer disks allowing us to customize handouts to fit our needs. In the spring quarter, the first eight-week small-group program was carried out with self-selected students and received highly favorable evaluations.

Curriculum Revision

We had already begun a behavioral sciences course for second-year dental students several years previously. This course was further revised so that the curriculum contained a blend of experiential and didactic teaching methods. It focused on stress and life-style issues, personalized stress assessments, stress management skills, interpersonal relations, communication, and behavioral science research on pain and anxiety. This course's philosophical position was that stress in dentistry is both a personal and interpersonal problem which requires a multidisciplinary perspective that has previously been lacking in dentistry. To further increase this course's importance, the number of behavioral science course hours/credits required in subsequent years was increased overall.

Research Program

To provide a systematic program of behavioral science research relevant to dental practice, a center for dental services research was established with a wellness component. The wellness program worked closely with the center directors to determine ways of cooperating in program expansion and in seeking additional funds and support. The center also served as an organizational umbrella for behavioral medicine research activities and grant applications.

In addition to ongoing basic and applied research, a number of program evaluation tools were also devised. These usually pertained to student reactions to or benefits from particular program activities or events. As men-

Figure 1

WELLNESS

WELLNESS

WHAT

IS

WELLNESS?

Presented by
School of Dentistry
Department of
Dental Public Health and Hygiene
University of California, San Francisco

WHAT IS WELLNESS?

The World Health Organization points out that health is "a state of complete physical, mental and social well-being and not merely the absence of disease or infirmity."

"Wellness" is a dynamic state of optimal health in this larger sense. It reflects personal and social integration. It includes psychological resilience, physical health, social support, and positive lifestyle habits in a context of self-acceptance and self-responsibility.

Wellness programs focus on many components of positive lifestyling, such as stress management, nutrition, physical fitness, weight control, smoking cessation, interpersonal communication skills, learning skills, and environmental sensitivity.

WHY WELLNESS IN THE DENTAL SCHOOL?

Increasingly, dental professionals perceive health in a broader sense and reflect this to patients. They enter into therapeutic partnerships which acknowledge patient responsibility as a key factor in achieving and maintaining health and well-being. Also, because dental professionals are often viewed as inflictors of pain, it is important that they understand how to alleviate stress, pain and anxiety reactions among their patients.

Stress-related disorders among both dental students and dental professionals are not uncommon. The Dental School faculty recognize the importance of minimizing stress and encouraging positive health behaviors and lifestyles.

Wellness promotion on a university campus increases the probability of student retention in academic programs and enhances future student success in the professional world. It also develops among students, faculty and staff a supportive climate which nurtures individual well-being, accelerated learning, personal growth, and professional excellence.

THE WELLNESS PROGRAM

The Wellness Program carries out research, education and service activities in health promotion. The Program was created in the Fall, 1983, under the Division of Behavioral Sciences and Wellness, Department of Dental Public Health and Hygiene, School of Dentistry. It serves as a focus for consultation and outreach to other university, business, and community groups.

The Wellness Program:

- Sponsors workshops, forums and classes in health promotion and wellness
- Provides a library of key wellness resource materials
- Offers consultation services to students and faculty
- Sponsors networking and support groups on campus
- Maintains a current list of key campus and community health resources

- Engages in ongoing research studies evaluating the effects of the current programs
- Works in cooperation with other university and community wellness programs

Current programs offered include:

- health awareness for health professionals
- stress management
- weight control
- nutrition
- physical fitness
- learning skills
- meditation and relaxation practices

The Wellness Program is offering classes, intensive small group sessions, and a forum series through the year. If you would like more information on any of these activities, or if you are interested in volunteering to lead a workshop or group, please call 666-5802 or stop by D-1118

Figure 2

WELLNESS

1984
ISSUES
IN WELLNESS

FORUM SERIES

Presented by
School of Dentistry
Department of
Dental Public Health and Hygiene
University of California, San Francisco

WELLNESS

ISSUES IN WELLNESS
FORUM SERIES

The World Health Organization points out that health is "a state of complete physical, mental and social well-being and not merely the absence of disease or infirmity." Issues in Wellness is designed to explore the wider and more comprehensive dimensions of health and well-being. Five monthly Forums will be held January through May. Each Forum will provide current background information, a key resource list, experiential techniques and a discussion period. The Forum Series is open to all UCSF faculty and students. Your participation and suggestions are enthusiastically welcomed.

THE FORUM FACULTY

Faculty includes Samuel J. Wycoff, D.M.D., M.P.H., Professor, Department of Dental Public Health and Hygiene; Jared I. Fine, D.D.S., M.P.H., Visiting Lecturer in Behavioral Sciences and Wellness; Lewis E. Graham II, Ph.D., Visiting Lecturer and Researcher in Behavioral Sciences and Wellness; and Cary E. Howard, Ph.D., Visiting Lecturer and Wellness Program Coordinator.

Issues in Wellness is an ongoing activity of the Wellness Program in the Division of Behavioral Sciences and Wellness, Department of Dental Public Health and Hygiene, School of Dentistry. For more information on the Forum Series or other Wellness Program activities, please call: 666-5802.

T H E   P R O G R A M

Forum I: Health Awareness for Health Professionals: Lifestyle and Well-Being

- Lifestyle and longevity — avoiding hazards of a profession
- Developing healthful beliefs and attitudes about responsibility for others and oneself
- Tailoring a satisfying lifestyle that encompasses personal health and well-being
- Recognizing changing roles among health care professionals
- Creating a cultural shift in health care awareness

Forum II: Health Awareness for Health Professionals: Life Stages, Death and Dying

- Life transitions as stages of growth
- Realizing life's limits: Confronting your own mortality
- Developing a philosophy of death and dying
- Understanding the psychological processes such as fear, anxiety and guilt which surround the dying process
- How to talk about death: Working with grieving patients
- How others have found meaning in life through near-death experiences

Forum III: Learning and Health: Memory, Recall and Mental Efficiency

- Understanding procrastination and inefficiency
- Motivating yourself to master difficult material
- Improving memory and recall abilities
- Applying effective time management principles

- Developing skills that enhance learning pleasure and reduce stress
- Keeping up with the information explosion in your field

Forum IV: Personal Wellness through Meditation and Cognitive Imagery

- Understanding differences in Eastern and Western spiritual traditions
- Examining the benefits of meditation
- Learning meditation techniques which reduce stress and enhance well-being
- Practicing cognitive imagery for relaxation, insight and personal clarity
- Participating in guided meditations and depth imageries

Forum V: Personal Wellness: Nutrition and Physical Activity

- Staying well in a sedentary world
- Integrating good nutrition and physical activity into daily life
- Adopting a diet and weight control program to meet individual needs
- Goal-setting that works: Applying the principle of gradualism in self-directed change
- Taking the time to take care of yourself

The Wellness Program is being made possible through a grant from the Ichinose Family Foundation, given by Benjamin Ichinose, D.D.S., and his family in appreciation for the education he received at UC Berkeley and UC San Francisco. Dr. Ichinose expresses special gratitude to Marybeth Monte, who helped and encouraged him in many ways at UCSF, and to his mentor William Elsasser, D.D.S.

tioned in the introduction, these data consistently indicated the program was succeeding in promoting health and authentically meeting perceived campus needs.

CONCLUSION

The University of California at San Francisco is exclusively a health sciences campus dedicated to training health professionals in a wide range of professional disciplines. The School of Dentistry faculty at U.C.S.F. recognizes the importance of minimizing stress and encouraging positive health behaviors and life-styles. Increasingly, dental health professionals perceive health in a broader framework and reflect this in their services to patients. They enter into therapeutic partnerships that acknowledge patient responsibility as a key factor in achieving and maintaining health and well-being. Also, because dental professionals are often viewed as inflictors of pain, it is important that they understand how to alleviate stress, pain, and anxiety reactions in their patients.

The goal of the wellness program described here has been to carry out research, education, and service activities in health promotion. In addition, it has served as a focus for consultation and outreach for other university, business, and community groups. Currently, funds are being sought to continue the development and expansion of the initial program. Our plans include developing transferable health awareness programs for dental students, designing a student-to-dentist transition program for fourth-year students, enlarging intervention strategies for wider campus use, developing a teacher training program for health promotion in the health sciences, and studying ongoing community practices to identify the key elements that contribute to business success among professional practitioners.

The ongoing paradox of medical education is that the process of education can also be detrimental to emotional, interpersonal, and physical well-being of health professionals in training. However, to be effective, the process of introducing health promotion and wellness must be gradual and must eventually penetrate every aspect of campus life. This takes time and requires restructuring institutional thinking so as to promote health instead of eroding it. For such programs to produce positive results, we believe they must be carefully planned with extensive input, systematically evaluated, implemented, and revised in a politically sensitive manner, and expanded over a long-term basis so that values and practices are gradually but markedly shifted.

Wellness promotion on a university campus increases the probability of student retention in academic programs and enhances future student success in the professional world. It also develops among students, faculty, and staff a supportive climate that nurtures individual well-being, accelerated learning, and personal growth through academic excellence. We believe these key results clearly serve the best interests of our universities, the health professions, and the public alike. Our experience has shown that health promotion programs that accomplish these results are possible when they are planned and carefully implemented with a clear understanding of the institutional context in which they unfold.

Index

Abortion, 245
Academic physicians, *see* Faculty
Accidents, 263
Actualization, 30-31, 60
Acupuncture, 143, 245
Adler, D. (Janus), 94
Administrators, 36-38
Advisor's role, 153-154
Affective disorders, 64-65, 93-94
Aging, problems of, 231
Alcohol abuse, 5-7, 63-64, 66, 188, 192, 231
    detoxification programs, 192
    Employee assistance programs and, 259-
        260
    insurance coverage and, 263
    medical students and, 148-150
    prevalence of, 222
    residents and, 73
    women physicians and, 65
Alpert, J.J., 212
American Academy of Family Practice, 17
American culture, 4, 113
    scientism and, 116-117
American Holistic Medical Association, 142
American Medical Association, 3-4, 17, 221-
    225, 232, 271
Angell, M., 89, 95, 98, 102-104
Anxiety, 187
    attacks, 164
    other people's pain and, 195
Architecture, 31-32
Ardell, P.B., 218
Arem, C. (Scadron), 90
Aronson, E., 20, 37, 135 (Pines)
Artiss, K.L., 177-178
Assertiveness training, 179, 247-248

Assessment skills, 250
Assue, C.M. (Small), 270
Atkins, E.C. (Talbott), 233
Authoritarian style, 118
Autonomy, 27-29, 60, 68, 186
    marriage relationship and, 130-131
Avery, M.E., 86
Axelrod, M. (Scadron), 90

Bailar, J.C., 64
Bailyn, L., 88
Baker, L. (Minuchin), 111
Barish, A.M., 218
Barker, W.H., 218
Barnett, R.C., 99, 102-103
Barondess, J.A., 98
Barr, R., 4
Baruch, G.K., 99, 102-103
Bauer, K.G., 260
Beavers-Timberlawn family evaluation scale,
    251-252
Beavin, J. (Watzlawick), 111
Becker, H.S., 72
Becker, J.S. (Gualtieri), 233
Behavioral sciences
    clinical behavioral scientists, 161-172
        modeling problem solving and, 168-170
        patient counseling and, 163-165
        training of, 170-171
    course for medical students, 272-273
    curriculum for nurse practitioners, 239-
        240, 249-250
    dentistry and, 286, 289
Beigel, A. (Glasscote), 57, 62
Belz, M., 116, 118
Benson, D. (Talbott), 5

297

Benson, E. (Talbott), 5
Benzer, D.G. (Herrington), 230
Berg, J.K., 4
Berke, R. (Goldstein), 135
Bespalec, D.A. (Goby), 6
Bielby, D.D., 102
Bigger, T.J. (Friedman), 74
Biofeedback, 143, 245, 286
Birnbaum, J.A., 99
Bishop, J.M., 183
Bissell, L., 6, 233
Bjorksten, O., 148-150
Black women physicians, 102
Blakeslee, S. (Cadden), 271
Blazer, D.G., 68
Board certification, 96
Bobula, J.D., 95
Bogdonoff, M.D., 270-271
Bojar, S., 73, 149
Bok, D., 182
Boorstin, D.J., 113
Borenstein, D.B., 157
Borus, J.F., 120, 127
Bosk, C.L., 74
Bouhoutsos, J., 187
Bowman, M.W., 87
Boyle, B.P., 47, 50, 73
Bradley, N.J. (Goby), 6
Bradlyn, A.S. (Kelly), 179
Bradshaw, J.S., 6
Braslow, J.D., 86-87, 96-99, 104
Breiner, S.J., 270
Bremer, W. (Tokarz), 4, 6, 178
Bressler, B., 118, 132
Brighton, J.R., 119, 231 (Vaillant)
Brill, P.L., 149
Brody, H., 111
Bromet, E.J. (Goldstein), 92, 101
Brown, J.P., 6
Brown, R.M. (Plaut), 156
Brown, S.L., 101
Bryson, J.B., 86, 88
Bryson, R.B., 86, 88
Bunker, J.P., 6
Bureaucracy, 38-39
Burgess, A.W., 190
Burnout, 11, 137-138, 197
  bureaucracy and, 38-39
  cognitive functioning and, 191
  communication problems and, 39
  definition of, 19, 135
  early manifestations of, 149-150
  faculty and, 147
  house-staff training environment and, 5

  impaired professionals and, 186
  job burnout model, 20-21
  job related rewards and, 37
  medical students and, 148-149
  personal unresolved issues and, 190
  physical environment and, 31-33
  positive outcome and, 135
  role strain and, 61
  self-actualization and, 30-31
  significance of the job and, 30
  social competence and, 22
  social work relations, 34-38
  variety in the work place and, 29
  women physicians and, 101-102
  work environment and, 21-23, 28, 41-42
  work overload and, 29-30
Burnstein, A.G., 73
Burr, B.C., 74
Burr, W.R., 121
Business skills, 285, 294
Buxton, W.D. (Green), 7

Cadden, J.J., 271
Calhoun, G.L., 218, 259
California Psychological Inventory, 73
Callan, C., 91, 95-99
Callis, R., 152-153
Cancer, 6
Cardiovascular disease, 63, 216
Career development, 41, 72
  family matters and, 121
  parent/child relationship and, 124-125
  women physicians and, 102
Career equality, 120-121
Carlson, G.A., 93-94
Carpenter, D.C., 218
Carroll, G.J. (Green), 7
Cartwright, L.K., 72, 91-93, 96, 98-99, 102
Cassel, E.J., 213-214
Center for Healing Arts, 138
Center for the Well-Being of Health
  Professionals, 17
Chan, K.B., 71
Change, stages of, dissatisfaction, 137-138
Chappel, J.N., 230
Chase, G.A. (Weisman), 86-87, 98
Chemical dependency, *see* Alcohol abuse:
  Drug abuse
Cherniss, C., 135, 137, 197
Children, *see also* Families
  the physician/parent and, 122-128
  sexuality and, 245
  time to listen to concerns of, 129
Chodoff, P., 63, 65

Clark, C.C., 186
Clayton, P.J., 50, 74
Clayton, P.J. (Welner), 92-93
Clinical behavioral scientists, 161-172
  expanded use of, 210
Clinical practice, 9, 11, 13
Co-workers, 34-36
Cohen, E.D., 94-96, 98, 104
Coker, R.E., 94
Colligan, M.J., 217, 259
Communication, 289, 291
  marriage and, 119-120, 130
  problems, 39
  skills, 242-244
Community, physicians' relationship to, 78
Computers, 209
Conelly, J.C., 230
Confidentiality, 151, 190, 231
  Employee assistance programs and, 264,
    266-267
Consultants, 164
Continuing education, 17
Control issues, 27, 29, 40, 200, 202
Cook, K., 157
Coombs, R.H., 10, 45, 47, 50, 52, 73, 163
Cooper, B.S., 216
Coping mechanisms, 52
  for stressed interns, 176, 178-181
  for stresses in family practice, 81
  women physicians and, 102
Core, N. (Pepitone), 93, 150
Cosentino, J.P. (Gualtieri), 233
Coser, R.L., 88
Cost containment, 57
Costanzo, P.R., 88
Council on Mental Health, American
    Medical Association, 222-223
Counseling
  medical students, 152-153, 156-158
  of patients, 163-165
Countertransference, 67-68, 191, *see also*
    Transference
Court cases
  *Board of Curators of the University of
    Missouri v. Horowitz*, 150, 152
  Stoller v. College of Medicine, 152
Cousins, N., 50
Craig, A.G., 93
Crisis, 199-200
  personal, 137, 139-142
Crites, J.O., 72
Crovitz, E., 101
Crowley, A.E., 98
Cultural expectations, 4, 113, 116-117

Cunningham, R., 258
Curriculum development, 235-252, *see also*
    Medical education
  behavioral science series, 239-240
  course format, 240-252
  dentistry wellness program, 291
  mission statement, 237-238

D and D syndrome, 123
Darley, S.A., 88, 91
Datson, R. (Lorr), 277
Davidson, R.C., 235
Davidson, V.A., 100, 104
Davis, M.A. (Welner), 92-93
Davis, R.M., 163
Death, 73, 177, 287, 288
  reactions to, 247-248
  viewed as preventable, 52
Decision making, 117
Defense mechanisms, 66, 189
Delusions, 189
Denial, 16, 66, 230-231, 233, 271
  patient's pain and, 195-197
  rigidity and, 189
  self-care and, 214
Dentistry wellness program, 282-295
Depauw, M. (Callis), 152-153
Dependency needs, 10, 118-119, 122
  physician/patient relationship and, 178
Depression, 4, 139, 187-188
  burnout and, 20
  interns and, 116
  medical students and, 148-150
  physicians's personality and, 63-66
  physicians's suicide and, 7-8
  residents and, 74
  women physicians and, 92-93
Desensitization program, 164
Detached concern, 61-62, 195-197
Detached marriage partner, 120
Detection of impairment, 223-224, 226
Detoxification program, 192
Diagnosis, 117, 168
  uncertainty in, 74
Dickstein, L.J., 156, 272, 274
Dimond, E.G., 87, 102
Disease, *see also* Health
  incidence of, 211-212
  new and redefined, 209
  origins of, 212-213
  systems view of, 111
Disengagement, 122-123, 128-129
Disraili, R., 284
Divorce, 98-99, 119-122, *see also* Marriage

Donnelly, J.C., 4, 179
Doub, N.H., 75
Doyle, B.B., 97, 100, 269
Drug abuse, 4-5, 7, 188, 192, 231
  insurance coverage and, 263
  medical students and, 148-150, 158
  as most frequent impairment, 233
  physician's personality and, 63-64, 66
  prevalence of, 222
  residents and, 73
  women physicians and, 65
Dubbert, P.M. (Kelly), 179
Ducker, D.G., 90-92, 94-99, 102-103
Duff, R.F., 12
Dykman, R.A., 94

E and D syndrome, 122-123
Earnings, 114-115
Ecker, M. (Lorber), 96, 98-99
Education, *see* Health education: Medical
  education
Edwards, M.T., 73, 148-149
Ego rewards, 10
Eisenberg, C., 88-89, 93-94, 97-98
Elkes, J., 273, 280, 286
Elliott, C.M., 86, 88, 94-96, 98
Elwood, J., 4
Emergency rooms, 115
Emotional deadening, 196
Emotional exhaustion, 20, 61, 202, 214
Emotional isolation, 51-53, 55, 118, 139,
  197, 272
Employee assistance programs, 258-267
  definition of, 260
  employee orientation and, 265
  internal vs. external staffing of, 266-267
Enmeshment, 122
Epstein, C.F., 88, 90, 98
Equality of power, 120-121
Equilibrium, 111
Errors, 189-190
Ethical Standards, American Personnel and
  Guidance Association, 150
Ethics, 178, 187
Etzioni, A., 56
Exercise, 132

Faculty, 47-48
  burnout and, 147
  career success and, 124
  counseling students and, 152-153, 156-158
  interventions for impaired students, 153-
    158
  lack of collegiality and, 271

role with impaired students, 150-153
  self-care curriculum development and, 238
  teaching the behavioral sciences, 165-167
  women physicians as, 97
Fadiman, J., 136, 198, 215
Families, 202-203, *see also* Children:
    Marriage
  background and impaired physicians, 66
  crisis and, 141
  disengaged, 122-123
  enmeshed, 122
  experienced as a source of pressure to
    give, 197-198
  interplay with society, 112
  issues for impaired physicians, 188
  life cycle, 116, 123
  physician's stress and, 79
  planning together time and, 129
  pressure on children to become doctors,
    117
  prevention of dysfunction in, 128-132
  self-care within, 211-212
  sharing reponsibility and, 131
  support for residents, 77
  women physicians and, 98-99
Family Educational Rights and Privacy Act
    of 1974, 150, 152
Family practice, 77-79, *see also* Practice
  acceptance of women in, 80
  clinical behavioral scientist and, 164-165,
    172
  definition of, 235
  positive aspects of, 81
  residents, 75-77
  teaching behavioral science and, 165-166
Family systems theory, 110-112
Family therapy, 249-252
Farber, B.A., 186
Farrell, K., 97
Fawzy, F.I., 163
Feedback, 37, 166, 171, 245
Feminine role, 101, 126, *see also* Women
    physicians
Fielding, J.E., 213, 215-216
Filley, A.C. (House), 36
Finances, 114-115
Fishman, R. (Welner), 92-93
Flach, D.H., 154-155, 271
Flach, F.F. (Cadden), 271
Folk medicine, 58
Ford, C.V., 196
Forer, B.R. (Bouhoutsos), 187
Fox, R., 61
Fox, R.C., 52

Freud, S., 67
Freudenberger, H.J., 135, 185-187
Friedman, R.C., 74
Frosch, W.A. (Ginsberg), 68
Fuller, M. (Kardener), 65, 68

Gaensbauer, T.J., 72
Gardner, E.R., 270
Garell, D. (Goldstein), 135
Garrard, J., 4
Geer, B., 72
Gehlbach, J.H., 87
Geller, A., 233
General systems theory, 110-111
Gerber, L.A., 112-113, 119-121, 129-130
Geyman, J.P., 98
Gilder, H. (Wallis), 97
Ginsberg, G.L., 68
Glass, D.C., 63
Glasscote, R., 57, 62
Glasser, M.L. (Flach), 154-155
Glick, I.D., 120-121, 127
Goby, M.J., 6
Goldstein, M., 135
Goldstein, M.Z., 92, 100, 101, 271
Goode, W., 88-89, 98
Gordon, J. (Hastings), 136, 198, 215
Gorlin, R., 177
Gough, H.G., 72
Gould, R., 134
Gray, J.D., 86, 99, 102
Green, R.C., 7
Greenberg, E.A. (Scadron), 90
Greenberg, M. (Bouhoutsos), 187
Grief, 248
Groesbeck, J., 200-201
Group dynamics, 168-170
Groves, J.E., 177
Gualtieri, A.C., 233
Guided imagery, 143
Guilt, 8, 52, 125
    dealing with patients and, 177
Gujarati, D.N. (House), 36
Gunderson, E.K., 213

Habits of Nervous Tension Scale, 270, 277
Haggerty, R.J. (Alpert), 212
Hall, D.T., 102
Hall, R.C.W., 270
Hall, R.M., 155
Hall, W.B., 72
Hanusa, B.H. (Goldstein), 92, 101
Harris, P.L., 149
Harris, S., 92, 104

Harrison, W.D., 22
Hass, R. (King), 64
Hastings, A., 136, 198, 215
Hawk, J.E., 75
Health, *see also* Disease
    alternative conceptions of, 237-238
    definition of, 210-211, 216
    psychological factors and, 182
    science of, 272
    systems view of, 111
Health Awareness Workshop, 272, 274-280
Health care system, 57-59, *see also* Hospitals
    built-in risks of, 215-216
    changes and, 209-210
    stressful occupations and, 258, 261
Health care teams, 161
Health education, 215, 218-219, 236, *see also*
    Medical education
Health Maintenance Organization (HMO),
    115
Health prevention, 279
Health promotion, 215-217, 236
    Wellness program and, 284-286, 294-295
Heckman, N.A., 86, 88
Heifez, L.J., 186
Heins, M., 86-87, 89-91, 94-100, 102-104
Henry, W.F., 74, 163
Herrington, R.E., 230
Hettler, W., 284
Higgins, E., 97
Hilberman, E., 100, 271
Hilfiker, D., 182
Hirschfeld, R.M.A., 63, 65
Hobbins, T.E. (Plaut), 156
Holguin, M. (Farrell), 97
Holistic health/medicine, 135-136, 140, 142-
    143, 198
    student curriculum for, 245-246
Hollingshead, A.B., 12
Holmes, T.H., 213
Holmstrom, L.L., 88, 99
Holroyd, J. (Bouhoutsos), 187
Homeostasis, 111
Hopkins Precursors Study, 269-270
Hospital acquired infection, 216
Hospitals, 257-258
    costs, 217
    Employee assistance programs and, 261-
    267
    rate of hospitalizations, 211
    stress and, 258-259, 261
    working environment and, 217-218
House, R.J., 36
House-staff programs, 4-5

Howard, R.B., 90
Howard, T. (Kay), 149-150
Human development, 246-247
Hunt, G.J. (Plaut), 156
Hypertension, 63
Hypnosis, 286

Identity crisis, 74, 101
Illness, *see* Disease: Psychosomatic illness
Impaired physicians, *see* Physicians, impaired
Infections, hospital acquired, 216
Insurance, 217, 262-263
Intermediary providers, 62-63
Interns, 174-183, *see also* Medical students: Residents
  needed changes in training of, 181-183
  pregnancy and, 125-126
  rite of passage and, 116
  self-expectations and, 176-177
  sleep deprivation and, 9, 46, 74, 174, 270
  work schedule and, 50
Intimacy, 130, 203
Isolation, 9, 51-53, 55, 118, 139, 197, 272

Jackson, D.D., 111, 120
Jackson, S., 197
Jacobs, J. (Heins), 89, 91, 94, 98
Jacobsen, G.R. (Herrington), 230
Jaffe, D., 135, 186, 198
Janus, C.L., 94
Janus, S.S., 94
Jennings, C., 217
Jensen, P.S., 178
Job satisfaction, 30, 60
  clinical behavioral scientists and, 170
  physician's dissatisfaction and, 137-138
  women physicians and, 92
Johnson, A.C., 258-259
Johnson, C.L., 86, 88, 99
Johnson, F.A., 86, 88, 99
Johnson, F.P. (Plaut), 156
Johnson, J.H. (Sarason), 213
Johnson, R.P., 230
Jolly, P., 97
Jones, L., 217, 257
Jones, R.E., 6, 93
Jones, R.W., 6
Jonsen, A., 176

Kafry, D. (Pines), 135
Kahn, R., 4
Kahn, R.L., 41
Kalin, R., 163

Kanas, N., 175
Kantner, T.R., 74
Kaplan, S.R., 98, 100, 102, 104
Kapp, M.B., 152
Kardener, S.H., 65, 68
Katz Social Adjustment Scale, 277
Katz, M.M., 277
Kay, J., 149-150
Keenan, C., 217
Kehrer, H., 96
Kelly, J.A., 179
Kessler, I.I., 75
King, H., 64
Kinnev, R.E., 260
Kitchen, L.W., 271
Klagsbrun, S., 203
Klein, R.H., 101
Klerman, G.L., 63, 65
Klipstein, E., 91, 95, 96-97, 98-99
Knott, D.H., 279
Kobos, J.C. (Burstein), 73
Kohn, E. (Glasscote), 57, 62
Konanc, J., 100
Konanc, J. (Hilberman), 271
Konior, G.S., 177
Kornfeld, D.S. (Friedman), 74
Korper, S.P., 94-96, 98, 104
Korr, I., 219
Kosa, J., 94, 212
Kotkin, M., 86, 88
Kotz, H.J., 213, 215-216
Kramer, M., 149
Kryter, K.D., 32

Labor unions, 263
Lake, K., 97, 104
Lancaster, R. (Lief), 73
Lander, L., 10
Larsen, R.C., 230
Lasell, R.L. (Goldstein), 92, 101
Lawyers, 186, 188, 190
Leadership style, 36
Lederer, W.I., 120
Leichner, P., 163
Lenhart, R.C., 147
Lerman, H. (Bouhoutsos), 187
Leserman, J., 87, 90
Levin, L.S., 211, 215-216
Levine, A.S., 177-178
Levine, D.M. (Weisman), 86-87, 98
Levinson, D., 134
Levit, E.J., 73
License revocation, 224
Licht, B.G. (Bryson), 88

Licht, M.H. (Bryson), 88
Lief, H.I., 51-52, 73, 271
Lief, V.F., 73
Life cycle, family, 116, 123
Life-style, 190-191, 236
  Employee assistance programs and, 261
  imbalanced, 50-51
  preventive health care and, 210
Light, D., 73
Linn, B.S., 270
Lippitt, R., 100, 102
Listening skills, 243
Little, R., 231
Loes, M.W., 163
Lopate, C., 99
Lopez, S. (Farrell), 97
Lorber, J.A., 89, 96, 98-100
Lorr, M., 277
Lorr Mood Scale, 277
Loucks, S. (Burstein), 73
Lovelace, J.C., 102
Lowenstein, P. (Nadelson), 89
Lyerly, S.B., 277

Magee, J.E., 123
Magee, M.C., 123
Malpractice, 59-60, 78, 114, 189
Mandelbaum, D.R., 86, 90, 94-98, 101-102
Market analysis, 57
Marriage, 64, 119-122, 196-197, 200, *see also*
  Divorce: Families
  crisis and, 141
  prevention of dysfunction in, 130-132
Marten, S. (Welner), 92-93
Martindale, L.J. (Rosen), 95
Maslach, C., 35, 40, 61, 197
Mason, J., 55
Massad, R.J., 112
Matteson, M.T., 97
Mausner, J., 7, 93
Mawardi, B.H., 98, 119, 182
May, D.S., 45, 51
McArthur, C. (Vaillant), 6, 63-64, 71, 178,
  231, 233, 270
McCue, J.D., 74-75, 101, 182
Medical education, 8-12, 63, 294, *see also*
  Curriculum development
  affective aspects of, 53-55
  assumptions in, 210-215
  behavioral scientist and, 162
  changes in, 181-183, 271-272
  continuing, 17
  costs of, 115
  dissatisfaction with, 270-271

  emotional isolation and, 51-53
  overwork and, 4-5
  preventive health and, 218-219
  prevention of physician impairment and,
    13-17
  status deprivation and, 46-49
  stress and, 11, 72-73
  values and, 236-237
Medical model, 13, 162, 210
Medical school professors, *see* Faculty
Medical students, *see also* Interns: Residents
  chemical dependency and, 5
  conflict of image/reality of work, 196-197
  coping with patient pain, 196
  emotionally constricted, 51-53
  expectations versus actual experience, 48-
    49
  exposure to burned-out physicians, 15
  faculty/student relationship, 153-158
  Health Awareness Workshop for, 272,
    274-280
  health risks and, 270, 280
  lack of collegiality and, 271
  marriage and, 120
  mental health programs for, 54-55
  percentage of female, 58
  poor clinical performance and, 151-152
  premedical education, 8
  primary prevention programs and, 223
  problems of, 148-150
  psychological characteristics predictive of
    mental illness in, 64
  reasonable work loads and, 154
  stress and, 5, 72-73, 270, 280
Meditation, 142-143, 286-288
Meitz, J.E. (Scadron), 90
Mensh, I.N. (Kardener), 65, 68
Mental exhaustion, 20
Mental Health Program for Physicians in
  Training, 157
Mental illness, 6, 66, 225-226, 233
  health care professionals and, 259
  prevalence of, 222
  residents and, 73
  women physicians and, 92-93
Mental status examination, 250
Mentor's role, 154-156
Meyer, J.H., 190
Midlife crisis, 68
Miller, C. (Bjorksten), 148-150
Miller, D.C., 93-94
Mind/body split, 240
Minuchin, S., 111
Mizner, G.L., 72

Modeling, 14
Modlin, H.C., 63
Montes, A., 63
Moore, D.F. (Small), 270
Moral decisions, 178
Mueller, C.B. (Levit), 73
Muldary, T.W., 101
Mullins, S.C., 120
Mumford, E., 104

Nackashi, J., 127-128
Nadelson, C.C., 86-87, 92, 97-101, 103-104, 126
Nagy, B.R., 185
Narcissism, 189
Nelson, E.G., 74, 163
Noise, work environment and, 32-33
Notman, M.T., 86-87, 92, 97-101, 103-104, 126
Numbing, 195-196, 198-199
Nurse practitioners, 235, 239, 249, 251
Nurses, 15, 34, 57, 148-149
  burnout and, 186
  mental illness and, 259
  and patient relationship, 203-204
  preventive health and, 219
Nutrition, 276, 287-288

Ogilvie, C., 219
Oski, F.A., 94
Osler, W., 182

Pain, 289, 294
  coping with, 195-196
  psychosomatic, 164
Paperwork, 38-39
Paraprofessionals, 57-58
Parent-child relationship, 122-130
Parmalee, R.D. (Powers), 94
Pasnau, R.O., 73, 163
Paternity leave, 127
Patient advocates, 14
Patients, 34, *see also* Physician/patient relationship
  affective aspects in the care of, 54-55
  counseling of, 163-165
  dying, 177
  expectations of health care providers, 60-61
  pain and, 195-196
  personality characteristics and, 67
  psychosocial problems and, 250
  rights, 58
  self-care curriculum and, 237-238

  sexual concerns of, 244
  sexual involvement with, 187, 200
  team approach and, 165
  women physicians and, 80
Pelletier, K., 261, 284
Pepitone-Arreola-Rockwell, F., 93, 150
Perez-Reyes, M. (Hilberman), 271
Perlow, A.D., 120
Permission-Limited Information-Specific Suggestions-Intensive Therapy Model, 244
Personnel policies, 263
Perun, P.J., 102
Peters, K. (Tokarz), 4, 6, 178
Pfifferling, J.H., 4, 5, 71, 148, 163
Physical exhaustion, 20
Physician assistants, 58, 239, 249, 251
Physician/patient relationship, 10, 12-13, 14, 114
  holistic health/medicine and, 136, 143
  patient compliance and, 165
  patient's responsibility and, 15-16
  patient's satisfaction and, 60
  physician's role in the, 61
  sexual involvement and, 68, 187, 200
  stressful for interns, 177-178
  transference/countertransference and, 67-68
  videotaping patient encounters, 171
Physicians, *see also* Women physicians
  availability, 114
  combining personal and professional life, 61, 77-79, 82-83
  competition for professional survival, 59
  confronting his own vulnerability, 200-201
  cultural expectations for, 4, 113-114
  early childhood role and, 201-202
  family dysfunction among, 112-113
  feelings about death, 52-53, 194-204
  finances and, 114-115
  healer's role and, 60-63
  health of, 214-215, 270
  myths about professional conduct, 196, 198
  rites of passage, 174
  self-care and, 219
  self-image of, 4, 6, 118
  self-needs and, 132, 143
  social/familial relationships and, 66-67
  socialization and, 10, 12-13, 62, 73-74
  socialization of female, 100-101
  stress and, *see* Stress
Physicians in Transition, 135
Physicians, impaired, *see also* Alcohol abuse;

Burnout; Depression; Drug abuse;
    Suicide
compared to emotionally "well," 45
costs of, 16
definition of, 3-4, 185, 225-226, 229-230,
    232-233
detection of, 223-224, 226
education values and, 11-12
factors contributing to, 186
family background and, 66
financial problems and, 227
imbalanced life-style and, 45, 50-51
number referred to state medical societies,
    230
as patients, 6, 199
personal crisis and, 137, 139-142
personality characteristics predictive of,
    63-66, 118-119
presenting symptoms and, 187-188
prevalence of, 222, 226, 233
prevention of, 13-17
professional organizations and, 221-227
profile of, 230-231
reasons for occupational choice, 191
recovery and, 191-192
self-expectations and, 186
treatment and, 188-191, 201-204, 224, 229
Pines, A., 20, 22, 31, 35, 37, 40, 61, 135,
    187
Pitts, F.N., 93
Plaut, S.M., 156
Pope, S. (Callis), 152-153
Povar, G.J., 116, 118
Power issues, 120-121, 189
Power, L., 94
Powers, P.S., 52
Practice, 74-75, *see also* Family practice
    changes in perspective in, 142-144
Premedical school, 72, *see also* Medical
    education
Presenting problem, 187-188, 231, 266
Preventive health care, 210
Price, S. (Janus), 94
Primary health educators, 14
Problem identification, 150-151
Problem-solving skills, 11-14, 163
    in the clinical environment, 168-170
Professionals, impaired, 186-187, 227, *see
    also* Nurses: Physicians, impaired
    presenting problems and, 187-188
Psychiatric illness, *see* Mental illness
Psychological testing, 166
Psychosomatic illness, 212, 245, 250
Psychosomatic pain, 164

Psychotherapy, 142, 199
    insurance coverage and, 263
Public health, 215-217, 279

Raber, M. (Glasscote), 57, 62
Rahe, R.H., 213
Rakel, D.C., 235
Ransom, D.C., 112
Raskin, M., 72
Rationalization, 66
Ray, G.J., 147
Reaction formation, 66, 118-119
Referrals, 156-157, 224, 229-230, 233-234
    Employee assistance programs and, 264,
        266
Reframing, 163
Regression, 67
Reidbord, S.P., 147
Relaxation techniques, 143, 164, 179-180,
    246, 276, 286
Relman, A.S., 87
Remen, N., 140
Repression, 66
Residents, 73-74, 169, *see also* Interns;
    Medical students
    chemical dependency and, 5
    evaluation of, 167
    expectations of self and, 163
    medical education and, 8-12
    pregnancy and, 125-126
    rite of passage and, 116
    role of behavioral scientist and, 162-163
    stress and, 75-77, 82, 163, 270
    work schedule and, 50
Retirement, 7
Rice, D.D., 216
Richardson, A.C. (Talbott), 233
Richardson, W.C., 212
Richelson, G., 186
Rights and Freedoms of Students, Joint
    Statement on, 150
Rinke, C.M., 89, 97, 100-101, 104
Robbins, A., 186
Robertson, J.J., 271
Rockwell, D. (Pepitone), 93, 150
Roeske, N.C.A., 57, 59, 63-65, 68, 97, 104
Rokoff, G., 88
Role ambiguity, 40-41, 63
Role boundaries, 62
Role conflict, 40, 88-91, 101, 121-122, 188
    choice of specialty and, 97-98
    male physicians and, 128
    positive aspects of, 103
    professional participation and, 94-95

suicide and, 93-94
women physician/mother and, 125-127
Role models, 115-116, 128
Role strain, 56-57, 61
  physician/patient relationship and, 178
  women physicians and, 83, 88, 91-92
Romm, S., 102
Rosch, P., 284
Rose, K.D., 94
Rosen, R.H., 95
Rosenberg, P.P., 271-272
Rosenlund, M.L., 94
Rosman, B.L. (Minuchin), 111
Rosow, I., 94
Ross, M., 7
Rossi, A., 88
Rothblum, E.D., 92
Rubin, H.L., 228
Ruhe, P., 90
Russell, A.T., 73, 163

Salary, 114-115
Salladay, S., 90
Sandler, B.R., 155
Sarason, I.G., 213
Scadron, A., 90, 97
Schaff, E., 50
Schedule of Recent Experiences, 213
Scheele, A., 12
Scheiber, S.C., 6-7, 97, 100, 163, 269
Scher, M., 94, 100
Schulz, R., 258-259
Schumacher, E.F., 236
Schwartz, A.H., 148
Scientism, 116-117
Scott, C.D., 75
Seagraves, R.T., 120
Self-actualization, 30-31, 60
Self-care, 83, 143, 198, 211, 214, 272
  curriculum, 235-252
  definition of, 215
Self-esteem, 68-69, 189, 192, 197
  parent/child relationship and, 124-125
Self-healing, 143
Self-hypnosis, 286
Self-image, 4, 6, 118
  medical students and, 8, 285
Senility, 226
Sensitizing techniques, 179
Separation anxiety, 131
Separation/individuation, 68
Service recipients, *see* Patients
Sex roles, 125, 128
Sexual deviance, 226

Sexual relationships
  physician/patient relationship and, 68, 187, 200
  student curriculum and, 244-245, 250
Shapiro, T. (Ginsberg), 68
Sharpe, J.C., 6
Shavshin, M. (Levit), 73
Shaw, M.E., 88
Sheridan, E.P., 186
Sheridan, K., 186
Shore, J.H., 233
Shortt, S.E.D., 3, 6-7
Siegel, B., 179
Siegel, J.M. (Sarason), 213
Sifneos, P.E., 190
Skinner, D.A., 86, 88
Slaby, A.E. (Schwartz), 148
Sleep deprivation, 9, 46, 174, 270
  psychological problems associated with, 74
Sluzki, C.E., 122
Small, G.W. (Coombs), 45
Small, I.F., 270
Small, J.G., 270
Smith, I.R. (Lorr), 277
Smith, M.F. (Flach), 154-155, 271
Smith, R.J., 233
Smith, S.V., 97
Smith, W.G. (Flach), 154-155, 271
Smith, W.W., 6
Smock, S. (Heins), 89, 91, 94, 98
Smoking, 132
Snitcher's law, 187
Sobel, D., 111, 284
Sobowale, N.C. (Vaillant), 6, 63-64, 71, 178, 233, 270
Social isolation, 9, 51-53, 55, 118, 139, 197, 272
Social workers, 57, 59
Southgate, M.T., 87
Space, work environment and, 32
Spruiell, V. (Lief), 73
St. John, J., 47
St. Lawrence, J.S. (Kelly), 179
Stalnaker, J.M., 94
Stanford Behavioral Medicine Group, 289
Stanford Heart Disease Prevention Program, 284
Stanton, B. (Burstein), 73
Starr, P., 57-58
State medical societies, 222-225, 228-234
State-trait anxiety inventory, 284
Status deprivation, 46-49
Status disorders, 41
Stein, M. (Heins), 89, 91, 94, 98

Steindler, E.M., 7, 233
Steinwachs, D.M. (Weisman), 86-87, 98
Stephens, L.L., 271
Steppacher, R.C., 7, 92, 93
Steward, T. (Bjorksten), 148-150
Steyer, R., 185
Stoller, R.J., 68
Stone, G., 171
Stress, 46, 71-72
  burnout and, 149
  communication problems and, 39
  coping mechanisms for, 81, 102, 176, 178-181
  costs of, 260-261
  divorce and, 122
  elements that contribute to, 112
  family practice physicians and, 77-79
  holistic health and, 136
  hospital environment and, 218, 258-259, 261
  interns and, 175-179
  management techniques for, 14, 285-287, 289
  medical students and, 5, 11, 72-73, 270, 280
  physical environment and, 31-33
  physician/patient relationship and, 67-68
  practice and, 74-75
  premedical school and, 72
  residents and, 75-77, 82, 163, 270
  role conflict and, 40
  student curriculum for, 246
  triggers of, 285
  unrewarding social encounters and, 45
  women physicians and, 80, 83, 87, 101
  work environment and, 22
  work relations and, 35-37
Substance abuse, *see* Alcohol abuse: Drug abuse
Suedfeld, P., 33
Suicide, 7-8, 118, 150
  physician's personality and, 63-64, 66
  women physicians and, 7, 65, 93-94
Supervisors, 36-38
Support groups, 13, 135, 138, 156, 175
  Health Awareness Workshop and, 279-280
  Student Hour, 272, 274
Support systems, 99-101, 204
Sutherland, S. (Bjorksten), 148-150
Swartzburg, J.L. (Schwartz), 148
Symonds, A., 65
Systems theory, 110-111

Tager, M.J., 217

Taintor, Z.C. (Russell), 73
Talbott, G., 5, 233
Teamwork, 35
Technological interventions, 12
Tennessee University Medical School, 15
Terris, M., 215-216
Thaler, H., 97
Therapeutic alliance, 190
Therapeutic model, 164
Third-party payers, 217
Thomas, C.B., 7, 63-64, 270, 277, 279
Thomas, L., 174
Time management, 16, 82, 179, 286
Tokarz, J.P., 4, 6, 178
Transference, 9-10, 67-68, *see also* Countertransference
Treadwell, T.W., 171
Triangulation, 123
Tuttelman, C., 72
Tweed, S., 150
Type A behavior, 64, 176

Unions, 263
Urgent-treatment centers, 115

Vaillant, G.E., 6-7, 63-64, 71, 119, 178, 231, 233, 270
Valko, F.J., 50, 74
Values clarification, 13
Vance, C.N., 155
Vastyan, E.A., 74
Videotaped student presentations, 241
Vincent, M.O., 188
Viner, J. (Tokarz), 4, 6
Visualization, 286-287
von Bertalanffy, L., 110

Wallis, L.A., 97
Walsh, M.R., 86
Ward, L.M., 33
Waring, E.M., 6
Warschawski, P., 75
Watzlawick, P., 111
Weed, L.L., 11
Weiman, C.G., 258
Weinstein, H.M., 150, 158
Weisenfelder, H. (Powers), 94
Weisman, C.S., 86-87, 98
Welch, G. (Kay), 149-150
Welch, R.L., 147
Wellness program, 282-295
Wellness Promotion Strategies Conference, 284
Welner, A., 92-93

Whitefield, C.L., 279
Williams, P.B., 94, 98
Wise, T.N., 179
Witte, M.H., 90, 97
Wochnick, E. (Welner), 92
Women physicians, *see also* Physicians
  in academic medicine, 97
  attitudes of colleagues and, 89-90
  burnout and, 101-102
  career interruptions and, 96
  changes in the medical profession and, 87
  factors leading to impairment in, 187-188
  families and, 198
  holistic health perspective and, 140
  job satisfaction and, 92
  marital and family status of, 98-99
  mental illness and, 92-93
  nonprofessional demands and, 88-89
  number of, 58, 86
  parent/child relationship and, 125-128
  physician/patient relationship and, 68
  professional participation and, 94-96
  professional success and, 96-97
  role strain and, 88, 91-92
  social support and, 99-101
  specialty choice and, 90, 97-98
  stress and, 80, 83, 87, 101

suicide and, 7, 65, 93-94
Work environment
  ability to adapt to, 63
  burnout and, 21-23, 28, 41-42
  case study (special education class), 23-26
  financial aspects of the, 114-115
  health promotion and, 217
  hospitals, 217-218
  organizational dimension of the, 38-41
  physical dimension of the, 28, 31-33
  psychological dimension of the, 27-31
  social dimension of the, 33-38
Work environment survey, 284
Workaholic, 116
World Health Organization, 216

Yankelovich, D., 279
Yates, J., 35, 37, 39
Yogev, S., 92, 104
Young, K. (Lief), 73

Zafros, G. (King), 64
Zeppa, R., 270
Ziegler, J.L., 175
Zimet, C.N., 73, 148-149
Zimring, C.M., 31
Zucker, H.D., 177